Thesis Writing for Master's and Ph.D. Program

Subhash Chandra Parija • Vikram Kate
Editors

Thesis Writing for Master's and Ph.D. Program

Springer

Editors
Subhash Chandra Parija
Sri Balaji Vidyapeeth (Deemed University)
Pondicherry
India

Vikram Kate
Department of Surgery
Jawaharlal Institute of Postgraduate Medical Education and Research (JIPMER)
Pondicherry
India

ISBN 978-981-13-0889-5 ISBN 978-981-13-0890-1 (eBook)
https://doi.org/10.1007/978-981-13-0890-1

Library of Congress Control Number: 2018956493

This Springer imprint is published by the registered company Springer Nature Singapore Pte Ltd.
The registered company address is: 152 Beach Road, #21-01/04 Gateway East, Singapore 189721, Singapore

Foreword

"If you can't explain it simply, then you haven't understood it well enough."—Albert Einstein

Writing and submitting one's thesis is a major part of any graduate program. An ideal graduate program is designed to stimulate and advance the student's scientific interest, and what better way to do so than to engage them in original research? This original research is ultimately presented at the end of their course in the form of a thesis. A thesis, therefore, is the written evidence of the efforts put in by the student for the length of their program. Hence, it becomes imperative that it is well written, scientifically accurate, and comprehensible. This is typically easier said than done! Everyone knows thesis writing is challenging, but only those who have undergone the experience can tell you exactly how hard it is, and such individuals make the best guides to support you in your own work.

In addition to writing the thesis, there are several associated activities that should be considered such as presenting your work at conferences and writing up a scientific paper. When considering all of this, it is little wonder that the prospect of thesis writing at times seems daunting and insurmountable. But it is, indeed, surmountable, as the authors of this book would tell you. Of course, thorough study and hard work are all important, but there is indispensable practical guidance that students require to ensure their thesis is of high quality.

This book admirably provides this guidance.

Prof. Parija and Prof. Kate have, between them, several years of experience in this field. Prof. Parija is an internationally renowned author of several papers in national and international journals and has authored ten textbooks. He has been awarded the B C Roy National Award of the Medical Council of India for his contribution to the development of Medical Microbiology. Prof. Kate, a recipient of "Distinguished DNB Teacher of Excellence Award" (2018) of the Association of National Board Accredited Institutions has contributed more than 35 chapters in reputed textbooks of surgical gastroenterology and surgery, besides a huge volume of research to his credit.

This book, over the course of 28 well-planned chapters, takes you through the process of thesis/dissertation writing in a clear and logical manner. The step-by-step approach, from the very basics such as choosing a topic, selecting objectives, and designing a protocol, through to the more complex aspects of writing up one's thesis, helps keep the narrative clear and focused. Importantly and, consistent with modern scholarship, information is provided regarding digital tools which can greatly assist in thesis writing and the issue of what to do after submitting one's thesis—namely, getting it published.

In all, this book forms a succinct and practical guide to the student. It dispels the mystery and fear that sometimes surrounds thesis writing and research in general, and instead extends a helping hand to the reader, serving as a guide for any student about to embark on a program of research that culminates in a thesis.

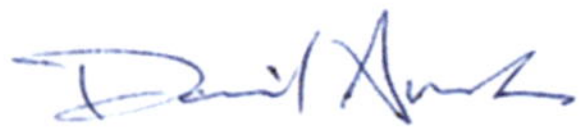

Professor David Austin
Faculty of Health
Deakin University
Melbourne, VIC, Australia

Preface

Thesis writing is one of the most crucial rites of passage in the postgraduate study period. Yet, for many, it remains the most arduous one as well. What is meant to be an exercise in gaining in-depth knowledge of research methodology often ends up as a slapdash production from the part of the harried graduate student. The difference, we believe, lies in a proper and methodical approach to thesis/dissertation writing. Right from the beginning of the research project, one must be clear with the topic, the objectives, and the methods. While choosing a topic, one must keep in mind several factors such as the appropriateness, the feasibility, and, above all, one's interest in that particular area. The importance of securing clearances from the appropriate monitoring bodies at the correct time cannot be stressed enough. This exercise also gives the students an invaluable opportunity to learn various aspects of statistics, and this will go a long way in their future careers.

In this book, we have made every attempt to cover the many facets of thesis/dissertation writing. From the very basics such as preparing a title page and abstract to the more complicated aspects of data management and analysis, we have traversed the length and breadth of the processes that go into writing a thesis. Practical aspects such as plagiarism and grammar checking have also been discussed. A separate section deals with thesis writing for Subspecialty and Doctor of Philosophy courses. Valuable inputs have been provided regarding the presentation of one's thesis in a conference and preparing a manuscript for publishing in journals.

The authors, who are experts in their respective fields, have lent their wisdom in the 28 chapters this book contains, for which we are deeply grateful. All of this information has been conveyed with nuance and lucidity so that it may best reach the intended audience.

We thank our publisher, Springer Nature, for their unwavering encouragement and support. We hope that you will find this book to be a trusty guide while traveling down the rocky road of writing one's thesis!

Pondicherry, India

Subhash Chandra Parija
Vikram Kate

Acknowledgments

First of all, our thanks go to the participants and the authors of this book. We would like to thank all the authors for their contribution to the scientific content and preparation of this book. We would like to express our deep gratitude to Dr. Ashutosh Mukherji, Dr. Archana Elangovan, Senior Resident, Department of Surgery, Dr. R. Kalayarasan, Dr. Suresh Kumar, Dr. Mohsina Subair, Dr. Anahita Kate, Dr. Divya Singh, and Dr. A. R. Pranavi, Junior Residents, Department of Surgery, for the editorial assistance, assembling the text, tables, graphs, and reference from the various authors into a coherent manuscript.

We are grateful to Dr. Niroj Kumar Sahoo, Former Junior Resident, Department of Ophthalmology, JIPMER, and Ms. Jaya Madhuri and Ms. Srijita Saha, MBBS students, JIPMER, for providing wonderful cartoons for the chapters, which made the book look more reader friendly. Last but not least, we would like to thank the publisher, Springer Nature, for the association and for helping to bring out this book for the readers.

Subhash Chandra Parija
Vikram Kate

Contents

Contributors

Santhosh John Abraham Head, Department of Surgery, Lourdes Hospital, Kochi, Kerala, India

C. Adithan Dean (Research), Sri Balaji Vidyapeeth, Pillaiyarkuppam, Pondicherry, India

Senthil Amudhan Associate Professor, Department of Epidemiology, National Institute of Mental Health and Neuro Sciences, Bangalore, India

Karthik Balachandran Assistant Professor, Department of Endocrinology, Sri Ramachandra Medical College and Research Institute, Chennai, India

Savio George Barreto Clinical Fellow, Hepatobiliary and Esophagogastric Unit, Division of Surgery and Perioperative Medicine, Flinders Medical Centre Bedford Park, Adelaide, South Australia

Puneet Dhar Professor and Head, Department of Gastrointestinal Surgery, Amrita Institute of Medical Sciences, Kochi, India

Lalgudi N Dorairajan Professor, Department of Urology, Jawaharlal Institute of Postgraduate Medical Education and Research, Pondicherry, India

Stuart Enoch Director of Education and Research, Doctors Academy Group (Intl), Cardiff, UK

Meenakshi Girish Associate Professor, Pediatrics, NKP Salve Institute of Medical Sciences, Nagpur, India

Divya Gupta Consultant Dermatologist, Oliva Skin and Hair Clinic, Bengaluru, India

Sanjay Gupta Director Professor and Head, Department of Surgery, University College of Medical Sciences, New Delhi, India

Ajay Haldar Assistant Professor, Department of Obstetrics and Gynaecology, All India Institute of Medical Sciences (AIIMS), Bhopal, India

K T Harichandrakumar Assistant Professor, Department of Biostatistics, Jawaharlal Institute of Postgraduate Medical Education and Research, Pondicherry, India

Sudhir Kumar Jain Director Professor, Department of Surgery, Maulana Azad Medical College and Lok Nayak Hospital, New Delhi, India

Rajive Mathew Jose Consultant in Plastic Surgery, University Hospital Birmingham, Birmingham, UK

Noyal Mariya Joseph Assistant Professor, Department of Microbiology, Jawaharlal Institute of Postgraduate Medical Education and Research, Pondicherry, India

Prashant Joshi Consultant Cardiothoracic Surgeon, Department of Cardiothoracic Surgery, Monash Health, Melbourne, Australia

Raja Kalayarasan Associate Professor, Department of Surgical Gastroenterology, Jawaharlal Institute of Post Graduate Medical Education and Research, Pondicherry, India

Sadishkumar Kamalanathan Additional Professor and Head, Department of Endocrinology, Jawaharlal Institute of Post Graduate Medical Education and Research, Pondicherry, India

Anahita Kate Fellow, Cornea and Anterior Segment, L.V. Prasad Eye Institute, Hyderabad, India

Nina V. Kate Senior Consultant Obstetrician and Programme Coordinator, National Board of Examinations, Rajiv Gandhi Government Women and Children Hospital, Pondicherry, India

Vikram Kate Professor and Head, Department of Surgery and Senior Consultant General and Gastrointestinal Surgeon, Jawaharlal Institute of Postgraduate Medical Education and Research, Pondicherry, India

Rohit Kaushik Junior Resident, Department of Surgery, Maulana Azad Medical College and Lok Nayak Hospital, New Delhi, India

Akhila Kavirayani Consultant Paediatric Rheumatologist, Nuffield Orthopaedic Centre, Oxford University Hospitals NHS Foundation Trust, Oxford, UK

Jharna Mandal Additional Professor, Department of Microbiology, Jawaharlal Institute of Postgraduate Medical Education and Research, Pondicherry, India

Ramanitharan Manikandan Additional Professor and Head, Department of Urology, Jawaharlal Institute of Postgraduate Medical Education and Research, Pondicherry, India

Johns Shaji Mathew Assistant Professor, Department of Gastrointestinal Surgery, Amrita Institute of Medical Sciences, Kochi, India

Ketan Mehra Senior Resident, Department of Urology, Jawaharlal Institute of Postgraduate Medical Education and Research, Pondicherry, India

Ashutosh Mukherji Additional Professor, Department of Radiation Oncology, Regional Cancer Centre, and Associate Dean Research, Jawaharlal Institute of Postgraduate Medical Education and Research, Pondicherry, India

Anand V. Pangarkar Honorary Associate Professor, Indira Gandhi Government Medical College, Nagpur, India

Meena A. Pangarkar Head of Department of Laboratory Medicine, National Cancer Institute, Nagpur, India

Nitin V Pangarkar Associate Professor, National University of Singapore, Singapore, Singapore

Rajesh Panwar Assistant Professor, Department of Gastrointestinal Surgery and Liver Transplantation, All India Institute of Medical Sciences, New Delhi, India

Madhuri Parija Senior Resident, Department of Orthopaedics, All India Institute of Medical Sciences (AIIMS), Bhopal, India

Subhash Chandra Parija Vice-Chancellor, Sri Balaji Vidyapeeth, (Deemed University), Pondicherry, India

Nisha V Parmar Specialist Dermatologist, Rashid Hospital, Dubai Health Authority, Dubai, UAE

Kariyarath Cheriyath Premarajan Professor and Head, Department of Preventive and Social Medicine, Jawaharlal Institute of Postgraduate Medical Education and Research, Pondicherry, India

A M Quraishi Professor, Department of Surgery, Government Medical College, Nagpur, India

M.K. Ravindran Professor and Head, Department of Emergency Medicine, Government Medical College, Kozhikode, Kerala, India

N Ravishankar Assistant Professor, Department of Statistics, Manipal University, Manipal, India

Antony Roy Former Senior Resident, Department of Orthopedics, Government Medical College, Kozhikode, Kerala, India

Peush Sahni Professor and Head, Department of Gastrointestinal Surgery and Liver Transplantation, All India Institute of Medical Sciences, New Delhi, India

William Y. Shi Department of Cardiothoracic Surgery, Monash Health, Melbourne, Australia

Zile Singh Professor and Head, Department of Community Medicine, Pondicherry Institute of Medical Sciences, Pondicherry, India

Kiruthika Sivasubramanian Consultant in Child and Adolescent Psychiatry, Black Country Foundation Trust, West Bromwich, UK

Julian A. Smith Department of Surgery (School of Clinical Sciences), Monash Medical Centre, Clayton, VIC, Australia

N. Sreekumaran Nair Professor and Head, Department of Biostatistics, Jawaharlal Institute of Postgraduate Medical Education and Research, Pondicherry, India

P. Stalin Associate Professor, Department of Community Medicine, Pondicherry Institute of Medical Sciences, Pondicherry, India

Mohsina Subair Senior Resident, Department of Plastic and Reconstructive Surgery, Postgraduate Institute Medical Education and Research, Chandigarh, India

A. Surendiran Associate Professor, Department of Pharmacology, Jawaharlal Institute of Postgraduate Medical Education and Research, Pondicherry, India

Sathasivam Sureshkumar Associate Professor, Department of Surgery, Jawaharlal Institute of Postgraduate Medical Education and Research, Pondicherry, India

Mahalakshmy Thulasingam Associate Professor, Department of Preventive and Social Medicine, Jawaharlal Institute of Postgraduate Medical Education and Research, Pondicherry, India

Mukta Wyawahare Additional Professor, Department of Medicine, Jawaharlal Institute of Postgraduate Medical Education and Research, Pondicherry, India

Balaji Zacharia Additional Professor, Department of Orthopedics, Government Medical College, Kozhikode, Kerala, India

About the Editors

Subhash Chandra Parija Vice-Chancellor, Sri Balaji Vidyapeeth (Deemed University), Pondicherry, India, with almost three and a half decades of teaching and research experience in medical microbiology. Prof. Parija is a Food and Agriculture Organization (FAO) expert and has been consulted to draft guidelines on food safety for parasites. He was on the MD Examination Boards at Colombo University, Sri Lanka, Sultan Qaboos University, Oman, and the University of Malaya, Malaysia. He was awarded a D.Sc. for his contributions in the field of Medical Parasitology by Madras University. The author of ten books, including the *Textbook of Medical Parasitology*, he has published more than 300 papers in prestigious national and international journals.

Prof. Parija has received more than 25 awards, including the Medical Council of India's Dr. BC Roy National Award and the National Academy of Medical Sciences' Dr. PN Chuttani Oration Award. He founded the Indian Academy of Tropical Parasitology (IATP), the only professional organization for Medical Parasitologists in India, and initiated the journal *Tropical Parasitology*. In collaboration with Prof. Vikram Kate, he edited the book *Writing and Publishing a Scientific Research Paper*, which was published by Springer Nature in 2017.

Vikram Kate is currently a Senior Professor, Head of the Department of Surgery, and Senior Consultant General and Gastrointestinal Surgeon at the Jawaharlal Institute of Postgraduate Medical Education and Research (JIPMER), Pondicherry. He has contributed more than 35 chapters in prominent surgical gastroenterology and surgery textbooks and has published over 140 papers. He is a Past President of the Indian Association of Surgical Gastroenterology and was awarded the Faculty of Surgical Trainers' Membership Diploma by the Royal College of Surgeons, Edinburgh. Further, he is currently serving as Editor-in-Chief of the *International Journal of Advanced Medical and Health Research*, the official journal of JIPMER.

Professor Kate is an examiner for the M.S./M.Ch./DNB and Ph.D. program for Surgery, Surgical Gastroenterology and Intercollegiate Membership of the Royal College of Surgeons, Edinburgh. He is a Fellow of the Royal College of Surgeons of England, Edinburgh and Glasgow (FRCS, FRCS Ed., FRCS Glasg.), and of the American College of Surgeons (FACS) and the American College of Gastroenterology (FACG). He has received numerous awards, including the Association of National Board accredited Institutions "Distinguished DNB Teacher of Excellence Award" (2018), Dr. Mathias Oration (2010) and Prof. N. Rangabashyam Oration (2015) from the Tamil Nadu and Pondicherry Chapter of the Association of Surgeons of India, and the Dr. S.K. Bhansali Memorial Oration (2017) of the Association of Surgeons of India.

Part I

Deciding on the Topic/Area of Research/ Approval

Thesis, Dissertation and Project

Subhash Chandra Parija and Vikram Kate

Research is to see what everybody else has seen, and to think what nobody else has thought.—Albert Szent-Gyorgyi

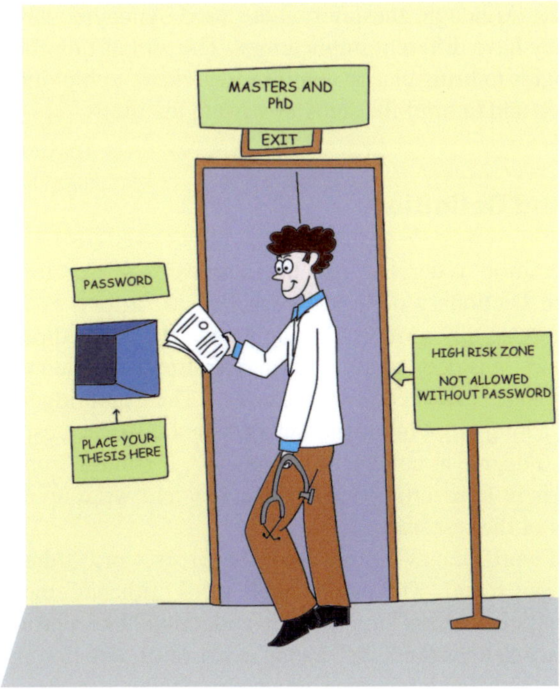

S. C. Parija
Vice-Chancellor, Sri Balaji Vidyapeeth, (Deemed University), Pondicherry, India

V. Kate (✉)
Professor and Head, Department of Surgery and Senior Consultant General and Gastrointestinal Surgeon, Jawaharlal Institute of Postgraduate Medical Education and Research, Pondicherry, India

S. C. Parija, V. Kate (eds.), *Thesis Writing for Master's and Ph.D. Program*,
https://doi.org/10.1007/978-981-13-0890-1_1

Key Points

- In most institutes and universities dissertation and thesis is a part of the curriculum and a mandatory requirement for the award of a postgraduate or doctoral degree.
- The process of doing literature review provides an in-depth knowledge in a particular field and helps postgraduates to familiarize with statistical concepts.
- The outcomes of thesis, dissertation and projects can be published as a research paper in scientific journals.
- Research career of the postgraduate can also be set off by the thesis and dissertation work.
- Thesis writing can be understood in a simplified manner by following the ten defined steps starting from choosing suitable research area to get the thesis published.

Terminologies like thesis, dissertation and project are common in academic and research practice. Although, these terms are used synonymously by students and some faculty they have different implications. The aim of this chapter is to explain these terminologies to bring clarity among researchers, to highlight the importance of doing research and to brief the steps of writing the thesis.

Etymology and Definition

The word 'dissertation' is derived from the Latin word "dissertare" which means 'to discuss'. Oxford Dictionary defines dissertation as 'a long essay on a particular subject or topic especially written for a university degree or diploma'. In Merriam Webster dictionary, it is defined as "an extended usually written treatment of a subject; specifically: one submitted for a doctorate". The Cambridge dictionary defines dissertation as "a long piece of writing on a particular subject, especially one that is done to receive a degree at college or university". It is clear from these definitions that the emphasis in a dissertation is on a review and write up on a subject rather than the novelty of the research.

The origin of word "thesis" comes from the Greek word "tithenai" which means "to place or to put forth". The early Greek word "tithenai" metamorphosed into 'thesis' which in Greek refers "to put forth something" like a proposal. The Oxford English dictionary defines thesis as "a long essay or dissertation involving personal research, written by a candidate for a university degree". In Merriam Webster dictionary it is defined as a "dissertation embodying results of original research and especially substantiating a specific view". The Cambridge dictionary defines thesis as "a long piece of writing on a subject, especially one based on original research and done for a higher college or university degree". In some countries, a dissertation is also referred to as a thesis. However, in contrast to dissertation thesis is an in-depth study of a topic that contributes novel information in the field of research.

The word project is derived from the Latin word "projectum" from the Latin verb "proicere" (before an action), which in turn comes from "pro" (precedence), and "iacere"(to do). Thus, the original meaning of the word "project" is to plan of something and not to the act of carrying out the plan. The Oxford English dictionary defines project as "a piece of research work undertaken by a school or college student". In Merriam Webster dictionary, it is defined as a planned undertaking: such as a formulated piece of research. The Cambridge dictionary defines project as "a study of a particular subject done over a period, especially by students".

The word project is often used in the engineering field and various government plans. A research project can be a short-term (less than a year) or long-term project. A short-term research project is usually undertaken by the undergraduate students and a long-term project is usually undertaken by faculty working in research institutes. A short-term research project is an abbreviated form of dissertation where the focus is on research methodology and not the outcome of research. In long-term research project, the focus is on the novelty of research in addition to the methodology like a thesis. The differences between a dissertation, thesis and a short-term research project is summarized in Table 1. It is important to understand these differences so that the researcher is aware of the purpose of research and its implications.

Table 1 Differences between a dissertation, thesis and a short-term research project

Parameter	Dissertation	Thesis	Short-term research project
Requirement	Completion of dissertation is a requirement to appear for the final exit exam but does not guarantee a postgraduate or master's degree (MD/MS) unless the candidate clears the final exam	On completion awarded a doctorate or Ph.D. degree	A student research project is not a mandatory requirement for the award of a degree
Duration	Usually 3 years including protocol preparation and final write up and it is a part-time assignment for medical students	Usually 3 years and the duration is extendable if the work is not complete. It is often a full time research course	Usually a short period ranging from 1 month to 2 year and it is a part-time assignment for medical students
Research methodology	Important	Extremely important	Important
Novelty of research	Not crucial	Extremely important. Aim of thesis is to add novel findings to existing literature	Not important
Hypothesis	Not mandatory	Mandatory requirement	May or may not be present
Research outcome	Not as important and does not determine the acceptance of dissertation	Extremely important for the acceptance of thesis	Not as important
Evaluation and defence	Usually perfunctory, in front of examiners (closed defence) at the time of exit examination	Oral defence (usually public) in front of eminent researchers is an important criterion for acceptance	Not mandatory

Need for Dissertation, Thesis and Research Projects

The main reasons and advantages of doing a dissertation, thesis and research projects is outlined below.

Academic Requirement

In most institutes and universities, dissertation and thesis is a part of the curriculum and a mandatory requirement for the award of postgraduate or doctoral degree [1]. For the faculty, a research project is a mandatory requirement for assessment based promotion in may academic institutes.

Learning Research Methodology

Short term research projects and dissertation helps undergraduate and postgraduate students to learn the art of doing research and understanding the research methodology. The process of doing literature review provides an in-depth knowledge in a particular field. It also helps postgraduates to familiarize with statistical concepts as well [2].

Critical Appraisal of Data

Dissertation and thesis help postgraduates to develop the art of collecting, recording and critically analysing the data instead of blindly accepting the results published in the literature. This translates to improved patient outcomes.

Publication

The outcomes of thesis, dissertation and projects can be published as a research paper in scientific journals. Publication helps to disseminate the findings of your research to other investigators to guide future research, provide reliable scientific information to patients and enhance academic career and job opportunity to the publisher.

Research Grants and Research Career

The dissertation or a thesis can be presented in national and international conferences which will bring recognition to the young researcher and may attract the potential funding agencies for providing research grant for continuing the research work or to carry out the subsequent advanced research in the similar research field, thus research career of the postgraduate can also be set off by the thesis and dissertation work [3].

Thesis Writing: How to Start?

The successful thesis writing can be represented in a ten steps work station which needs to be followed in an order to complete the dissertation work. Figure 1 shows the flow chart representing the Steps of Thesis writing.

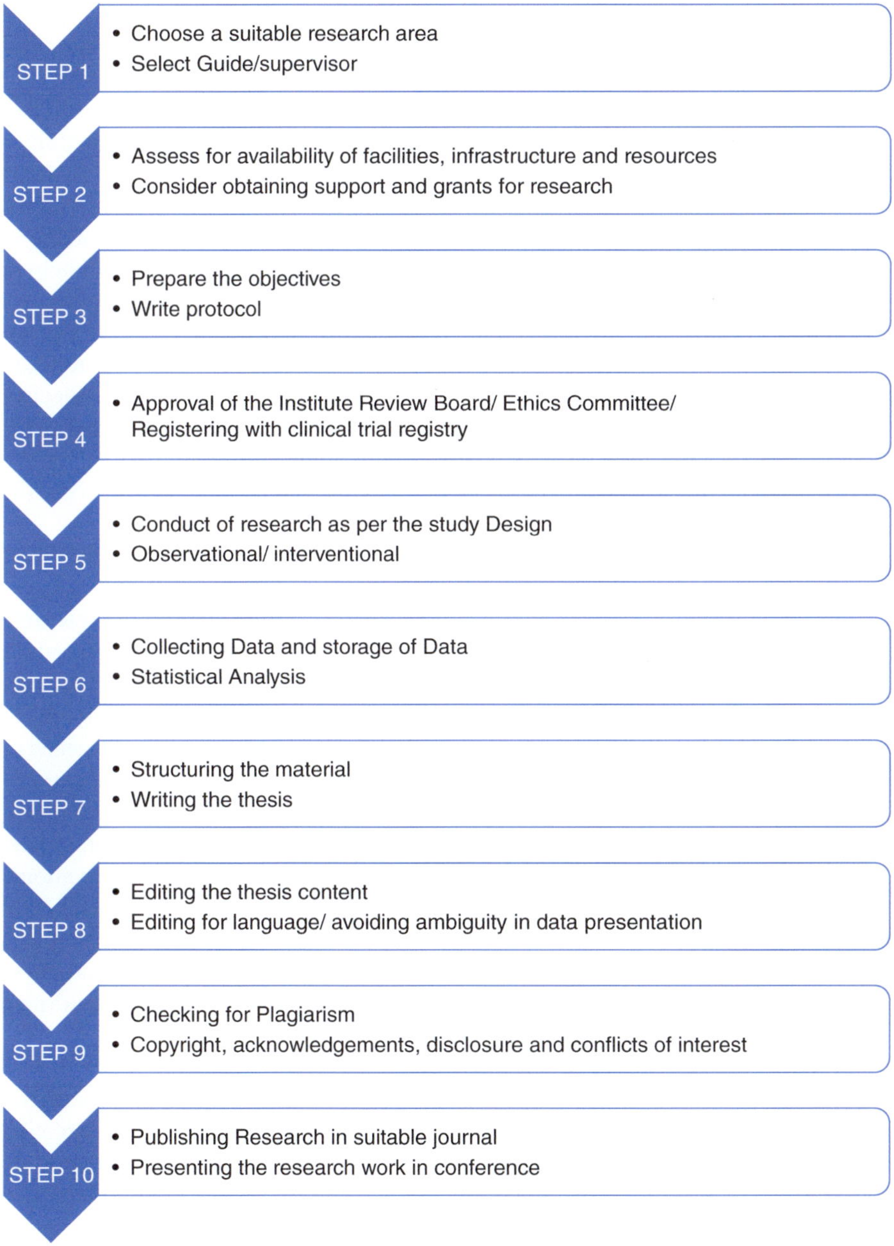

Fig. 1 Flow chart representing the steps of thesis writing

Step 1: Choose a suitable research area and Select Guide/Supervisor

The first step in thesis writing is to choose the appropriate research area. The research topic should be thirst area of the particular specialty in which the students doing his/her master degree and should be relevant to the existing knowledge gap. Selecting the guide/supervisor is of vital importance since the conduct and completion of the research requires tremendous help from the guide. Guide also helps in identifying the suitable topic with their experience.

Step 2: Assess for availability of facilities, infrastructure and resources and consider obtaining support and grants for research

The research work planned should always be assessed with respect to available infrastructure and facility to meet the required resources [1, 2]. Conducting a research work for which the existing infrastructure is inadequate will lead to delay in completing the thesis. If the required facility is not available, it can be obtained through research grants from appropriate funding agencies [3]. The suggestions of guide/supervisor can be taken for processing the research grant, which will help in avoiding the unnecessary rejections from multiple funding agencies.

Step 3: Prepare the objectives and write the protocol

Once the potential research thirst area is identified and available resources are ensured, the actual thesis writing begins with defining the objectives. The objective should be specific, measurable, achievable/attainable, realistic/relevant and time-bound. Once the objectives are defined the suitable study design for carrying out the research should be decided and protocol for the same should be prepared as per the standard instruction of institutional review board [4–6].

Step 4: Approval of the Institute Review Board/Ethics Committee/ Registering with clinical trial registry

Obtaining ethics committee approval is mandatory before starting the research. Necessary modifications should be made as per the suggestions given by the ethics committee to avoid ethical and legal issues during and after the completion of research [4–6]. All the clinical trials should be registered prospectively in an approved trial registry and trial register number should be specified in all means of presentation of the thesis work including conference presentation and publication.

Step 5: Conduct of research as per the study design

After the necessary approval from institute review board and ethics committee, the research should be carried out according to the study design chosen. Observational and interventional study should be carried out according to the details specified in the protocol and necessary consent should be obtained from all the participants before enrolment [5, 6]. The proforma including all the required variable and information helps in recording the findings and outcome which can later be transformed to an electronic data collecting tool to avoid loss of important data.

Step 6: Collecting and Storing the Data, Statistical Analysis

The data collection is the most vital part as the outcome of the study depends on the effective and proper data collection. Storage of collected data till the completion of sample size/required number of study subject is as tedious job. Many methods are available for data storage including electronic and print applications. Electronic data storing applications such as REDCap, EpiData, EpiInfo etc. helps to maintain large volume of data and also supports in analysis due to ease of decoding the necessary variables [7]. Statistical analysis provides reliable and meaningful results out of large raw data which should be understandable by the target audience. The results can be represented in tables, figures, charts and line diagrams etc.

Step 7: Structuring the material and Writing the thesis

Writing up of a research finding for thesis purpose is different from the standard journal publication format with respect to style, content, data presentation, formatting and submission [8, 9]. The thesis should include the front page detailing the credentials of the student, guide and the institute along with the certification of original work done by the student. The acknowledgement, abbreviations list and the content list follows the certification. Main content of the thesis should be incorporated in the order of Abstract, Introduction, Review of literature, Aim and objective, Materials and methods, Results, Discussion, Summary and Conclusion [8, 9]. The tables, figures, necessary certificates such as ethics committee certificate, institute review board certificates, consent form, patient information sheet, master data chart etc. should be attached as annexure following the main thesis content.

Step 8: Editing the thesis content, Editing for language and avoiding ambiguity in data presentation

Editing the thesis content makes it easier for the reviewer and the target audience to understand the conceptualization better. Non-native English speaking candidates may require assistance for language editing which is available for a reasonable fee from professional agencies. Language editing also helps in publication in the international academic journals.

Step 9: Checking for Plagiarism, Copyright, acknowledgements, disclosure and conflicts of interest

Copying whole or a part of other's work is considered plagiarism and is viewed as a serious misconduct by all the academic publishers [10]. Detection of plagiarism may lead to rejection of the research work, penalty and also black listing in majority of the publication network. Hence it is vital to carry out plagiarism checking of the research work written which will help in correcting the unintentional plagiarized content, which may happen especially when writing large volume of review of literature. Similarly, copyright issue should be anticipated when using photographs, classifications, flow diagram, tables etc. from the published resources and the same should be clarified from the concerned publishers and necessary permission should be obtained prior to submitting the research work. Financial disclosure and declaration of conflict of interest has become mandatory nowadays when publishing the research work. Acknowledging the same should be done to avoid legal issues related to publishing the research work.

Step 10: Publishing Research in suitable journal and presenting the research work in conference

The quote "If it wasn't published, it wasn't done" explains the importance of presenting and publishing the research work [9]. Any outcome or finding irrespective of positive or negative results should be presented in the conferences and published in standard scientific research journals so as to reach the target population. Limitation of the research is not a limitation for publication. Certain weakness of the research work can arise due to logistic constraints and limited infrastructure and should be brought out in the publication so that the said limitations can be addressed in further studies [9]. Presentation in conferences and publishing the research work also brings recognition for the researcher and possible invitation from the funding agencies to carry advanced research work in the field.

Case Scenarios

1. A student studying his master degree in medicine wanted to do thesis on the role of presence a particular viral antibody and prognosis of pneumonia. Which of the following should be done first to carry the thesis work?
   (a) Get approval from Institute Review Board/Ethics Committee
   (b) Check the availability of such testing facility in the present Institute
   (c) Write the protocol
   (d) Select appropriate study design
2. After writing the thesis, the student wants to publish the research work. Which of the following is not correct?
   (a) Check for plagiarism
   (b) Edit for language and content
   (c) Avoid specifying limitations of the research work
   (d) Disclose financial and conflict of interest

References

1. Roberts CM. The dissertation journey. 2nd ed. New York: Corwin; 2010.
2. Evans D, Gruba P, Zobel J. How to write a better thesis. 3rd ed. New York: Springer; 2014.
3. Turner S, Davidson P, Stanton L, Cawdeary V. Features of successful bids for funding of applied health research: a cohort study. Health Res Policy Syst. 2014;12:54.
4. Terrel SR. Writing a proposal for your dissertation: guidelines and examples. New York: The Guilford Press; 2016.
5. Duane L, Michael C. Graduate student learning outcomes at the masters and doctoral level. In: Assessment and review of graduate programs. 2nd ed. Washington: Council of Graduate Schools; 2011.
6. Gliner JA, Morgan GA, Leech NL. Research methods in applied settings: an integrated approach to design and analysis. 3rd ed. New York: Routledge; 2017.
7. Perrier L, Blondal E, Ayala AP, et al. Research data management in academic institutions, a scoping review. PLoS One. 2017;12:e0178261.
8. Kate V, Sureshkumar S, Mohsina S. Abstract and key words. In: Parija SC, Kate V, editors. Parija and Kate's research book series -I—*Writing and publishing a scientific research paper*. New Delhi: Springer; 2017. p. 27–37.
9. Parija SC, Kate V. Why write a research scientificpaper? In: Parija SC, Kate V, editors. Parija and Kate's research book series -I—*Writing and publishing a scientific research paper*. New Delhi: Springer; 2017. p. 3–8.
10. Gasparyan AY, Nurmashev B, Seksenbayev B, Trukhachev VI, Kostyukova EI, Kitas GD. Plagiarism in the context of education and evolving detection strategies. J Korean Med Sci. 2017;32:1220–7.

Objectives of Writing Thesis

Meena A. Pangarkar, Nitin V. Pangarkar, and Anand V. Pangarkar

I hope to write someday something worth plagiarizing.—unknown

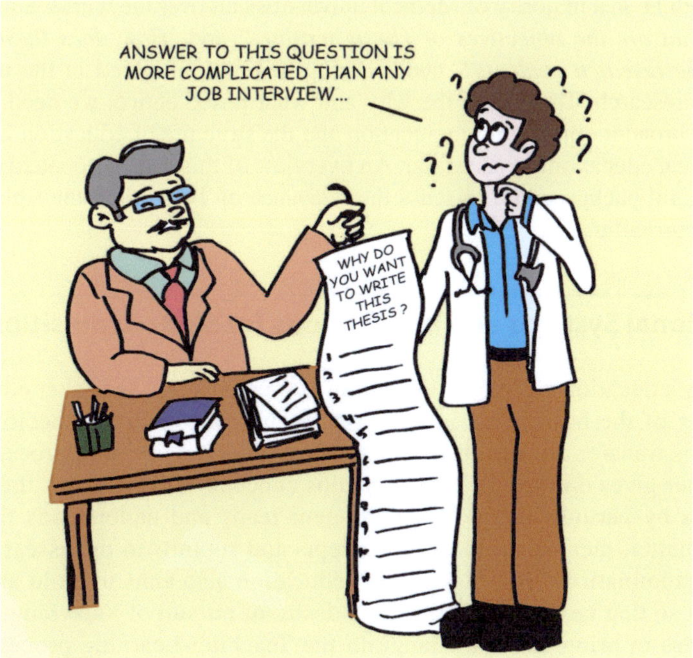

M. A. Pangarkar (✉)
Head of Department of Laboratory Medicine, National Cancer Institute, Nagpur, India

N. V. Pangarkar
Associate Professor, National University of Singapore, Singapore, Singapore

A. V. Pangarkar
Honorary Associate Professor, Indira Gandhi Government Medical College, Nagpur, India

S. C. Parija, V. Kate (eds.), *Thesis Writing for Master's and Ph.D. Program*,
https://doi.org/10.1007/978-981-13-0890-1_2

Key Points

- The aim of writing thesis or dissertation is to develop a research mindset, which promotes scientific curiosity.
- Thesis writing helps in the development of project management skills, to build up the scientific report writing skills and to build up the credibility amongst peers and scientific community.
- Well-executed theses could often be presented in conferences and/or published in journals.
- Conduct of a scientific inquiry, in a structured manner, will help the student pursue a research career in future.

Introduction

Thesis writing is a pre-requisite for the award of a post-graduate degree such as M.D. or Ph.D. in a majority of Medical universities all over the world. So, the questions '*What are the objectives of Thesis writing?*' and '*How does thesis writing benefit the research students*?' need to be posed and answered in the interest of scientific research. To analyse the why and what posed above, we need to understand the broader objectives of education and the structure of education in general, and medical education, in particular. An overview of this broader context equips us with a useful background to discuss the relevance of Theses and their place in the medical curriculum.

Educational Systems and Implications for Skills Acquisition

Primarily, education has multiple aims and objectives. At the higher educational level, one of the basic aims is imparting technical or subject-specific knowledge. This transfer of knowledge is usually a didactic, one-way process, where the teacher gives out information, explains concepts and evaluates the learning outcomes by various methods. The student reads and understands the taught subject matter, memorises the key concepts and submits to the assessments by writing examinations. But higher level education also aims to mold and evolve a student so that he develops a lifelong desire of pursuit of knowledge. Thus, a need arises to bring about a change in the Teaching-Learning process, laying more emphasis on self-learning. The goals of this pursuit of knowledge include developing an inquisitive mindset, acquiring intellectual skills like comprehension, analysis, synthesis and integration of a large body of information, application of these skills in working life to do problem-solving, developing effective communication skills and ability to do teamwork. Another critical goal is to build a strong ethical foundation which helps to gain credibility amongst academia and society [1, 2].

The Indian medical education system is structured in two tiers- Graduate and Post graduate levels. The Medical Graduates' Teaching—Learning involves extensive study of different subjects e.g. Anatomy, Physiology, Pathology, Medicine, Surgery, to name a few, with a great emphasis on written and oral examinations. This model leaves some gaps in terms of developing a broader perspective and imparting non-technical skills. Modern Medicine and the healthcare industry evolution are putting a great emphasis on 'Evidence based Medicine'. Consequently, newer skills are in demand, e.g. efficient information processing, analytical ability, organization of 'Big Data' and effective communication.

Viewed in the above context, 'Thesis writing' acts as a vital tool which helps to bridge the gap between acquiring the academic and nonacademic skill sets [3].

Thesis Writing: A Win-Win Proposition

Writing a thesis is novel for most students. It is also "painful" because it requires a substantial amount of focused work on a topic. The novelty and the magnitude of the task imply that most students will find it challenging to write a thesis. Thesis supervision also poses challenges to the advisors who have to guide inexperienced researchers and help them towards successful completion of the thesis. Given the "costs" or challenges of writing and supervising a thesis, there have to be tangible and intangible benefits for the thesis tradition to continue, in the foreseeable future.

The educational aims of writing a thesis are manifold

The first aim is developing a research mindset which promotes scientific curiosity, so that the student not only gathers information but also learns to question it [4]. Developing an independent thought process is a critical requirement for any research worker. In an age where a lot of information is available to us, at the click of a mouse button, research ability may be confused with "googling". But research requires sifting and synthesis of the vast information that is available on the internet and other sources and developing ones' perspective by understanding that information.

Conduct of a scientific inquiry, in a structured manner, will help the student to pursue a Ph.D., and a research career in future. As the society needs clinical physicians to treat patients, it also needs researchers who will understand disease patterns and incidences, etiopathogenetic factors, do basic research and help translate this research into clinical work. A developing country like India may have different priorities than developed countries such as the US and researchers grounded in the local context can help understand the challenges better as well as tackle those challenges more cost efficiently and effectively.

The second aim of thesis writing is development of project management skills. Since writing a thesis requires design and implementation of a research project, mostly based on the students' initiative, it requires a different set of skills from attending semester-long and year-long traditional courses. Even more importantly, it requires candidates to develop some testable propositions or models, design a method to test those models and arrive at conclusions. Both skills are useful in their professional careers, regardless of whether they become practicing physicians, academicians, administrators or researchers. Learning to be a self-starter and pacing yourself to finish a substantial piece of work that meets rigorous standards, needs efficient time management skills, and a realistic assessment of achievable targets.

Like all research projects, thesis writing is an uncertain process. One can start walking in a particular direction only to discover that it is a "dead end". Navigating this uncertain process successfully, without externally imposed deadlines such as assignment due dates or examinations provides tremendous learning opportunities, which are bound to be useful to students later in their careers.

The third aim is to help buildup the scientific report writing skills of the student. [4]

A lucid and simple introduction of the thesis helps in understanding the whole study. Incorporation and explanation of technical jargon at the beginning itself makes the reader comfortable while delving deeper into the study. Integration of the collected data and sequential organization of the observations on this data, help to avoid being overwhelmed by the large volume of collected data. Analysis and logical interpretation of all the observations form the backbone of the research project. This is reflected in the discussion section of the thesis, which in essence tells you all about the outcomes of the whole project [4].

The fourth aim is to build up the credibility amongst peers and scientific community by imparting an ethical dimension to the budding scientists. While reviewing all the published research on the topic of thesis, one comes across the huge contributions made by many workers in the field. Plagiarism is a constant temptation while doing research, to take short-cuts, cut corners and to take undue credit. By learning to use all this information responsibly, by acknowledging the contribution of previous researchers in the bibliography section, the student strengthens his/ her moral integrity [4].

The fifth aim is to gain a publication record. Well-executed theses could often be presented in conferences and/or published in journals. For candidates wishing to pursue a career in academics, these publications could serve as a head start. Even for candidates who don't pursue an academic career, a conference presentation and/or a journal paper could add to legitimacy. Additionally, the process of submitting to a journal or presenting at a conference is a learning experience by itself. A conference presentation involves preparing a manuscript and a concise presentation to communicate the significance of the research and its findings. A conference presentation also involves a question and answer session where the candidate could face challenging questions about the research and its significance. Responding to this scrutiny, to defend the findings with scientific arguments and analyses, is a skill by itself. This process tests not only the candidate's knowledge of his/ her work but also his ability to think on his/her feet. To publish an article in a journal requires undergoing an even more rigorous process in terms of satisfying the editor and peer reviewers while addressing their comments adequately, sometimes through multiple rounds of revision. (Fig. 1)

Fig. 1 Five skillsets developed by the research student during writing a thesis

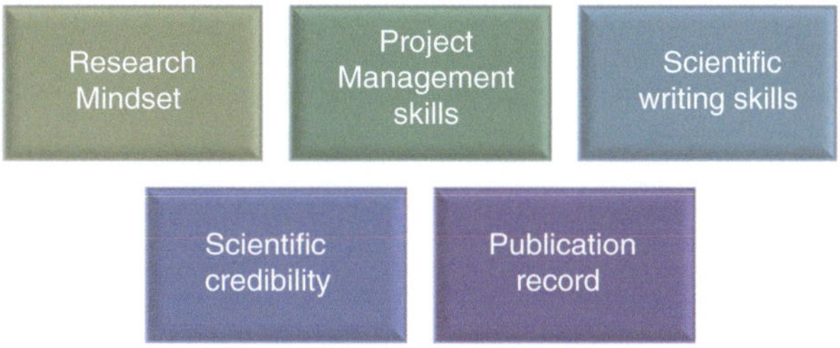

To achieve the above Aims, six specific objectives can be formulated:

Objectives

1. To formulate a specific question addressing an area/subject in the context of available/current knowledge. This involves a comprehensive review of all the published work related to the topic of interest, thus imparting a breadth and depth to the research student's knowledge.
2. To identify appropriate research techniques, which are needed to address the posed question so as to find a solution. An understanding of different research methodologies is necessary, to be able to decide which method is suitable for the research question. The availability of adequate financial and technological resources has to be ensured to bring the project to fruition.
3. To collect adequate clinical material and data on which to demonstrate the application of research techniques. This objective makes the student discern the criteria of sample size, and judge the adequacy and validity of clinical data.
4. To report the findings in a cogent, coherent way, subjecting them to appropriate statistical analysis employing relevant statistical tests. Distilling and making sense of the voluminous data develops the skills of organization and collation of a large amount of information.
5. To apply logical thought process to draw general conclusions and/or suggest other hypotheses to further study. The skills of derivation and deduction are honed, leading to evolution of newer concepts in the subject.
6. To submit the work to rigorous scrutiny by presentations in oral/poster formats in scientific meets and conferences and disseminate the research findings amongst the scientific community by publication of the work in peer-reviewed journals. This is the most tangible and visible outcome of the thesis writing, whereby the researcher creates a track record, and strengthens the foundation of the individual's scientific career (Fig. 2).

Thesis writing not only benefits the research student but also the Mentor or Guide. From a supervisor's perspective, there are numerous benefits of mentoring research students. Thesis supervisors may be able to initiate new projects. Many supervisors may have identified interesting directions for further research but simply do not have the time to devote to the new project. With greater time resources, and fresh perspectives to address these issues, research students can be the ideal

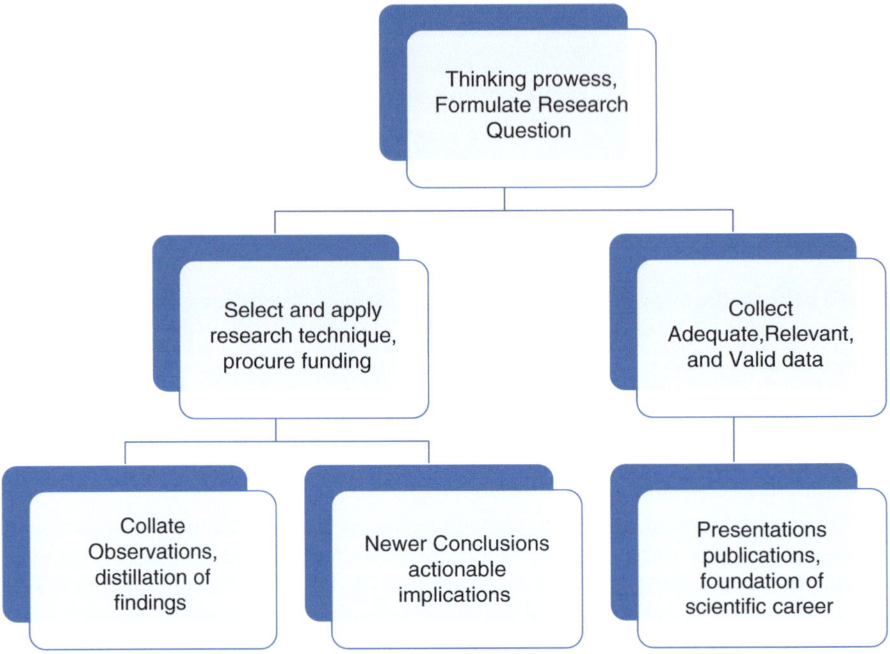

Fig. 2 Flow chart for planning the research work

partners to help their supervisors jump-start projects, or speed-up and advance others that have stalled.

Supervisors can also develop long-term relationships with mentees. Publishing joint research based on the theses may only be the first step in building this relationship and a long-term relationship can be fruitful and productive for both the mentee as well as the supervisor. Additionally, supervisors can have the added satisfaction of seeing their mentees successfully complete a substantial piece of work. There is the gratification of watching your students grow professionally and come up with insights and new knowledge [5].

Lastly the whole scientific community of the world is made richer because of the numerous theses undertaken in all the universities. 'The Butterfly effect' of Thesis writing continually expands the boundaries of science by a combination of original ideas and new knowledge, brought forth by research work [6].

Conclusion

Writing a thesis is a complementary approach to the examination based traditional courses in Indian medical education. It fulfills the course requirement for the award of a Masters or Doctoral Degree. This academic achievement leads to peer recognition in the scientific community. Further, the thesis writing process equips the students with a broad range of skills, which stand them in good stead throughout their future career. The Guides/Mentors also derive significant benefits utilizing the resources and vehicles of post graduate students. Thus, a continual, congenial ecosystem is built up, which enables scientific pursuits to benefit, improve and sustain the human community. While thesis writing is not without pain, adjustments and sacrifices, I believe the rewards justify the pain [7, 8].

Case Scenarios

1. Frame A Research Question
   (a) Prevalence of a disease in defined area.
   (b) Comparison of a new diagnostic test to established tests.
   (c) Test the etiological role of a factor in causation of a disease.
   (d) Effectiveness of a new drug in treatment of a disease.
2. How many data points are needed to derive statistically significant conclusions
   (a) Percentage of population.
   (b) Equal number of new and established test results.
   (c) Case to control numbers ratio.

References

1. Anglin GJ, Ross SM, Morrison GR. Inquiry in instructional design and technology: getting started. In: Anglin GJ, editor. Instructional technology: past, present and future. 2nd ed. Englewood: Libraries Unlimited; 1995.
2. Zaidi S, Nasir M. Teaching and learning methods in medicine. Springer; 2015.
3. Honors Thesis. The interdisciplinary program in archaeology. [Document on the Internet]. Washington University in St. Louis: 2017 [cited 2017 Nov 5]. http://www.archaeology.artsci.wustl.edu.
4. Borges A. Should you write an honors thesis? Ácademics. [Document on the Internet]. Intern with HER CAMPUS 2014 [cited 2017 Nov 5]. http://www.hercampus.com/life.
5. Himeles D. Thesis writing benefits. [Document on the Internet]. CLASSROOM; Leaf Group Ltd. 2017 [cited 2017 Nov 5]. http://www.classroom.synonym.com.
6. Lorenz E. Deterministic Non Periodic flow. J Atmos Sci. 1963;20(2):130–41.
7. Giesler M, Boeker M, Fabry G, Biller S. Importance and benefits of the doctoral thesis for medical graduates. GMS J Med Educ. 2016;33(1):Doc 8.
8. Larick D, Carter M. Graduate student learning outcomes at the masters and doctoral level. In: Assessment and review of graduate programs. 2nd ed. Council of Graduate Schools: Washington; 2011.

Choosing a Suitable Research Area and Supervisor

Prashant Joshi

"It is our choices, Harry, that show what we truly are, far more than our abilities."—J.K. Rowling

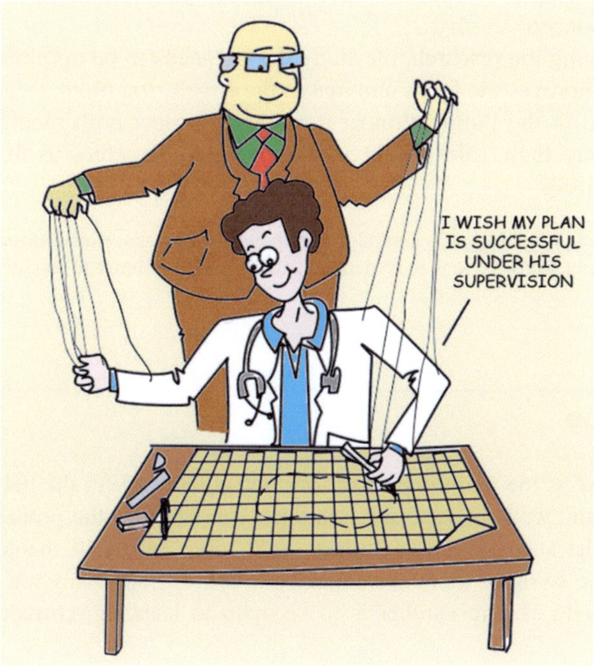

P. Joshi
Consultant Cardiothoracic Surgeon, Department of Cardiothoracic Surgery, Monash Health, Melbourne, Australia

S. C. Parija, V. Kate (eds.), *Thesis Writing for Master's and Ph.D. Program*,
https://doi.org/10.1007/978-981-13-0890-1_3

Key Points

- Most research topics are selected with ease using a lot of common sense.
- Meticulously selected research topics are easy to work on and more likely to finish in the given time frame.
- It is vital to know the time frame and resources available right from the start to accomplish the research project.
- A good mentor can not only facilitate the research project but also, eventually, help in getting published.
- The research topics are everywhere. From within one's own thoughts to the existing status of healthcare there are infinite possibilities of useful research topics that could advance the field of medical science.
- Finding a suitable mentor, with expertise and interest in the selected research topic is as important as selecting the research topic itself.
- Some research projects need more than one mentor.
- Mentorship is a learned skill.
- Both the mentor as well as the mentee works together with compassion, dedication and develop/evolve the new idea. Both are 'involved' in the new concept and make the concept 'evolve'.
- For publishing the research, the study design needs to be optimised. Narrowing the topic improves the focus and makes the conclusion more accurate.
- To succeed in the publication of a research project both mentor and mentee have to play their roles while molding their characters to fit in with their responsibilities.

> In the search for certainty, it is natural, to begin with our present experiences, and in some sense, no doubt, knowledge is to be derived from them [1]—Bertrand Russel (Problems of Philosophy)

Introduction

Common sense is the main ingredient of good science. With the help of it, a carefully chosen and well-focused research topic can simplify the process and make it interesting. The successful selection of right topic and right mentor depends on several factors, some of them are under your control, but many are not. However, what one can do as a researcher is to be open to learning, corrections and even failures.

A meticulously selected topic is carried through to its publication with ease and the entire experience becomes an enjoyable journey. On publication, the article attracts many readers and keeps on appearing repeatedly in the references of many future studies. If the study turns out to be a ground breaking work, it does not merely remain the matter of name and fame, but often creates career opportunities for the authors.

How to Choose a Suitable Research Topic

The process of choosing a suitable research topic can be summarised in a single word—"re-search". Even though it is possible to summarise it in a word, finding a good topic is probably one of the most difficult things about research. And it is an evolving process. However, prior to embarking upon this, the researchers must ask two simple questions to themselves.

1. What is the given time frame?
2. What resources are at my disposal?

Basic Principles for Finding Suitable Topic

1. Seek help, find a mentor: This has been elaborated in detail under the heading, 'Choosing a Mentor'.
2. At the onset of selecting a suitable topic for research, try to look for a question, a project or a field of your interest. It is always easy to write about the topic of your interest, e.g. Surgery, Medicine, Maternal Health, Nutrition, Mental Health, Preventive Medicine, Infectious Disease, Nursing, Physiotherapy, etc.

Where to Find the Topics of Interest?

It is likely that there is a particular health issue that inspired you to enter the profession which you have chosen for your career. At some point in your career, it might have struck you that certain issues surrounding current standard of care or the outcomes are not up to the mark and might benefit from a renewed strategy. This is where a research topic might be unfolding itself.

There could be different approaches, management strategies or surgical techniques that need verification as to the superiority of one over the other in terms of prognosis, life expectancy and event-free survival benefits. This is a breeding ground for research topics. Review of topics covered in textbooks could generate a lot of research potential when they are read between the lines. Good texts in the books often mention about the pitfalls in the diagnosis and management of many ailments and conditions. Selecting a topic aimed at answering those questions can advance the health science as a whole. These are the fields where most of the medical research is blooming.

The table of contents of National Health Statistics is also a very important source for choosing a topic of interest that could make an impact on National Health Policies. Health Care Management issues in an institution, the cost control measures required by the health organizations are all extremely potent sources of research topics.

Many times, the experience comes handy for those who have already worked in specialized fields. Their insight into the specialty provokes the thoughts for methods to improvise the existing systems, techniques or even medicines. For those who had no such opportunity, maybe there is a particular disease or a clinical condition that stirs a curiosity in you, through your own experience or that of your family or friends.

Sometimes, topics of combined or social interests, such as health issues involving a particular racial or ethnic group that one would like to learn more about could bring the need for research into light. For example, are there any disparities between different ethnic groups in terms of access to the health services compared to the mainstream population.

Controversial issues: Sometimes some controversial issues are interesting to explore. For instance, Comparison of different techniques of inguinal hernia repair, comparison of different strategies for treating multi-vessel coronary artery disease in octogenarians, etc. There might be a recent article or news in multimedia that could be of interest to the community, such as primary preventive measures, best secondary or tertiary preventive measures.

3. The Ultimate Source: By and large the best source for specific research topics is the recent research studies. A good research article, at the end, identifies the implications or recommendations for future research. The epigraph at the beginning of this chapter by the great philosopher, Bertrand Russel, is so apt in this context that wishfully, it could be set in neon lights for this 'search'.

Virtues of Writing Down as the Search Begins

In order to maximise the output from your effort, get into a habit of writing as soon as the idea is conceived. By developing this habit, you might be able to write multiple papers based on different dimensions of the topic. However, to have that ability, you have to identify your key idea first.

What's an idea? An Idea is defined in many ways. But one definition stands out which says, "The idea is a reusable insight, useful to the reader." Remember, at the outset that your initial idea might vary during the first phase of choosing the suitable topic itself. It might even span out into three ideas. Keep your mind open to the possibility of writing three different papers.

Most importantly, selection of the suitable research topic is strongly influenced by time frame and availability of resources, as has been emphasized at the beginning of this section.

Narrowing the Topic/Choosing Specific Research Focus

To succeed in publishing the research, optimising the study design is the single most important factor, whether the project is a basic science experiment, a clinical trial, or a population-based study.

The beginners in this field often pick a broad, general topic, thinking that big topics are easier to research. But some topics are just too big to research, for example, eating disorders, physical fitness etc. The problems with big topics are multiple. They are overwhelmingly difficult to acquire the data and design a proper protocol. Therefore, avoid time-consuming studies with multiple investigators involvement, at least in the beginning, where your role might become minimal. On the other hand, the study should not be too simplistic, like, writing a case report, as it is not a research. Also, developing a new tool or technique could be more satisfying. However, this could be a monumental task and might require more inspiration than most research and eventually, it might end up being less productive.

How to Narrow the Topic

One simple way of narrowing a research topic is to try to look for a project that is driven by a hypothesis or a well-defined observational study.

In order to add focus to the design, look at the study and ask yourself five simple single worded questions about it, *Who*? *What*? *Where*? *When*? and *How*?

Firstly, ask yourself, *who* might benefit from the study? Try to focus on particular age group or a group with certain risk factors who are at risk or likely to improve on the proposed intervention or management plan.

Secondly, ask, *what* kind of effects are anticipated? e.g. reduce blood pressure; affect a measurable level of serum or urine bio-marker; prolong the survival; avoid the recurrence of the problem; reduce adverse events such as end-organ dysfunction; diminish stay in the Intensive Care Unit; improve the quality of life or significantly affect the hardest end-point which is to cheat death.

Thirdly, ask yourself *where?* Can your hypothesis be tested on a single event, specific group, limited period, one cause or effect, one argument or a viewpoint?

The fourth step would be to ask, *when*? Patients studied in a specific time interval significantly reduces the size of the study. However, it must be remembered at this stage that for a meaningful conclusion the sample size has to be adequate.

And finally, *how*? This is the time to work on the protocol of the study.

There are different study designs to consider. The Classic example would be the Null hypothesis.

Medical research has many dimensions that have evolved over the past two decades after clinical trials have exploded into this field. There are legal, regulatory, ethical, statistical, procedural and clinical dimensions which influence the field of medical research and have changed the structure of the research methodology, which were not prevalent to anyone who entered medicine decades earlier. It is important for the researcher to implicate these dimensions into the study design and give an excellent amount of depth to the chosen research topic (Fig. 1 and Table 1).

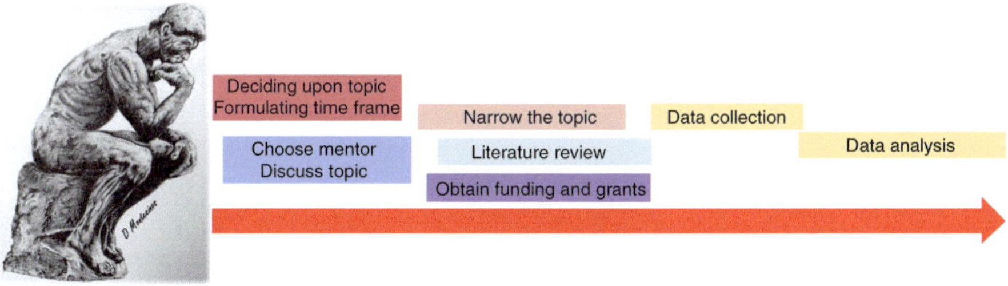

Fig. 1 Flow chart depicting the process of commencing research project with the help of a mentor(s)

Table 1 Key factors: choosing a research topic

Look for the right people who could help you
Find area/field or project of your own interest
Find a well-defined project that is within your capacity
Project should be worth doing. The question should be worth answering
Balance your thoughts, your interests and your independence with those of others

Choosing a Research Mentor

Several studies underline the importance of a Mentor in clinical research [2–5]. To understand why we need a mentor in research, a glance at the illustration in the figure, that has been adopted from Cohen et al., might be of help. Each has to balance a number of imperatives in personal and professional lives. Your personal needs must be balanced with relationships with others [6]. At the same time, professional development and responsibilities must be balanced with personal, in the interest of all parties involved. The major function of mentoring is to aid in developing four individual components and help you in keeping them in balance.

In this context, it is interesting to read how Keyser and Zukerman have separately defined the phenomenon or process of Mentoring. According to Keyser, " Mentoring is a dynamic reciprocal relationship environment between an advanced career incumbent (mentor) and a beginner (protégée), aimed at promoting the development of both." [5] And as per Zukerman, "Mentoring is a complex multidimensional process through which emerging scientists acquire the norms and standards, values and attitudes, and knowledge, skills and behaviours to develop into successful independent researcher." [7]

It is important to recognize the fact that the relationship between the mentor and the mentee needs to be based on compassion, always positively charged and constructive. Occasionally, that might not be the case. The needs and interests of each party often change. Accordingly, the ability to work in effective partnership may change. More often than not, a mentor-mentee relationship fails, when the mentor is not able to separate his or her needs from those of his mentee [8]

Mentorship: A Learned Skill

There are studies to demonstrate that mentorship is an acquired skill. It works better when supported by the institution in addition to the interest taken by the mentor in his mentee and the project [9] (Table 2).

Responsibilities of a Successful Mentee

It is understood that both the mentor and his mentee must be committed and interested.

Table 2 Essential elements of a successful mentor

Interested in serving as a mentor and is compassionate.
Flexible to commit time and effort.
Able to recognize and even keep aside, at times, the personal interests of those of the mentee.
Has the expertise in the area in which he/she is acting as a mentor

Table 3 Characteristic features of a successful mentee

Capable of clearly defining the support and help he/she needs
Recognises the fact that only one person may not be able to help in meeting all the mentoring needs
Recognises the fact that only one person may not be able to help in meeting all the mentoring needs
Recognises the fact that only one person may not be able to help in meeting all the mentoring needs
Recognises the fact that the needs for mentoring do change all the time
Recognises the fact that only one person may not be able to help in meeting all the mentoring needs
Able to accept the constructive criticism and work through it
Interested in working with mentor for help
Commitment to make an effort to enable the relationship to develop and function

Scheduled regular meetings are essential for planning and implementation.

Formulate questions well in advance of such meetings related to technology, research methodology, data analysis, funding, and other resources that your mentor can help you answer.

The concerns regarding time management, ethical aspects and even dealing with difficult colleagues and supervisors, should be sorted out with discussion.

A mentor should be able to help you address questions regarding research related networking, even promotions and jobs.

You might need more than one mentor to accomplish all objectives (Table 3).

Conclusion

With regard to both, choosing a project and finding mentors, enlightened self-interest is the key. This exercise is certainly going to provide the researcher with immense personal satisfaction and develop cognitive skills that are universally helpful. It is a labour of love, after all. Just like many things in life, even if you don't get it right the first time, never give up, because you almost always get there!

Case Scenarios

1. You are a third-year resident working in the department of cardiology where you are routinely exposed to different protocols of managing anti-platelet therapy

after coronary stenting and there are several conflicting protocols adopted by different Specialist Cardiologists in the department.
   (a) What would you think about the superiority of one protocol over the other in the population that you are treating at your institution.
   (b) What is the evidence in the literature for preventing stent thrombosis.
2. You are a junior consultant in general medicine working in a small district hospital where certain ethnic group of patients has significantly worse outcome despite identical prescription for a proven clinical condition.
   (a) How would you narrow the research topic?
   (b) What factors would you think are responsible for different outcomes in two ethnic groups?

References

1. Russel B. Problems of philosophy. Radford: Wilder Publications; 2008.
2. Howell E, Kravet S, Wright SM. An innovative approach to supporting hospital physicians towards academic success. J Hops Med. 2008;3:314–8.
3. Hussey-Jones J, Berstein L, Higgins S, Malebranche D, Paranjape A, Geano I, et al. Repaving the road to academic success: the IMeREG approach to peer mentoring. Acad Med. 2006;81:674–9.
4. Sambunjak D, Straus SE, Marusik A. Mentoring in academic medicine: a systematic review. JAMA. 2006;296:1103–15.
5. Keyser DJ, Lakosi JM, Lara-Cinisomo S, Schultz DJ, Williams VL, Zellers DF, et al. Advancing institutional efforts to support research mentorship: a conceptual framework and self assessment tool. Acad Med. 2008;83:217–25.
6. Cohen MS, Jacobs JP, Quintessenza JA, Chai PJ, Lindberg HL, Dickey J, et al. Mentorship, learning curves, and balance. Cardiol Young. 2007;17:164–74.
7. Zukerman H. Scientific elite: nobel laureates in the United States. New York: Free Press; 1977.
8. Bettmann M. Choosing a research project and a research mentor. Circulation. 2009;119:1832–5.
9. Wright DE, Titus SL, Cornelison JB. Mentoring and research misconduct: an analysis of research mentoring in closed ORI cases. Sci Eng Ethics. 2008;14:323–36.

Assessing Availability of Facilities, Infrastructure and Resources

Puneet Dhar and Johns Shaji Mathew

"It is much easier to put existing resources to better use, than to develop resources where they do not exist."——George Soros

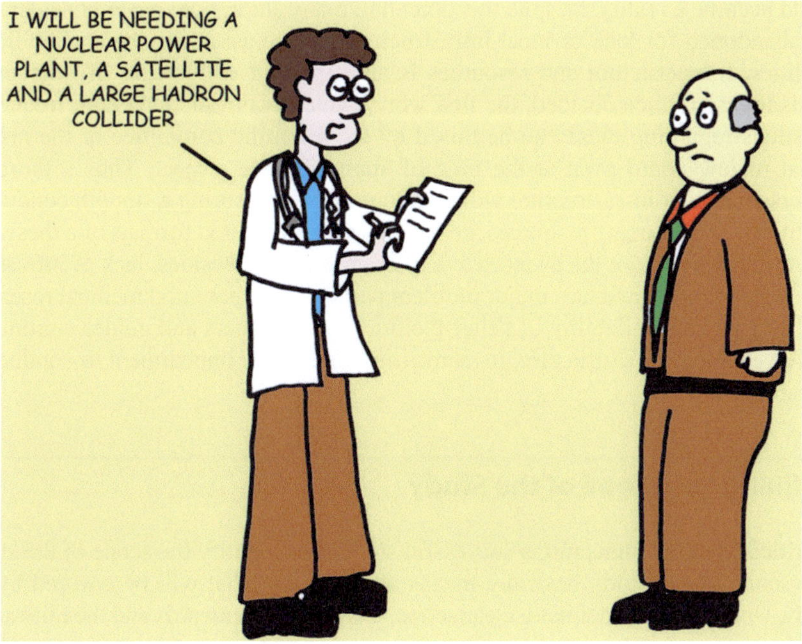

P. Dhar (✉)
Professor and Head, Department of Gastrointestinal Surgery,
Amrita Institute of Medical Sciences, Kochi, India

J. S. Mathew
Assistant Professor, Department of Gastrointestinal Surgery,
Amrita Institute of Medical Sciences, Kochi, India

S. C. Parija, V. Kate (eds.), *Thesis Writing for Master's and Ph.D. Program*,
https://doi.org/10.1007/978-981-13-0890-1_4

Key Points

- Introduction and Defining the scope of the study
- Making a timeline
- Lab and other facilities in your own institution. Personnel to help
- Multidisciplinary work, and outsourcing within the country
- Facilities for data maintenance and management
- International collaboration
- Animal research

Introduction

A Thesis should not be the last stop in education—rather it is the runway to begin lifelong meaningful research whether it is in clinical or basic sciences! With rapid expansion of the internet and ancillary tools for acquiring and disseminating information, the possibilities of doing world-class studies in the remotest corners of the world became a reality. Despite this potential, many studies are never considered or are abandoned for lack of local infrastructure. Hence assessing the availability of facilities, infrastructure and resources is an important component of finalising a thesis topic, or once decided, the first worry which confronts us! Quite frequently questions regarding these can be raised by the scientific committee or the institutional review board even at the time of approving the project. Thus a thorough understanding of infrastructure will go a long way in ensuring a smooth conduct of the thesis. Whilst many resources are available for structured formats of a thesis [1], few resources explore the avenues to explore resources! Besides, lack of infrastructure is frequently cited as a major problem perceived by potential medical researchers [2]. Despite availability of better facilities—researchers and guides continue to perceive lack of infrastructure, resources and time as an impediment to conducting research [3].

Defining the Scope of the Study

A critical step in conducting a successful study is to identify the scope of the study. The scope of the study basically means all the things that will be covered by the study. Unless a study defines a clear scope, it will creep outwards and the milestones skip out of reach. The scope helps researches to stay focussed on the issue at hand and not divert resources away from the problem at hand.

1. Identify the problem and creation of a problem statement. The first step is to identify the problem which needs to be studied. The problem(s) are identified by individuals with a deeper knowledge of the field. Once the problem is identified, data regarding its prevalence needs to be collected especially whether other researchers around the world have found this problem and how did they

circumvent it. Such individuals can be contacted, to have a better understanding of the problem. In addition, a thorough understanding of the field of study is also important.

2. Setting the boundaries: Fence in all the things that will be covered by the research. Clearly define what end points are hoped to be achieved by the study. The researchers must enlighten themselves on all the background aspects of the project and the objectives proposed to be achieved. In addition, it would be wise to identify potential limitations of the study beforehand itself. There must be clear instructions to stick to the previously agreed objectives and not stray into areas which are not primarily covered by the research. Such activities are common as the researcher stumbles upon a new finding and devotes time and energy into that, thereby losing track of the main picture. One must not lose the forest for the trees.
3. Creating a strategy: Once the milestones are defined, a strategy for achieving these must be in place. A general proposal on how to reach the milestones and whether these are reasonable and easily achievable. It is important alongside to ensure that budget and resource allocation has been looked into.

Timeline Creation

A well-designed project implementation schedule clarifies and describes what the project should deliver and within what time-frames. It is the beating heart of every project—captures the essence of the what the project will achieve.

Dividing the project into multiple phases/multiple discrete subtasks may prove useful. Audit and control implementation of each project phase is to define checkpoints (the key milestones) to be conducted on a regular basis during the implementation process. Responsibilities must be clearly allocated. It is possible that the project faces unanticipated delays and may fall out of sync with the timeline. Revision of the time line can be accepted provided it does not stretch too far from the initial estimates.

Facilities, Infrastructure and Resources

A major issue in choosing a research project or topic is the feasibility. Of course funding is a major limiting factor. Equally important is to ensure that the facilities exist to carry out the thesis or project; and resources are available or can be arranged by the researcher or the guide.

Resources include work area, equipment, library access, and human resources (leader, peers, technical assistants and availability of students) [4]. Colleagues serve as a source of knowledge, skill, expertise, emotional support, stimulation and reinforcement, thereby providing the right milieu of research "culture". It has been shown that research productivity improved in a better environment especially with productive colleagues around! [5].

Choice of the institution and guide is clearly critical even apart from intellectual input—prior training in research methodology is extremely useful, as is the ability to be able to get work done cohesively within the department as well as elsewhere. Access of the guide to her own exclusive lab or the ability to arrange protected time in a different lab, can make the study easier to perform. The presence of adequate infrastructure to carry out the project is paramount to the conduct of the research. Should the need arise, this could even be from a different establishment or institution.

This assessment would include help and liaising with laboratories, other ancillary departments and also the technical staff who are able to provide dedicated time for the thesis. Availability under the same roof, is undoubtedly an asset and likely to increase productivity, but its absence should not hinder the research quality. In assessment of infrastructure it is extremely important to look for solutions, and not just list out potential problems. A good research guide who is actively involved in the field of study could help the candidate search for additional research facilities in other centres.

For facilities in your own Institution—In case the research project entails a substantial component outside the core competency of the researcher or her guide, it is mandatory to ensure a rapport with all the departments involved. Invariably other departments would look on most extraneous work as an additional unnecessary burden to their routine work. There are many ways to work around this. The most popular is to include the key persons as co-guides, especially if it is a major component of the thesis. If this is not possible, then at least an understanding could be effected, that these persons could be involved as authors, should a publication emerge from the study. Sometimes the suggestion that they would get help from us, should it be needed for their own research projects, may work, (almost as a quid pro quo!). At the very least, all help from personnel or departments must be acknowledged. If the thesis project indeed involves a substantial extra effort from other departments such as a laboratory, which may actually hamper their own work, then it is the responsibility of the researcher to either offer to help in the said work (as possible in Example one below) or organise and authorise extra qualified personnel for the additional work and this may need to be budgeted as well. Frequently other researchers may be working on different subjects but studying the same aspect covered by the ancillary department (e.g., a specific gene analysis in different tumors—uterine cancer from gynaecology and pancreatic cancer by a GI researcher), and a mutually acceptable way can be worked out to share costs and efforts.

Occasionally the additional department or laboratory involved may accept the extra work, but may not be able to absorb the financial implications for the use of facilities or extra expensive reagents etc. Here the onus of organising funding for this, rests with the researcher. With respect to laboratory tests, technological advances have made it possible to have modular kits to do the same tests or experiments, which can circumvent the extra effort and sometimes may reduce costs as investigations need to be batched together.

There are national and international efforts to have centralised core reference and research centres to encourage research locally or regionally and must be sought out and encouraged. It does require a few bureaucratic hurdles to be smoothened out initially, but it is well worth the effort eventually. Examples are Sanger Institute, Sheffield RNAi Screening Facility and cancer Research in UK [6], the various NIH funded centres in USA and the national reference labs all over India.

It is important to ensure that the lab or other extra personnel involved in the study, commit to extending the use of the facility for the entire expected duration of the study. This may be important to secure in departments with frequent transfers.

It is also useful to assure that the resources or database does not have competing studies involved. For example, a small endoscopic biopsy may be competing for genetic or immunohistochemical studies in one thesis and be required for electron microscopy for another topic of research! Some of these problems can be surmounted for instance in this example, by taking extra biopsies after due Ethics clearance and patient consent.

Multidisciplinary Work, and Outsourcing

Occasionally the study may primarily involve a different department—e.g., doing a meta-analysis or systematic review may utilise a statistician more than the primary researcher who may do little else other than literature review. It may then be worthwhile for the researcher to actually get trained in those modules and seek assistance only if and when required. Many online courses exist for a variety of research tools including statistics and many of them are free or highly subsidised. There can be a huge disparity in the perception of statistical help provided by their supervisors and the expectations by the researchers as shown in a recent German study [3].

It must be remembered that in certain instances it may be easier to outsource some of the components of the study to external professionals who are doing this regularly either for their own research or commercially. Examples include genetic sequencing, specialised immunochemistry, electron microscopy etc., where economies of scale may even render the test less expensive! Thus access to infrastructure and facilities can still be dictated by funding available!

If resources are used outside own institution, then it is suggested that rather than an informal arrangements, a proper Memorandum of understanding be organised with clear demarcation of extents and ownership of material data and primary sources etc. It is also good to keep the institutional ethics committee or scientific committees overseeing research and the management in the loop to avoid any ethical issues or those of trust. Suspicions are minimised if all this is sorted out up front before commencement of the study to minimise bureaucratic hurdles later on. It must be stressed that although most researchers try to look for completing their work within the confines of their own institution, all collaborations across specialties or departments or centres tend to have a better scientific and citation impact and are instinctively trusted.

Facilities for Data Management

Integrity and Maintenance of source documentation is of paramount importance, and nowhere is it more palpable, should a need arise in case of an audit (e.g., by the funding agency!!). Many Research organisations have begun to use electronic data capture options and use of electronic online databases. Although these were initially used mostly for sponsored research, they can be utilised in investigator initiated studies as well. Advantages are similar—of being able to capture data or indeed collaborate with different personnel, guide and coinvestigators etc.! Alternatively physical records may be maintained. Whatever technique is used, access must be convenient and privacy must be ensured and subject consent should be obtained for using the data subsequently. It may perhaps be easier to keep copies of original records, especially if possibility of loss of data is there, as in automatic archival or destruction of records after a set given period. In case of use of electronic data, on the contrary, the requirement may be instead to provision of WiFi access and other portable or Bluetooth enabled type gadgets! Access to communication modes is also important as dedicated or available computing devices etc. Thus it can be seen that a strategic vision is frequently required and many studies flounder for lack of it!! There is no doubt that in days to come use of electronic resources are going to improve data management exponentially [7]. Figure 1 shows the research plan and strategies adopted to implement it.

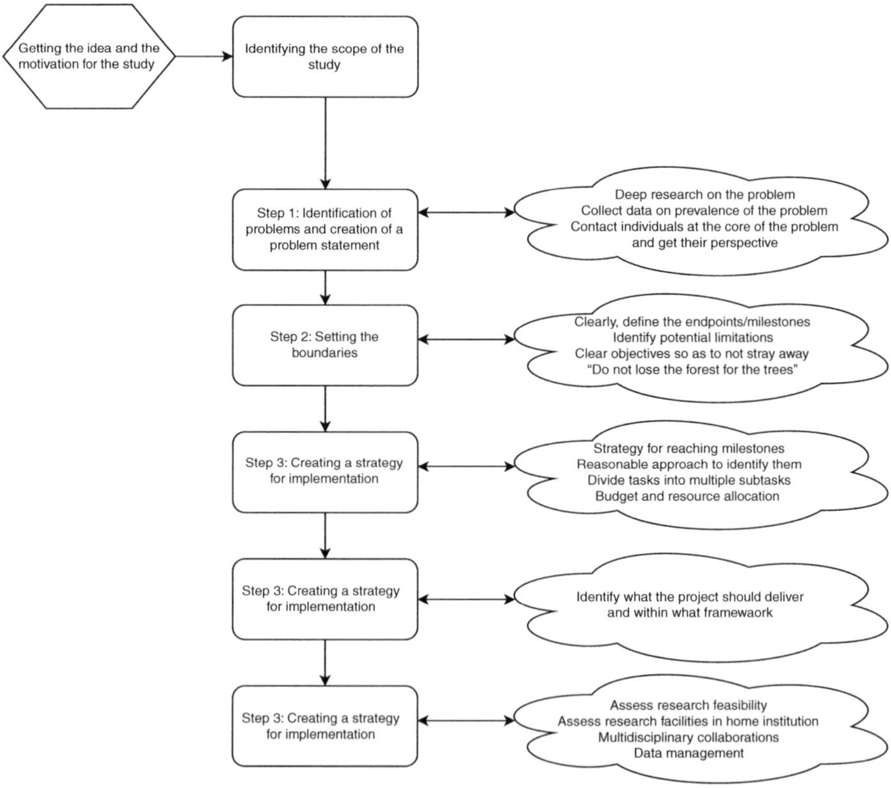

Fig. 1 Research plan and strategy to implement it

International Collaboration

Studies tend not to be as easy to conduct across countries (Unlike sponsored pharmaceutical trials!) with all the logistic hurdles that are likely with the addition of each country. For instance it is difficult to get permission to transport biological tissues outside the country. Hence it is important to be aware of all international regulation before embarking on these. Reliable communication which maintains privacy is of course even more important here.

Animal Research Facilities

Stringent regulations and animal rights activists make it easier in many countries to do research on human subjects rather than animals! Although they make a fair point in terms of need, applicability and easier slipping of norms, the ethics of such studies must be carefully looked into and are beyond the purview of this review! If used, it is important to adhere to humane principles and ensure all rules for animal protection are stringently followed.

Case Scenarios

1. A Researcher is working on prognostic value of lymphocyte subsets in a type of cancer. It involves identification of cases using aspiration cytology followed by subsequent core biopsy for immunohistochemistry. The pathology lab was extremely busy in clinical identification, typing reporting etc, and was left with little time to do the extra work. What are the possible options for the clinical researcher and possible issues involved:
   (a) Arrange for an extra lab technician who could do the additional work
   (b) "Request" or continuously "instruct" the lab that research work is equally important as clinical work!
   (c) Offer to do some part of the lab work that a clinician can do better and doesn't need too much of technical knowhow.
   (d) Monetary incentive to technicians or Change the topic
   (e) Outsource to a less busy Laboratory elsewhere
2. In a study to assess postoperative quality of life (QOL) after rectal cancer surgery, discuss the potential infrastructural problems.

References

1. Ahmad HR. How to write a doctoral thesis. Pak J Med Sci. 2016;32(2):270–3.
2. Kabra SK, Verma IC. Thesis during MD: must or bust. Ind J Paediatr. 2007;74:868–9.
3. Can E, Richter F, Valchanova R, Dewey M. Supervisors' perspective on medical thesis projects and dropout rates: survey among thesis supervisors at a large German university hospital. BMJ Open. 2016;6:e012726.
4. Bland CJ, Ruffin MT. Characteristics of a productive research environment: literature review. Acad Med. 1992;67(6):385–97.

5. Braxton JM. Departmental colleagues and individual faculty publication productivity. Rev High Educ. 1983;6:125–8.
6. Harriet Teare. Building the ideal environment for medical research. Cancer Research UK (Monograph on Cancer Research UK's analysis of the components required to conduct world-class research across the UK). September 2011.
7. Joseph CLM, Ownby DR, Zoratti E, Johnson D, Considine S, Renee Bourgeois R. Recruitment experience for a pragmatic randomized controlled trial: using EMR initiatives and minimizing research infrastructure. Clin Res Regul Aff. 2016;33(2–4):25–32.

Obtaining Support and Grants for Research

William Y. Shi and Julian A. Smith

Successful research attracts the bigger grant which makes further research impossible.—C. Northcot Parkinson

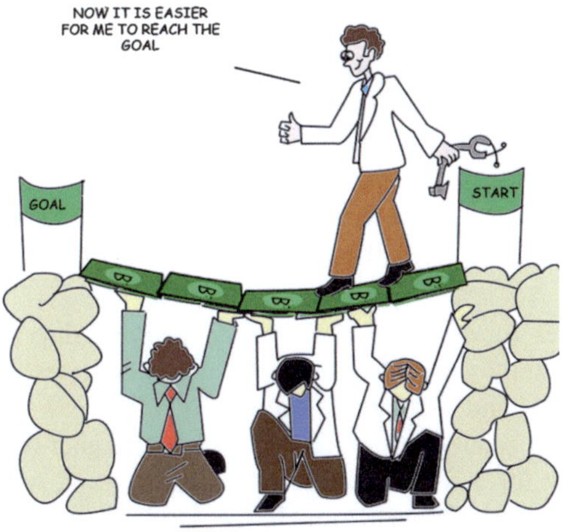

W. Y. Shi
Department of Cardiothoracic Surgery, Monash Health, Melbourne, Australia

J. A. Smith (✉)
Department of Surgery (School of Clinical Sciences), Monash Medical Centre, Clayton, VIC, Australia
e-mail: Julian.Smith@monash.edu

S. C. Parija, V. Kate (eds.), *Thesis Writing for Master's and Ph.D. Program*,
https://doi.org/10.1007/978-981-13-0890-1_5

Key Points

- Multiple sources of funding for research exist. Publically-funded research bodies serve as ideal starting points for investigators.
- A strong understanding of the research project is required prior to preparing funding applications.
- Grant applications must be tailored to the funding body's priorities.
- An experienced, multidisciplinary team is essential for securing funding for larger, more complex research projects.
- Important criteria used to judge grant applications include originality, generalizability, feasibility and methodological strength in addition to the track record of the investigators.

Introduction

Obtaining funding for medical research is a crucial and constant part of academic life. In essence, it is an exercise in communication. A well designed, pertinent research project may fail to achieve funding if inadequate attention is dedicated to its grant proposal. The grant application process can be complex, and requires substantial preparation by the investigator. This chapter outlines the process of obtaining grants for research and provides some basic strategies for success.

Grants and Fellowships/Scholarships

The main principles for securing either a grant, fellowship or scholarship is the same. Grants are generally awarded to support a particular research project or initiative while fellowships and scholarships generally refer to awards for individuals.

Aspiring clinician academics seeking to pursue a higher degree such as an MD or PhD. may apply for a fellowship or scholarship grant, which may support an applicant while they take a hiatus from clinical work and pursue full-time research. Some fellowship or scholarship awards require a proportion of the funds to be provided by the supervising university department.

Initial Preparation

As part of planning of any research project, an investigator should identify a topic of particular interest to themselves. The individual should strive to understand in detail the existing knowledge and literature concerning the topic, and importantly, where a knowledge gap exists which may be addressed by the research project. Researchers should also understand the methodology of the proposed study, including basic details concerning data collection, statistical analysis methods and how the results are to be presented. A firm understanding from the outset will facilitate the writing of a convincing grant proposal.

Almost all research is conducted as part of an academic or clinical unit, under the supervision of a senior investigator. This may be in an academic medical center in a university department, in a medical research institute or in a combination of each. To an extent, the research project should align with the interests, expertise and the available resources of the department or institution. Researchers looking for appropriate groups to join should review the department's publication, funding and supervision records, and discuss their expectations with current or past researchers.

Sources of Funding

There are a myriad of granting bodies, both public and private. Younger investigators or those entering a new area of study should determine the major opportunities for funding via their research supervisors, colleagues and other mentors.

In many countries, there exist large publically-funded research bodies which serve as the major sources of funding for medical researchers. Examples include the National Institutes of Health (USA) [1], National Institute for Health Research (UK) [2] and the National Health and Medical Research Council (Australia) [3]. In addition, there are also a host of specialty-specific organizations which provide resources. Examples in the cardiovascular science field include the National Heart, Lung and Blood Institute (USA) [4], British Heart Foundation (UK) [5] and the Heart Foundation of Australia [6].

Furthermore, medical specialty colleges and societies also offer grants of varying amounts. In Australia and New Zealand for example, the Royal Australasian College of Surgeons (RACS) is a major funder of surgical researchers (both trainees and established academic surgeons) and enables successful applicants to engage in full-time research to work towards a higher degree such as an M.D. or Ph.D. [7]. The RACS also provides awards for established academic surgeons to further develop their academic portfolio.

Researchers can also utilize databases devoted to research funding. Examples include Research Professional [8], Community of Science (COS) funding opportunities [9] and SPIN InfoEd International [10]. Most major universities also have a research and grants office that investigators can liaise with to find additional funding opportunities.

Private companies and the medical industry sector can also provide sources of funding for smaller studies. These can be identified by establishing relationships with industry representatives or industry-employed colleagues and determining a project which is of interest to the company. Some medical insurance agencies will also provide scholarship-type grants to those pursuing a higher research degree. Medical device companies may provide small traveling fellowship awards in order to allow clinicians to travel and learn new techniques which are associated with the company's products.

Many funding bodies, especially those who award fellowship/scholarship grants, will only consider applicants who do not concurrently hold another major scholarship or award. The applicant may need to enquire directly with the funding body to determine eligibility criteria and explore the possibility of co-funding arrangements in order to maximize opportunities. Two scholarship bodies will generally not contribute funds such that the sum exceeds the amount of a single award.

Writing a Grant Application

Successful grant applicants are those able to understand the sponsor's viewpoint and articulate the priorities of a funding body in their proposal. It is said that grant applicants often focus on their own need for resources, rather than matching their project with the funding body's priority. In the medical research arena, however, the basic principle underpinning most funding agencies is that of improving scientific knowledge and patient care.

The process of writing a grant application differs depending on the funding body. While smaller bodies will require only a few pages detailing the rationale for a project, larger, more prestigious bodies often require greater than 50 written pages for a given proposal. Major funding bodies will generally provide a template for an application. Practically-speaking, preparing a major grant application takes weeks to months. The major publically-funded sources usually have a "funding calendar" which researchers should become familiar with as these bodies receive applications once per year by a specified deadline.

Once a research idea is generated, multiple meetings and discussions are usually required involving senior supervisors and collaborators to better define the methodology, expected outcomes and logistics of a study. Grants usually require a sign-off from a Head of Department as well as a Finance Officer or representative from an institution's grants office. As such, in the authors' experience, the writing of the grant should be completed approximately 3–4 weeks prior to the submission deadline.

Researchers should familiarize themselves with the mission statements and aims of the funding body. Successful grants from previous applicants should be reviewed. Many university academics will have experience in the assessment of grants and should be approached for feedback and advice. Experts in the relevant field should be approached for advice regarding the feasibility and utility of the study. Universities also provide courses and workshops focused on grant writing. While different funding bodies will provide unique templates, the basic components of all grant applications are similar. These are discussed below.

Applicant Profile and Track Record

Almost all major funding bodies will assess a grant proposal based on the applicant(s) academic profile and track record. Items such as publications, presentations scholarships, prizes, previous successful grant applications are evaluated. Enrolment in a higher degree program such as a Masters, M.D., or Ph.D.—to which the grant will contribute—may also serve as an important factor. A personal statement, including the applicant's career aims is also usually required.

Funding bodies aim to select those who demonstrate the desire to sustain their academic practice, and this needs to be communicated clearly in applications. For clinician researchers, it is advantageous to emphasize how a project aligns with and will help shape their area of future practice and expertise.

Supervisors and the Research Team

Applicants must convey that their host institution is one which can provide the resources to complete the study. For example, if proposing a clinical project involving recruitment of study subjects, it is useful to present the volume of work performed by a clinical unit and the expected number of subjects. Research taking place at a high volume center with a particular expertise in a clinical area is more likely to engender the confidence of a funding body.

Similarly, for laboratory-based studies, applicants should demonstrate that the department has access to facilities with a track record of undertaking specific experiments. In cases of novel experimental research projects, it is useful to briefly present pilot data originating from the department to demonstrate feasibility. Where facilities are not available, it may be necessary to form collaborative arrangements with another department and these should be specified in the proposal.

The expertise and track record of a research team, namely the project supervisor(s) is an important factor for grant assessors. For projects of a larger scale, it may be necessary and advantageous to construct a multidisciplinary group to ensure all facets of a complex project are addressed. For example, in the authors' experience, multicenter clinical research projects in cardiac surgery often involve not only surgeons but also physicians, anesthetists, laboratory scientists, nursing staff and statisticians. Some funding bodies will require co-investigators to provide a curriculum vitae, a personal statement and describe their expertise in relation to the specific project.

Indeed, studies investigating predictors of grant application success have suggested that a multidisciplinary research team, the presence of a statistician, epidemiologist, health economist and even a consumer along with the completion of a pilot study are factors associated with a greater likelihood of success in obtaining funding [11].

The Project

When reviewing grant proposals, grant assessors focus on a number of key attributes. These are usually: significance and impact, originality, generalizability, feasibility (including the expertise of the research team) and sufficiency of available resources.

The impact of any study on the relevant field needs to be significant enough in order to be competitive at securing funding. Funding bodies wish to sponsor research which is "cutting-edge". However, projects must also have a broad application. Studies, while novel, may not provide wide-ranging clinical and scientific utility, and thus fail to secure funding. Investigators should ensure the scope of the project also needs to be realistic. Projects which will consume substantial resources and time—in particular those which may encounter slow recruitment of subjects—can be met with skepticism. A realistic timeline of the study needs to be constructed and conveyed in proposals.

An abstract is almost always required. A lay abstract or summary is also sometimes required as many panels assessing applications now have a lay person from the community. Abstracts are often the most read portion of an application and may serve as a reminder of the project for assessors prior to an interview. A succinct, articulate and well-structured abstract is invaluable.

The project's rationale, hypothesis and aims are always required. These must be presented so as to convey a deep understanding of the scientific literature and the gap in knowledge. This section is crucial as it conveys to the funding body that the research topic is pertinent and worthy of selection.

Following this, the proposed research plan is described in detail. This section must be rigorous, detailed, well-structured and logical. This section should detail how the study will fulfill the aims of the project. A description of the study sample, recruitment, data collection, statistical methods where relevant must be provided. In clinical studies, it is vital to specify and clearly define the endpoints being studied and sample size calculations are often required. A statisticians input here is often valuable. It is imperative that this section is completed meticulously, as grant assessors are experienced researchers and even minor flaws in methodology can jeopardize the validity of the project and therefore the grant application.

In clinical studies, investigators often report what is considered "hard endpoints" such as mortality and other adverse events which are deemed to be more relevant in clinical practice. However, these endpoints also tend to be rare, and when using these events as end-points, the sample population often needs to be very large—sometimes prohibitively so—in order to obtain adequate statistical power. In such scenarios, it may be prudent to use so-called "surrogate" markers as primary endpoints. These may include biochemical markers or investigative parameters which are more sensitive to an intervention. While using "hard" clinical endpoints may be more appealing for clinicians, formulating a well-designed study with adequate sample calculations will make it more likely to achieve funding.

Major funding bodies provide a section for budgeting. These sections are often very specific and include salaries for research personnel (which is specified by institutional pay schedules), equipment, animal research, travel and educational support. Some scenarios may dictate subcontracts or cost-sharing with a collaborating institution. The budget should be accompanied with rigorous justification. An institution's finance officer can serve as a valuable resource in budgeting.

Grant Review Process

Smaller grants may be reviewed by a panel within the funding body. Larger funding bodies send proposals for external peer review, convening a panel of reviewers with the relevant expertise. The reviewers will score the proposal using predefined criteria. As an example, the National Health and Medical Research Council of Australia has a peer review process whereby proposals are scored based on scientific quality (50%), significance/innovation (25%) and team quality and capability (25%), with each component being given a score of 1–7 [12]. For its major fellowship awards, the NHMRC makes selections based on track record (60%), potential for further career development (10%), career development strategy (10%), quality of research proposal (10%) and the quality of the research environment (10%) [13].

Some funding bodies will return with a request for revisions or rebuttal responding to queries and concerns the reviewers have raised. Here, it is important to acknowledge the reviewers' points and modify or justify parts of the study the reviewers have highlighted. The rebuttal is then resubmitted with a final verdict delivered by the review panel.

For fellowship/scholarship applications, the sponsor will often request to interview the candidate. This allows the panel to assess the applicant's understanding of their project and their academic potential. For applicants, rigorous preparation is key to ensure a solid understanding of the project is conveyed to the interview panel. Candidates may also be judged on their understanding of general research principles and career ambitions. Figure 1 shows the timeline of grant application.

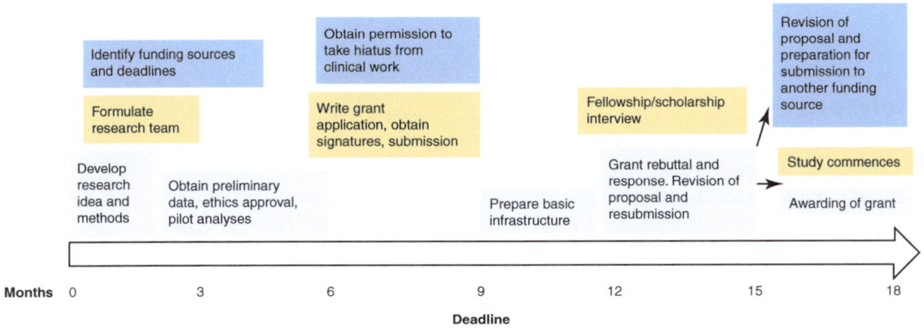

Fig. 1 Timeline of the grant application. The time taken to obtain funding will vary widely depending on the size and complexity of the research project

Conclusion

Applying for research grants, fellowships and scholarships is a key component of academic medicine. The process requires not only a deep understanding of research but also the ability to articulate its originality, significance and feasibility. Indeed, it represents an exercise in communication. The process also requires meticulous preparation, and the ability to collaborate as part of a multidisciplinary team. Success in obtaining one grant will greatly enhance the chances of success in subsequent applications.

Case Scenarios

1. You are an early-career surgical trainee who has developed an interest in a particular subspecialty area. Through clinical training, the direction of mentors and attendance at scientific meetings, you have come to realize a potential knowledge gap in the specialty area which interests you. You are aware of a well-regarded research unit in a local institution and your colleagues, seniors and mentors have suggested you take a hiatus from full-time clinical training and pursue a higher degree.
   (a) What are some options for funding your hiatus period?
   (b) Who can assist you in the fellowship/scholarship application process?
2. You are a junior consultant surgeon working in a university hospital. You have identified a particular area of you and our colleagues' practice where there is no data in the literature to guide clinical care. Your colleagues and Head of Unit support your desire to construct a clinical trial, however, funding is required.
   (a) What factors in your project methodology are most likely to make it successful in obtaining funding?
   (b) What characteristics of the host institution and research team members are evaluated by grant assessors?
   (c) If facilities are not available in your center, what alternative arrangements can be made and specified in your grant proposal?

References

1. National Institutes of Health. https://www.nih.gov/.
2. National Institute for Health Research. https://www.nihr.ac.uk/,.
3. National Health and Medical Research Council. https://www.nhmrc.gov.au/.
4. National Heart Lung and Blood Institute (NHLBI). https://www.nhlbi.nih.gov/.
5. British Heart Foundation. https://www.bhf.org.uk/.
6. The Heart Foundation. https://www.heartfoundation.org.au/.
7. Smith JA. Benefits of the Royal Australasian College of surgeons scholarship program highlighted. ANZ J Surg. 2016;86:855.
8. Research Professional. https://www.researchprofessional.com/.
9. Pivot (COS). https://pivot.cos.com/.
10. InfoEd SPIN. https://spin.infoedglobal.com/.

11. Turner S, Davidson P, Stanton L, Cawdeary V. Features of successful bids for funding of applied health research: a cohort study. Health Res Policy Syst. 2014;12:54.
12. NHMRC funding rules Section B) Attachment A—NHMRC project grants category descriptors. https://www.nhmrc.gov.au/book/nhmrc-funding-rules/section-b-project-grants/b1-objective-project-grants-scheme.
13. NHMRC funding rules F9) Fellowship Packages and Awards F10) Assessment Process Attachment C: Selection Criteria and Scoring Matrix. https://www.nhmrc.gov.au/book/nhmrc-funding-rules/f9-fellowship-packages-and-awards/f10-assessment-process/f11-administrati-3.

How to Write a Protocol

Mukta Wyawahare, Raja Kalayarasan, and Anahita Kate

Failing to plan is planning to fail.—Alan Lakiel

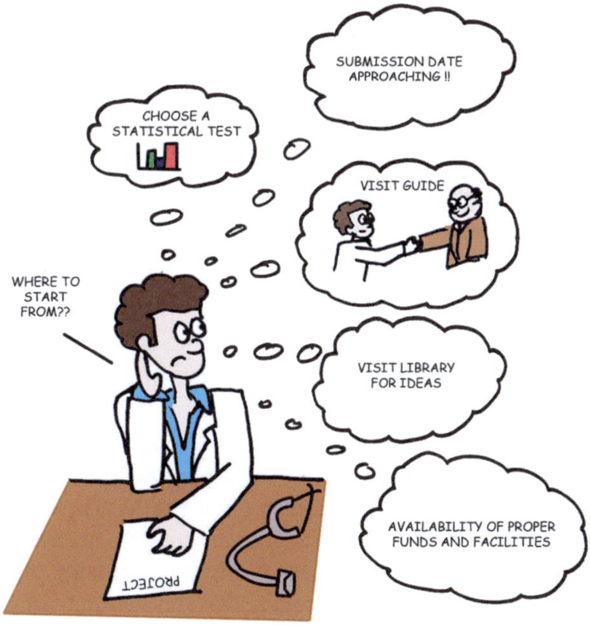

M. Wyawahare (✉)
Additional Professor, Department of Medicine, Jawaharlal Institute of Postgraduate Medical Education and Research, Pondicherry, India

R. Kalayarasan
Associate Professor, Department of Surgical Gastroenterology, Jawaharlal Institute of Post Graduate Medical Education and Research, Pondicherry, India

A. Kate
Fellow, Cornea and Anterior Segment, L.V. Prasad Eye Institute, Hyderabad, India

S. C. Parija, V. Kate (eds.), *Thesis Writing for Master's and Ph.D. Program*,
https://doi.org/10.1007/978-981-13-0890-1_6

Key Points

- Thesis protocol acts as a blue print and should list the important details of your research
- In the first section of the thesis protocol general information about the researcher and study should be mentioned
- In the second section of the thesis protocol technical details of the study should be written
- A descriptive title is commonly used for a thesis protocol
- Aims and objectives of the study are not synonymous
- Inclusion and exclusion criteria should be supplementary and not complementary
- A pilot study should be performed when the investigator is not sure about the feasibility of the proposed research

What Is a Thesis Protocol?

Thesis Protocol is a document formulated to provide the reader a concise plan of the proposed research. In addition to giving a panoramic view to the research project, a written protocol enables clarity of thoughts and allows introspection into all possible aspects of the study. A thesis protocol acts as a road map and should list the various details that constitute a vital component of the thesis. It is reviewed and approved by members of the Institute scientific committee and Ethical board. Once approved, the student must adhere to the protocol of his/her thesis. Various Institute bodies usually have a prefixed format for the same.

Need for a Protocol

All research bodies require clearance from their scientific and ethic committees for a project to commence, which in turn would necessitate the drafting of a protocol. If the project is a clinical trial, the same protocol would also have to be registered with the clinical trial registry. Various funding groups also need the submission of a protocol to evaluate the same for grant assistance. Furthermore, the protocol acts as a blueprint, a standard operating procedure, that the investigator can fall back on while performing the research.

Components of a Thesis Protocol

The thesis protocol broadly has two major sections [1–3]. **The first section** has general information, which includes the following:

- Name and address of the candidate, Guide and Co guide with their contact information
- Name of the course (MD/MS/DM/MCh/Ph.D.) and branch. Month and year of admission to the course and appearing for the final examination.

- Study duration—It should include the follow-up period if it is a part of the study
- Details about setting in which the study will be done e.g. institutional/inter-institutional/international
- Details of funding

The **second section** consists of technical details of the study, under the following headings, all of which should be written in the future tense. It consists of the following parts:

- Title
- Background of the study
- Research question
- Aims and objectives
- Brief review
- Methodology
- Any previous work
- Case record form

Title

It should be concise (preferably not more than 15 words), specific and informative. It should mention the study design (case-control/randomized trial), population that is going to be studied, the intervention intended, the employment of controls if any and the expected outcome. A descriptive title is commonly used for a thesis protocol. Interrogative title (introducing the subject in the form of question) should be preferably avoided for a thesis protocol. Use of acronyms, linguistic jargons, sensationalism, irony and puns in the title should be avoided.

Examples of titles to avoided and how to improve it:

Poor title (Interrogative title): Is esomeprazole a better drug than pantoprazole in treating bleeding duodenal ulcer?

Recommended title (Descriptive title): A comparative study of esomeprazole and pantoprazole in bleeding duodenal ulcer—a prospective randomized study.

Poor title (idioms and phrases): Synbiotics in pancreatic surgery: A Hobson's choice.

Recommended title: Evaluation of the role of synbiotics in patients undergoing surgery for pancreatic diseases.

Background of the Study

It should begin by providing an insight into what is known about the problem and is followed by brief description of previous studies done in the same field to highlight the lacunae in the existing knowledge. This, in turn, will justify the rationale behind the present study. The novelty of the study to be undertaken should also be discussed. A detailed review of literature is not required.

Research Question or a Hypothesis

A research question is a question for which the researcher wants to find an answer, by conducting the study. The question should be framed such that both the planned intervention and the population to which it is being applied, are mentioned. A research hypothesis should be in the form of a sentence that states the expected outcome of the study.

Example:

Research question: Is drain fluid amylase measurement on post-operative day one a predictor of pancreatic fistula after pancreatic surgery?

Research hypothesis: Postoperative day one drain fluid amylase predict pancreatic fistula after pancreatic surgery.

Aims and Objectives

Often the students are confused with the terms aims and objectives and use them interchangeably. The aim is regarded as a general statement of what a researcher hopes to achieve and is usually written using an infinite verb. Objectives usually more than one is often expressed through an active sentence to state the specific steps taken to achieve the aim. Objectives should be specific, measurable and achievable.

Example

Thesis title: Evaluation of micronutrient deficiency in patients undergoing bariatric surgery—a prospective observational study.

Aim:

To evaluate micronutrient level and the prevalence of micronutrient deficiency among the morbidly obese patients undergoing bariatric surgery in a tertiary care hospital.

Objectives:

To determine the baseline micronutrient level among the morbidly obese patients undergoing bariatric surgery.

To assess the changes in the level of micronutrients and bone health during the post-operative period of 1 year.

To identify the factors associated with the level of micronutrients among morbidly obese patients undergoing bariatric surgery.

A Brief Review of the Literature

In this section, the student should cite earlier studies and critically analyze them in terms of variations in methodology and research outcomes. Limitations of earlier studies and how the present research will add to the existing knowledge should be briefly explained. Seminal studies, RCTs and systematic reviews should not be missed out.

Methods

The methodology to be followed for the study should be elucidated in terms of the procurement of the study subjects, data collection, details of intervention, their frequency and duration, drug dosages, formulations, schedule and duration. Details of instruments used are also required. The duration of the study period should also be mentioned. Standardized and/or documented procedures/techniques should be described and bibliographic references, if not provided earlier should be provided. A graphic outline of the study design and procedures using a flow diagram must be provided. This should include the timing of assessments. The research protocol must give a clear indication of what follow up will be provided to the research participants and the duration of the same. This may include a follow-up, especially for adverse events, even after data collection for the research study is completed. The methodology should be self-explanatory and replicable by another researcher.

Study Design

Observational or Interventional (Experimental) (Fig. 1). In the observational study, the researcher just observes and analyses the events and has no control over the occurrence of the events [4]. Observational studies could be either descriptive or analytical. In descriptive studies, the researcher describes the prevalence/distribution of a health problem in relation to person, place and time. A descriptive study can be carried out as a cross-sectional or a longitudinal study. In the cross-sectional study, the study population is contacted or examined at one point in time to obtain the required information. Cross-sectional study is generally used to determine the

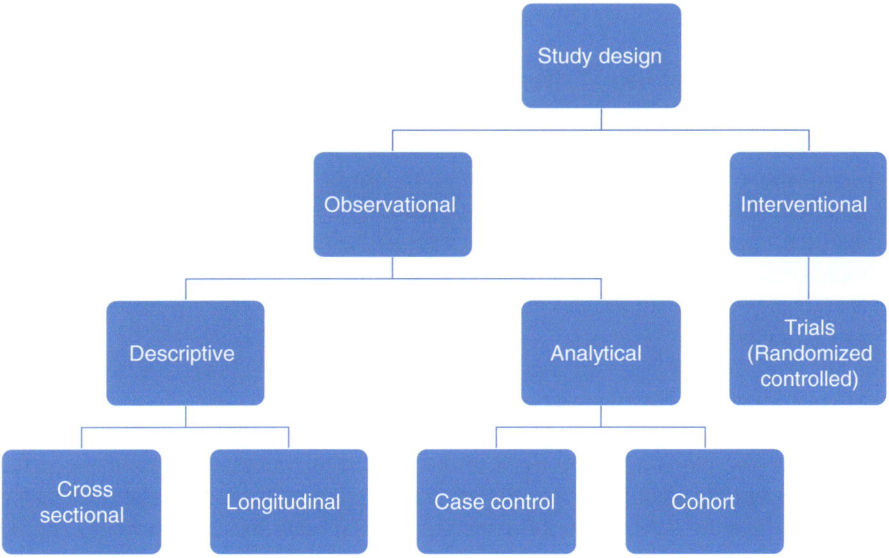

Fig. 1 Study design

prevalence of a health problem like anemia at one point in time. In a longitudinal study, a group of individuals (cohort) is followed over a period with frequent contact or examination to obtain the required information. An example of a longitudinal study is the determination of weight gain in pregnant women.

In the analytical study, the researcher attempts to determine the possible etiological or associated factors in addition to describing the health issue. Analytical studies are carried out as a case-control or cohort study. Case-control study is a retrospective study where the researcher goes back from the disease to the cause. The classical example of a case- control study is to determine whether smoking causes lung cancer the researcher selects patients with lung cancer and study the smoking pattern in them and compare it with those without lung cancer to arrive at a conclusion. In a cohort study, the researcher proceeds from cause to effect in a prospective manner. An example of a cohort study is to determine whether smoking causes lung cancer, a cohort of healthy people with the habit of smoking and another cohort of healthy people without smoking habit are followed for the occurrence of lung cancer and the incidence is compared to arrive at a conclusion.

In contrast to the descriptive study, in an interventional (experimental) study the researcher intervenes and has control over the events. Randomization and selection of study population play an important role in experimental studies. Interventional studies are generally performed to determine the efficacy of a new drug or procedure.

Study Setting

Hospital or community-based setting should be mentioned.

Study Participants

Whether the study involves humans or animals should be mentioned.

Inclusion and Exclusion Criteria

The criteria for eligibility to participate in the trial should be clearly listed as inclusion criteria. It should include disease condition, age group to be studied and in the case of animal studies the exact species and subspecies of experimental animals. Exclusion criteria often include characteristics or co-morbidities, which may confound the results and hence need to be excluded. Inclusion and exclusion criteria should be supplementary and not complementary. For example, a study on patients over 60 years of age should not mention all those below 60 years as exclusion criteria as it is obvious.

Sample Size, the Number in each Group

Details of the statistical method (power of the study, the level of significance) used for sample size calculation, along with the prior study details used to arrive at the calculated sample, should be mentioned. The number of participants in each group should be specified. Allowance for incomplete data and loss to follow up should also be accounted for in the calculation.

Sampling Method

Of the various sampling techniques (Random/Systematic/Stratified/Convenience/Judgmental/Snowball/Quota Sampling), the method used in the current study should be mentioned.

Randomization Techniques

Technique of randomization (Simple, Block, Minimization or Response-adaptive randomization, etc.) should be specified for a randomized controlled trial.

Ethical Considerations

Level of risk to the participant (less than minimal risk/minimal risk/more than minimal risk) to the study subjects should be mentioned (based on ICMR Code on Ethical Guidelines), for the ethical committee's assessment [5]. Patient information sheet and consent forms, both in the local language and English, should be enclosed. If the participant is a minor, then Parent consent/Assent forms should be enclosed.

List of Variables and Measurement Methods

The primary and secondary outcome measures should be defined, and the statistical tools for their estimation should be precisely mentioned.

Data Collection Methods and Periodicity

A timeline of participant's visits should be framed. The various parameters assessed at the baseline and at follow up visits should be given here.

List of Variable Wise Statistical Tests

Names of the statistical tests (parametric/nonparametric) being used for dependent and independent variables are given in this section.

References

A list of 10–15 relevant references should be written in Vancouver (ICJME) style of referencing.

Any Previous Work Done

A research thesis should not be started without getting an appropriate clearance is obtained from the ethics committee. However, the candidate can mention here about the preliminary collection of information from literature, seeing feasibility based on past records available.

Case Record Form (CRF)

Once ethical approval is obtained, participants can be recruited into the study. The data should be collected in CRF, which should have all the parameters mentioned in the methodology section of the protocol. Participant's details, history, examination, lab reports and follow up assessments should be written in an unambiguous manner in the CRF. The data collected will be used for statistical analysis. CRF is also called as patient proforma and is enclosed with the protocol.

Pilot Study

A pilot study is a small version of the proposed study to determine the feasibility and logistics of a proposed large-scale study [6]. In general, it is done before phase III randomized trials to avoid the potentially disastrous consequences of conducting a non-feasible large study. Occasionally postgraduates might need to do a pilot study to know whether the topic selected for the thesis is feasible. Pilot study helps to determine the feasibility of the processes (like recruitment/compliance rate) that are key to the success of the main study. Also, time and resource (budget) problems, information regarding treatment safety and safe dose level can be obtained from the pilot study. Although the pilot study is small-scale study, it is a complete study by itself in contrast to an exploratory study which is an incomplete study. The researcher should ensure that the study subjects of pilot study are not included in the main study.

To formulate a protocol that is both succinct and delivers the idea across it is essential to avoid flowery language and to stick to short and simple sentences. Also, maintaining the font size and ensuring accurate grammar goes a long way. Prior to submitting the protocol, it helps to have it reviewed by peers as well as experienced individuals and altering the needed revisions before tendering the document in (Fig. 2).

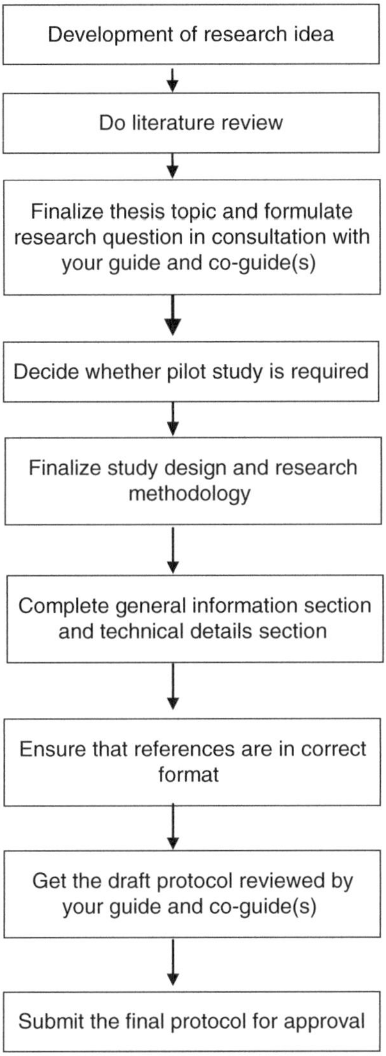

Fig. 2 Algorithm for writing a thesis protocol

Case Scenarios

1. You are planning to do a prospective study on the predictive value of different fistula risk scores to accurately predict clinically relevant postoperative pancreatic fistula. You have titled the study as "Fistula risk score and clinically relevant POPF—close, but not cigar." Comment on the title.
   Key: Avoid using acronyms and linguistic jargons in the title. The study design is not mentioned.
2. You are planning to do a thesis on a novel laboratory test. You are not sure about the feasibility of the study process like resource requirements. Before choosing the study as your thesis topic, what should be your approach?
   Key: to do a pilot study.

References

1. WHO | *Recommended format for a research protocol* [Internet]. Who.int. 2017 [cited 31st July 2017]. http://www.who.int/rpc/research_ethics/format_rp/en/.
2. *Guidelines for Writing a Research Protocol* | ORRP [Internet]. Orrp.osu.edu. 2017 [cited 31st July 2017]. http://orrp.osu.edu/irb/investigator-guidance/exempt.pdf.
3. Betkerur J. Guidelines for writing a research project synopsis or protocol. Indian J Dermatol Venereol Leprol. 2008;74:687–90.
4. Thiese MS. Observational and interventional study design types; an overview. Biochem Med (Zagreb). 2014;24:199–210.
5. New Delhi: Indian Council of Medical Research; 2006. Ethical Guidelines for Biomedical Research on Human Subjects.
6. Thabane L, Ma J, Chu R, Cheng J, Ismaila A, Rios LP, et al. A tutorial on pilot studies: the what, why and how. BMC Med Res Methodol. 2010;10(1)

Approval of the Institute Review Board, Ethics Committee and Registering with the Clinical Trial Registry

Zile Singh and P. Stalin

Ethics is knowing the difference between what you have a right to do and what is right to do.—Potter Stewart

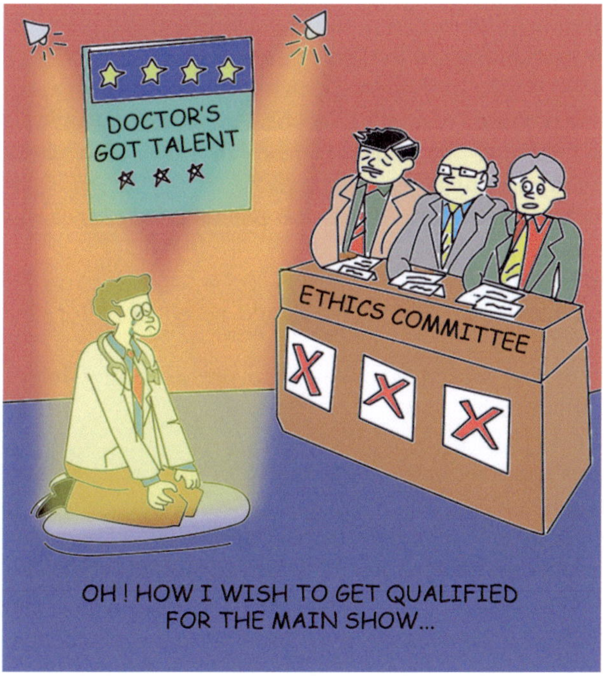

Z. Singh (✉)
Professor and Head, Department of Community Medicine,
Pondicherry Institute of Medical Sciences, Pondicherry, India

P. Stalin
Associate Professor, Department of Community Medicine,
Pondicherry Institute of Medical Sciences, Pondicherry, India

S. C. Parija, V. Kate (eds.), *Thesis Writing for Master's and Ph.D. Program*,
https://doi.org/10.1007/978-981-13-0890-1_7

Key Points

- Submission of research protocol with necessary documents to the Institutional Ethics Committee (IEC) for approval.
- Proposals with more than minimal risk where invasive and/or non-invasive procedures are carried out should be submitted for full ethics Committee Review.
- Patient information sheet and written informed consent forms should be submitted in both English and local language for ethics committee review.
- Registration of clinical trials at Clinical Trial Registry of India.
- World Health Organization has developed International Clinical Trial Registry Platform (ICTRP), which is a network of Primary Clinical Trial Registers.

Introduction

In order to ensure the welfare and the rights of the participants, researchers conducting bio-medical research involving human participants should submit their proposals to the Institutional Ethics Committee/Review Board and get their approval.

The main responsibilities of the Ethics Committees are:

- To review the proposed research protocols before the project initiation.
- To regularly monitor the approved research projects to check whether the researchers are adhering to their protocol.
- To ensure that the researchers follow the general principles of ethics:
  - Is the research essential?
  - It should be voluntary.
  - The agreement from community should be obtained for community-based research.
  - Consent of the participants should be obtained after informing them all aspects of research.
  - There should be no exploitation.
  - Research should not be conducted in ways that create social disharmony in the community.
  - Confidentiality and privacy of the participants should be ensured.
  - Taking proper precautions should minimize all types of risks.
  - Researchers should be professionally competent, accountable and transparent.
  - Research should serve maximum public interest and justice.
  - The Institution should assume responsibility for facilitating and arranging research.
  - The research findings should be in public domain without affecting privacy.
  - The responsibility of sponsors, researchers, institutions and participants to be specified.
  - Researchers should conduct the study as per the protocol.
  - Environmental protection should be ensured by the researchers [1].

Types of Reviews

Exemption from Review

Research proposals related to medical education such as measuring the efficacy of teaching-learning methods, approaches and strategies, which have less than minimal, risk to the study participants can be exempted from review. It also includes analysis of data available in the public domain, quality control studies and program evaluation etc.

Expedited Review

Due to the minimal risk involved in the research proposals based on already collected non-identifiable information such as clinical, laboratory and treatment data from patients, it can be reviewed quickly. Expedited review can also be done in situations like disasters, outbreaks etc.

Full Committee Review

Proposals with more than minimal risk where invasive and/or non-invasive procedures are carried out should be reviewed fully by all the members, especially if the study participants belong to vulnerable/ marginalized groups. The full committee should ratify the research proposals, which have undergone exempted from review or expedited review [1].

Proper Submission to Ethics/Regulatory Board

Information and Documents Required for Submission to IEC

According to the guidelines laid by Indian Council of Medical Research (ICMR), following documents should be submitted along with research proposals:

1. Researcher's name and his contact details.
2. Details of the study settings.
3. Approval obtained from the Head of the Department/Institution.
4. Research proposal with all necessary details such as justification, objectives and methods etc.
5. Plans to solve the identified ethical issues of the study.
6. Study tools such as case proforma; data extraction sheet should be attached as annexure.
7. Patient information sheet and written informed consent forms should be submitted in both English and local language.
8. In case of clinical trials involving new drugs/ techniques, all relevant data from previous animal and human studies both within and outside the country should be provided.
9. All the investigators should submit their curriculum vitae with the list of relevant and recent publications.

10. Clearance certificate from regulatory bodies should be submitted, if required.
11. Details of study budget, source of funding and insurances (if applicable) to be furnished.
12. Declaration form stating that investigators will follow the relevant national and international guidelines and report any Serious Adverse Events (SAE) to IEC.
13. Conflicts of interest should be stated, if applicable.
14. Study participants should be provided with all the information regarding compensation, arrangements for indemnity and insurance coverage etc.
15. In case of submission of the same protocol to other Ethics Committee in the past, their decisions and comments should be provided. If the investigators had made changes in the protocol based on their comments, details of the modifications should be mentioned.
16. Irrespective of the study results, researcher's plan for publication while maintaining the confidentiality and privacy of the study participants should be submitted.
17. Miscellaneous documents, if any.

Procedure for Application to the IEC

- Research proposals in the prescribed format duly signed by the investigators should be forwarded by the department's head to the Ethics Committee.
- Hard copies of the research proposals along with enclosures of all required documents should be submitted in numbers as required by the IEC.
- IEC will inform the researcher about the date of meeting and call him/her to attend it for any clarifications.
- After the meeting, IEC will share the decision about the proposal.
- In case of revision, investigator should modify the proposal according to the comments/suggestions received from the Ethics Committee and resubmit it within the given period of time.
- Fees, if any should be paid to the Ethics Committee [2].

Define Need for Study, Novelty/Requirement/Review of Literature

Need for Study

It is the responsibility of the researcher to justify the need for the study. Need for the study should be well written so that it tells us about the background, reasons and possible way forward for the health problem. It is similar to the introduction section of a research article. It should give information about the need and relevance of the study. The burden, distribution and determinants of the problem should be described at global, national, regional and local levels. Findings from recent similar published studies should be summarized briefly [3].

Novelty

Novelty means state of being new or unique or something different from what already exists related to the field of research topic. Many times, researchers are duplicating the studies conducted in some other states/regions/countries. Such duplications are commonly seen among the papers published by the faculty and postgraduates in some teaching institutions. Sometimes, the primary purpose of doing research gets metamorphosed to just fulfilling the requirement of postgraduate courses and faculty promotions. Rather, investigators should desire to find out the gaps in knowledge and practice in medicine and conduct research to fill such gaps.

Review of Literature

The review of literature should contain relevant and recent information about the proposed research topic. It helps to frame the objective(s) being studied. Literature review indicates that the investigator has studied the research works already done in the field. Therefore, the reader would be able to understand the problem related to the research topic, to appreciate the need for the present study and to accept the study methods chosen for that particular study.

Review of literature will help the researchers in the following ways

- To avoid duplication of the research work already done on the topic.
- To refine the problem statement of the health condition.
- To analyze the various methods and procedures followed in the previous studies.
- To develop discussions about the research topic.

Good review of literature should convince the readers about the researcher's acquaintance of the topic [4].

Prepare to Defend Methodology

Investigators should choose appropriate methods to achieve the objectives of the study and to take care of the internal and external validity of the study. The investigator should ensure the following:

- Choose the appropriate study design, which can answer the research questions.
- In case of randomized controlled trials, methods used for randomization, generation & concealment of allocation sequence and blinding (single/double) should be mentioned.
- To minimize random errors, sample size should be calculated using the appropriate formula. Values of the parameters used in the calculation need to be mentioned explicitly.

- In order to avoid selection bias, inclusion and exclusion criteria for the study participants should be specified clearly and ideal sampling method should be followed for selecting the study participants from the study population.
- Details about the data collection/extraction tools such as mode of administration (self/interviewer), type (structured/semi-structured/unstructured) and domains should be provided. List of variables to be studied should be provided in the protocol. If new tools/scales are used, information regarding the validity of the tools should be specified.
- Details about the interviewer/data collectors/extractors such as the number, qualification and designation should be mentioned. If many individuals are involved in data collection, measures to minimize the inter-observer variations should be described.
- Data entry procedure should be specified. Details of statistical analytical plan such as the software, types of statistical tests and level of statistical significance (p-value) should be provided.

Correctly Identify Ethical Issues, If Any

All the researchers should follow the basic principles of ethics such as voluntariness, beneficence, harmlessness and justice.

General Considerations

- The aims of the study should be informed to the study participants. Even after informing and getting the consent from individual participants, the level of awareness about their rights might be less. Hence, investigators should remain conscious about their duties and responsibilities towards the participants.
- In community-based research, the researcher should obtain the consent of the community through their representatives such as village head, political leaders *etc*. During this process, the people may give consent due to societal pressures. Therefore, investigators should make efforts to prevent it.
- Sometimes financial inducements are used to get consent from individuals and communities, especially in developing countries. Such practices should not be allowed. However, the investigators should provide compensation to the participants for their loss of wages and travel expenses as applicable.
- Participants should be explained in detail about all levels of risks, which includes less than minimal (e.g., Research on teaching-learning methods), minimal (e.g., Collection of information from study participants by interview method) and more than minimal (e.g., Collection of blood samples). Harms to the participants should be avoided or minimized.
- It is the responsibility of the investigator to maintain absolute confidentiality of data collected from the study participants as it may have effect on issues like patient's privacy, safety and national security.

- Investigators while writing the protocol should take into account culturally sensitive issues and address them appropriately.
- Study participants should be informed about the storage of their data and biological samples and written consent should be obtained. It is also important to specify the duration of storage. If participants don't give consent for storage, the biological samples should be discarded after carrying out the investigations.

Special Considerations

- In clinical trials, usage of placebo drugs and sham surgery should be minimized. It is unethical to refuse the available treatment to the study participants in the control arm.
- In case of drug trials, sponsor and ethics committee should be notified of all serious adverse events within 24 hours and within 7 days respectively.
- After the successful vaccine trial, the vaccine should also be provided to the control group. The study participants especially children may cross the age of vaccination at the end of the trial. In such instances, alternative vaccine should be provided to the control arm, if possible.
- In order to achieve the study objectives and for the community benefit, researchers deceive the participants by providing incomplete or incorrect information. Such studies involving deception should undergo full committee review.
- In case of multi-centric study, the protocol may be modified according to the local needs and should be approved by the institutional ethics committee of the individual sites [1].

Clinical Trial Registry Upload

In India, all clinical trials should be registered through online in the Clinical Trials Registry - India (CTRI). It is free and should be done before the initiation of the study. Completed and ongoing trials can also be registered retrospectively. However, it is better to register as early as possible. The public can freely access these registered trials.

Why Is It Important for Registration?

- As per the regulations of the Drugs Controller General of India, it is mandatory for registering the trials in the CTRI from 15th June 2009.
- In 2008, the World Medical Association, while revising the Declaration of Helsinki, mentions, "Every clinical trial must be registered in a publicly accessible database before recruitment of the first subject."
- Registration number of the clinical trial should be submitted for publication of the results in some journals.

Which Clinical Trials Are Required to be Registered?

Research studies in which interventions such as drugs; treatment procedures, health education etc. are used for modifying the health status of human participants. CTRI recommends that observational trials may also be registered.

The following information needs to be entered into the registry:

- Study titles (For both public and scientific)
- Name and contact details of the principal investigator
- Contact persons (For both public and scientific query)
- Source of funding/sponsors
- Objectives of the study
- Disease/ health condition studied
- Study settings
- Study design
- Study period
- Study participants—eligibility criteria
- Sample size calculation
- Details of randomization including sequence generation and concealment
- Interventions to be used in control and intervention arms
- Primary and secondary outcome/s
- Blinding especially for outcome measurement
- Details of the Institutional Ethics Committee
- Status of IEC clearance
- Clearance certificate from DCGI
- Phase of Trial
- Date of initiation
- Brief Summary

What Is the Procedure for Registration?

- In the Home Page of the CTRI (www.ctri.nic.in), initial registration should be done by the researchers. After registration, registrant will receive the username and password. NEW USER form should be filled and submitted online.
- The registrant should login to the CTRI site using their username and password. In order to fill the Trial Registration Form, TRIAL REGISTRATION should be clicked.
- The form consists of several Parts. All the parts of the form have to be filled for the submission.
- Certificates of Approval obtained from Institutional Ethics Committee and Drug Control General of India should be submitted online by the registrant. The public cannot access these documents.

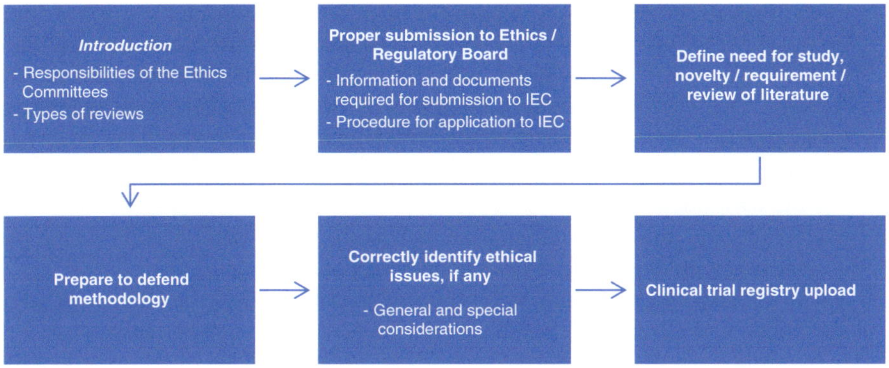

Fig. 1 Plan for submission of protocol from Ethics Committee to registration of the trial

- After submission, the CTRI scientists for their validity and relevance will review the details of the trial. They will also scrutinize the approval certificates obtained from IEC and DCGI.
- Principal investigators and corresponding author will receive the verification emails.
- After completion of the above steps, the trial will be registered and trial details can be viewed from the public domain [5].

Plan for submission of protocol from Ethics Committee to registration of the trial is shown in Fig. 1.

International Clinical Trial Registries

In order to ensure that health policy makers can access the research being conducted throughout the world, World Health Organization has developed International Clinical Trial Registry Platform (ICTRP), which is a network of Primary Clinical Trial Registers. Some of the primary registers are listed below [6].

- Australian New Zealand Clinical Trials Registry (ANZCTR).
- Chinese Clinical Trial Registry (ChiCTR).
- EU Clinical Trials Register (EU-CTR).
- German Clinical Trials Register (DRKS).
- Japan Primary Registries Network (JPRN).

Case Scenarios

1. Department of Community Medicine of a medical college is planning to train their 6th semester medical students in community-based research methodology through Re-orientation of Medical Education (ROME) posting. The project

titled "Prevalence of Oral Pre-malignant Lesions among Adults in a Rural Area of Tamil Nadu" is assigned to one of the groups of students in which study participants are required to be interviewed and examined by the students after proper training. This project proposal is submitted to the institutional ethics committee for approval.
   (a) What is the level of risk to the study participants involved in the above training cum research?
   (b) Which type of review (exemption, expedited or full review) should be done for this project proposal? Give your justification.
2. You are conducting a randomized controlled trial to measure the efficacy of yoga and meditation in reducing the blood pressure level among hypertension patients in an urban area of Puducherry. Before the initiation of the research, you have obtained the approval of your institutional research and ethics committee. Now, you are going to start the intervention of yoga and meditation after successfully completing the baseline survey.
   (a) At this point, you have come to know about the Clinical Trial Registry of India. Is it possible to register your trial at this stage?
   (b) Why is it important to register the trial under CTRI?

References

1. Ethical guidelines for biomedical and health research involving human participants. New Delhi: Indian Council of Medical Research; 2017.
2. Guidelines for preparing Standard Operating Procedures (SOP) for Institutional Ethics Committee for Human Research. Indian Council of Medical Research. http://icmr.nic.in/ethics_SOP.pdf. Accessed on 21st June 2017.
3. Recommended format for a Research Protocol. Research Policy. World Health Organization. http://www.who.int/rpc/research_ethics/format_rp/en/. Accessed on 30 June 2017.
4. Implementation research toolkit. Workbook on special Programme for research and training in tropical diseases. Geneva: World Health Organization; 2014.
5. Frequently Asked Questions. Clinical Trials Registry of India. National Institute of Medical Statistics. Indian Council of Medical Research. http://ctri.nic.in/Clinicaltrials/faq.php. Accessed on 10 July 2017.
6. Primary Registries. International Clinical Trials Registry Platform (ICTRP). World Health Organization. http://www.who.int/ictrp/network/primary/en/. Accessed on 17 October 2017.

Part II

Conduct of Research and Analysis

Plan and Conduct of Research: Observational and Interventional Study Designs

Vikram Kate, Sathasivam Sureshkumar, and Mohsina Subair

I strive for two things in designs: simplicity and clarity, great design is born out of these things—Lindon Leader

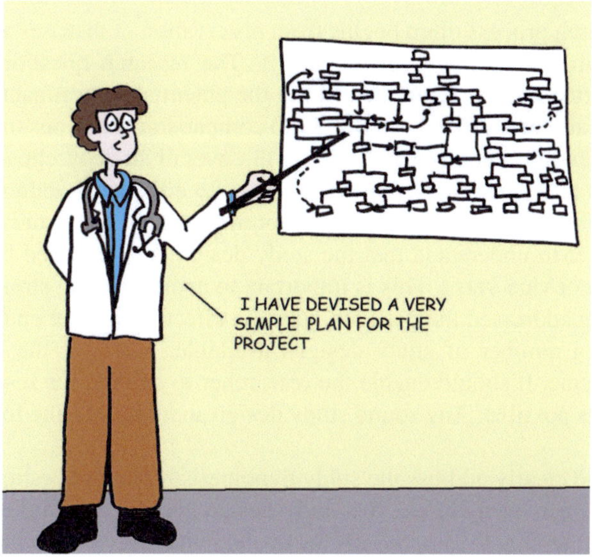

V. Kate (✉)
Professor and Head, Department of Surgery and Senior Consultant General and Gastrointestinal Surgeon, Jawaharlal Institute of Postgraduate Medical Education and Research, Pondicherry, India

S. Sureshkumar
Associate Professor, Department of Surgery, Jawaharlal Institute of Postgraduate Medical Education and Research, Pondicherry, India

M. Subair
Senior Resident, Department of Plastic and Reconstructive Surgery, Postgraduate Institute Medical Education and Research, Chandigarh, India

S. C. Parija, V. Kate (eds.), *Thesis Writing for Master's and Ph.D. Program*,
https://doi.org/10.1007/978-981-13-0890-1_8

Key Points

- The study design is the overall strategy chosen to logically assimilate the different study components so as to effectively address the research question and is determined by the research question and not vice-versa.
- Study designs in medical research can be broadly classified as basic, observational and interventional studies. Observational studies can be further divided into descriptive and analytic studies.
- Case-control study proceeds from outcome to exposure, whereas cohort study proceeds from exposure to outcome.
- RCTs can be divided as parallel arm, cross-over and factorial studies based on design and as superiority and non-inferiority based on hypothesis.
- The keystones in the decision making process for suitable study design is "reducing bias" and "increasing efficiency".
- Although RCTs and controlled cohort studies provide higher level of evidence, the best study design is the one that answers the research question most explicitly.

Medical research process often begins from observation of diseases and identifying particular characteristics associated with it. The research questions that can be posed are myriad ranging from identifying the potential determinants of a disease, analysis of a cause and effect relationship to comparison of various treatment strategies or interventions. The study design is the overall strategy chosen to logically assimilate the different study components so as to effectively address the research question [1]. It should include a road map for the conduct of the study. It is essential for a researcher to understand that the study design is determined by the research question and not vice-versa. This is important to avoid drawing strong conclusions and not having addressed the research question effectively at the end of the study.

There are a number of study designs available, however, the basic function remains the same. It should enable the researcher to address the research question as explicitly as possible. Any sound study design should fulfill the following [2]:

- Identify and clearly address the study hypothesis/research question
- Although a part of methods, the study design chosen should describe the data required for testing the hypothesis adequately and clearly state the data acquisition procedure
- Describe the appropriate analytical tests to be carried out on the data to check the hypothesis.

Types of Study Designs

The study designs in medical research can be broadly classified as follows [3]:

- *Basic studies*: This includes various cell, genetic and animal experiments aimed at establishing a cause and outcome relationship.
- *Observational studies*: These are non-interventional and non-experimental studies. They can be further classified as Descriptive and Analytical studies.

- *Experimental/Interventional studies*: These involve comparison of effect of a treatment or interventions with controls. These are further classified as clinical trials or field trials.

The observational and interventional study designs will be discussed in detail in this chapter. A broad outline of classification of study designs is shown in Fig. 1. Basic studies will not be included as it is out of scope for this chapter.

Observational Studies

These are non-interventional studies that aim at assessing the association between a particular exposure and outcome [4]. These are referred to as "observational studies" because the researcher simply observes—who is exposed/unexposed and who develops the outcome or not or vice-versa. These studies help in providing relevant insights into the disease process and its determinants without facing the practical and ethical difficulties of establishing a project. The major limitation of these designs is the presence of various confounding factors that its conclusions are less

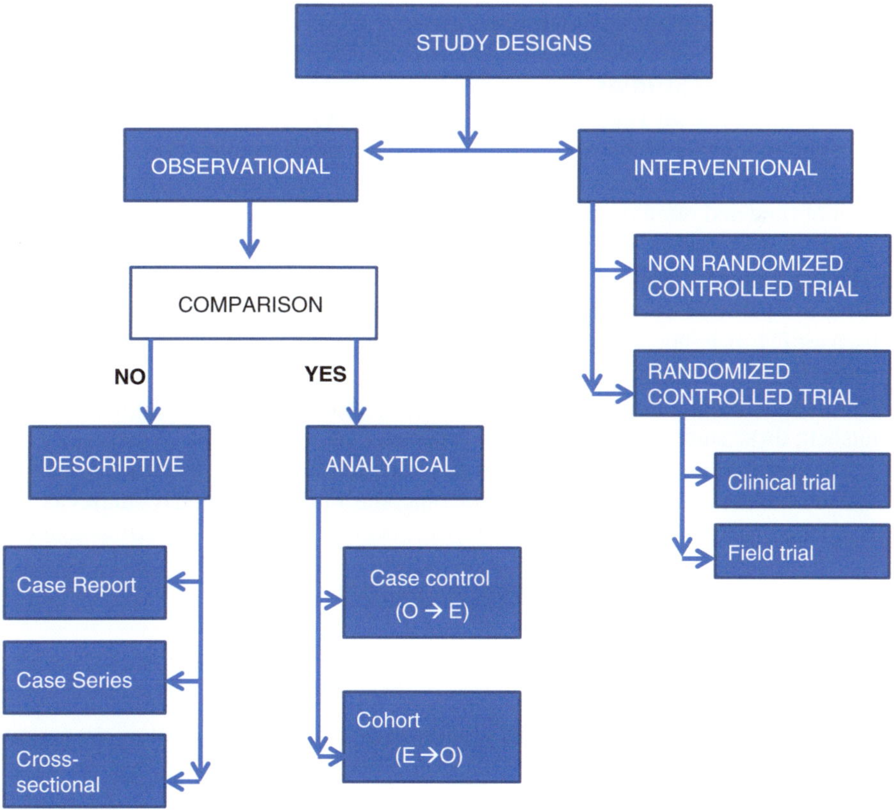

Fig. 1 Types of study designs. *O* outcome, *E* exposure

emphatic than non-interventional designs. Observational studies can be further classified as Descriptive and Analytical studies.

Descriptive Studies

In these studies, the researcher just describes the situation or events. It pursues answers to the "who, what, when, where, and how" questions pertaining to a disease or an event. It does not provide answers to "why" between various linked events. However, these studies can help in generating hypothesis that can be tested by further studies [3]. *Descriptive studies include case reports or series, cross-sectional and longitudinal studies.*

Case Report and Case Series

Case reports give detailed description of the disease potential causal effects and treatment outcomes in one or few patients, often less than 10 in number [1]. When the description involves >10 patients, it is referred to as case series [1]. These reports are the simplest research forms and do not help in determining the incidence of the disease or a causal effect. However, these serve as forerunners for generating hypothesis for the other study designs.

Cross-Sectional Studies

These are also known as prevalence studies. These studies describe the current situation pertaining to a particular disease and its outcome at a point of time in a certain population [5]. These studies analyses both the exposure and outcome at the same point of time and often do not have a follow-up period. Hence, a temporal relationship between exposure and outcome cannot be established. It is important to include a representative sample in these studies as there is high likelihood of selection bias. These are particularly useful to estimate the prevalence of long-standing common diseases [5]. It is not suitable for diseases such as cancers which need long-term follow-up. These studies are simple to conduct and incur low costs. These studies help in generating a hypothesis, but cannot explain the occurrence of an event. In nutshell, these studies can be called as "snapshot" of a population.

The distributive statistics such as mean, rate and frequency distributions can be inferred from these studies. The major outcome in cross-sectional studies is the prevalence, which is calculated as:

$$\text{Prevalence} = \frac{\text{Number of cases at one point of time}}{\text{Population at the same point of time}}$$

Longitudinal Studies

These are similar to cross-sectional studies except for having a follow-up period. These studies follow the same subjects over a period of time and assess particular events and potential risk factors and document the changes that have occurred over time. These help to define the trends in the disease as well as establish the direction of causal relationship if any. These are also known as "panel study" [6]. However, these require longer duration and costs when compared to cross-sectional studies. Cohort studies also follow a similar pattern of following up subjects; however, the inclusion is defined based on a particular exposure, which is not the case in longitudinal studies. In short, all cohort studies can be longitudinal studies, but not vice-versa. Often researchers use cross-sectional to identify links or associations and then follow it up with longitudinal studies to see for a cause and effect relationship.

Analytical Studies

Analytical studies are type of observational studies that aim to test the hypothesis generated by descriptive studies [4]. These studies are superior to descriptive studies in minimizing bias either by using a control group or by the process of prospective enrollment. *The analytical observational studies include case-control and cohort studies.*

Case-Control Study

It is a type of observational study similar to a retrospective case-series, but with an addition of a control group [1]. In these studies, patients with a disease or outcome (cases) are compared with those who do not have (controls), for the frequency of presence of a potential risk factor (exposure) in the past to determine the association between the outcome and exposure. The study proceeds retrospectively from outcome to exposure. The starting point is the identification of the cases and controls and answers the question about exposure (Fig. 2).

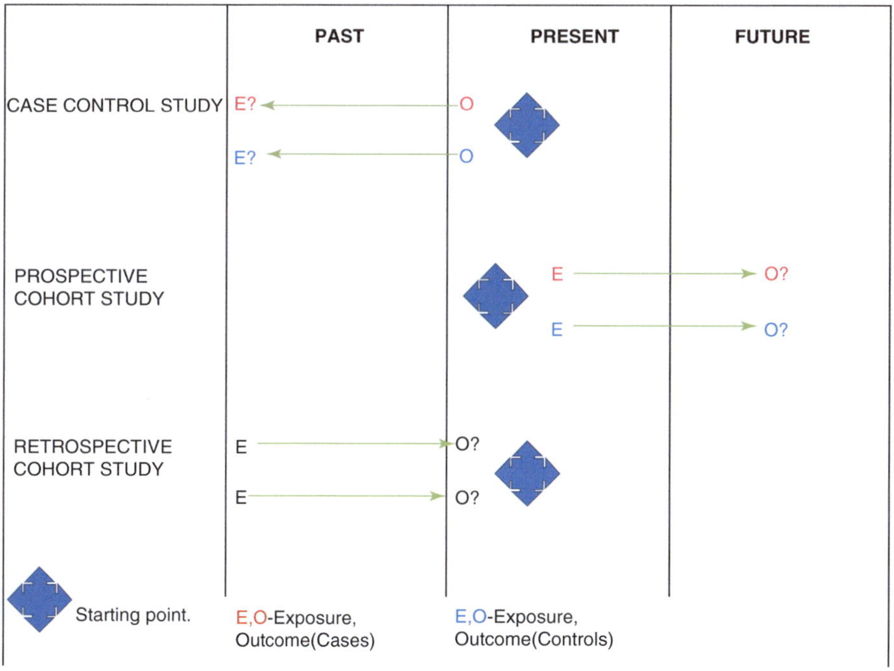

Fig. 2 Figure showing the temporal sequence of various study designs. *O* outcome, *E* exposure

The increased number by inclusion of controls will help in reducing the bias. A matched case-control design is one in which the cases and controls are matched in all factors except the one being investigated and further reduces the risk of bias. These studies are particularly useful for rare diseases or diseases with long latency [7]. These require relatively lesser time as the disease has already occurred and can look at multiple risk factors simultaneously. The real effect of potential risk factors can be demonstrated more conclusively in the presence of controls. However, as the study is a retrospective design, it is heavily dependent on memory and might affect the data quality [7]. Moreover, cases are likely to recall better than controls and hence may lead to recall bias.

In a case-control study, the magnitude of association between exposure and outcome can be measured in terms of Odds Ratio which is defined as follows [8]:

$$\text{Odds Ratio} = \frac{\text{Odds in exposed group}}{\text{Odds in unexposed group}}.$$

An example of a case-control study with calculation of OR is shown in the box:

Example: To Study the Association Between Diet Low in Fibre (Exposure) on Colon Cancer (Outcome)

	Disease+	Disease−	Total
Exposure+	35(a)	15(b)	50
Exposure-	5(c)	10(d)	15

People with and without disease identified and probed for exposure in past → Case-control study

OR = a/b ÷ c/d = ad/bc

OR = 35 × 10/15 × 5 = 4.6

Cohort Study

It is also known as "follow-up" study. These are prospective studies in which a particular group defined based on research question (cohort) is followed over time and are assessed for exposure and outcomes during the study period [9]. The study proceeds from exposure to outcome (Fig. 2). The cohort study can be carried out retrospectively also known as "Historical Cohort study" where the researcher goes back in time and follows up the cohort from exposure to outcome [4] (Fig. 2). In this design, the incidence of the disease in exposed or unexposed group can be calculated. The cohort study design closely resembles an interventional study as patients are classified as exposed/unexposed; however, in this study design, the allocation is not controlled by the researcher as opposed to the interventional studies where the researcher controls the allocation.

This is suitable for a disease with shorter course and the temporal sequence of the events can be studied more effectively. It allows multiple outcomes to be studied simultaneously. It is easier to match within a cohort for confounding variables than in case-control study. However, larger numbers needed and longer time required is the potential disadvantages.

In a cohort study, the magnitude of association is assessed in terms of relative-risk [10]. It is also known as the risk-ratio and is calculated as:

$$RR = \frac{\text{Incidence in exposed}}{\text{Incidence in non - exposed}}$$

RR of 1 indicates no observed association between outcome and exposure, >1 indicates a positive association and <1 indicates a negative association.

In a cohort study, it is possible to determine the attributable risk or excess risk, which indicates the extent to which the outcome can be attributed to the exposure [10].

$$\text{Attributable risk} = \text{Incidence in exposed} - \text{Incidence in non-exposed}$$

$$\text{Attributable risk percentage} = \frac{100 \times \left(\text{Incidence in exposed} - \text{Incidence in non-exposed}\right)}{\text{Incidence in exposed}}$$

Population attributable risk (PAR) refers to the expected reduction in the incidence if the whole population under study was unexposed compared to the current exposure pattern.

$$\text{PAR} = \text{Incidence in total population} - \text{Incidence in non-exposed}$$

The relative risk measures the strength of association, whereas attributable risk measures the impact of association in the health of population.

These calculations are demonstrated in the example: To study the association of alcoholism and liver disease, a cohort of people were followed up for development of liver disease.

	Developed disease	No disease	Total
Alcoholic	70	6930	7000
Non-alcoholic	3	2997	3000

(Relative risk = 70/7000 ÷ 3/3000 = 10/1 = 10. It indicates the risk of developing the disease is ten-times more in alcoholic when compared to non-alcoholics).

Attributable risk percentage = 100 x {(70/7000 – 3/3000) ÷ 70/7000} = 90% *(It indicates 90% of the cases of liver diseases are attributed to alcoholism)*

PAR % = 73/10,000 – 3/3000 = 63% *(It indicates 63% of cases in the population can be avoided by stopping alcoholism)*

As per the ethical guidelines, any studies involving human subjects including the observational studies have to be submitted for approval of Ethics Committee [11].

Study Design Assessing the Diagnostic Accuracy

This study design is chosen when a new test or investigation is evaluated for its accuracy in detecting/diagnosing/predicting the disease/condition/prognosis etc. When a new diagnostic test is evaluated, it is usually compared with the current gold standard for the particular disease or condition. The diagnostic accuracy is studied with the three intended purposes which include replacement; where the new test is expected to replace the current investigation, the add-on; in which the test is expected to be as accurate as the current gold standard and the triage; in which the new test is used to choose patients who will be subjected to the current gold standard. Majority of the study on diagnostic accuracy is done with the intent of replacement of current gold standard and hence expected to have superior sensitivity, specificity and low cost. It should be born in mind that the diagnostic accuracy of a test depends on multiple factors including, the population characteristics, disease prevalence and disease spectrum [12].

When this study is carried out, the diagnostic accuracy is measured as a discriminative ability (to differentiate health/disease, between two stage of the disease etc) or a predictive ability (to predict the possibility of acquiring/having a disease) using the following quantifying measures.

- Sensitivity and specificity
- Positive and negative predicative values (PPV, NPV)
- Likelihood ratio
- Diagnostic odds ratio (DOR)
- The area under the ROC curve (AUC)

The 2 × 2 table serves to calculate the true and false positive and negative values.

	Population with disease	Population without disease
Test positive	True positive (TP)	False positive (FP)
Test negative	False negative (FN)	True negative (TN)

The statistical assessment of the said measures are calculated as below

Description of measures used to assess the diagnostic utility of the test	Terminology used for the Statistical measure	Method of calculation
Proportion of population who have disease among the total test positive	Sensitivity	TP/(TP + FN)
Proportion of population who do not have the disease among the total test negative	Specificity	TN/(FP + TN)

Proportion of population who tested positive and have the disease	Positive predictive value	TP/(TP + FP)
Proportion of population who tested negative and who do not have the disease	Negative predictive value	TN/(FN + TN)
The likelihood of positive test in population with disease as compared to likelihood of positive test in population without the disease	Positive likelihood ratio	Sensitivity/ (1 − specificity)
The likelihood of negative test in population with disease as compared to likelihood of negative test in population without the disease	Negative likelihood ratio	(1 − sensitivity)/ specificity
Proportion of population correctly identified as either having or not having the disease	Accuracy	(TP + TN)/ (TP + FP + FN + TN)
Ratio of the odds of positivity in population with disease compared to the odds in population without disease	Diagnostic odds ratio	(TP/FN)/(FP/TN)

Receiver operating characteristic curve (ROC) made using the paired values of sensitivity and specificity for each cut off, plotting the sensitivity on the Y-axis and 1 − specificity on the X-axis. The AUC and the shape of the curve are used to predict the discriminative ability of the diagnostic test. The AUC ranges from 0 to 1 where 0.9–1 is considered as the best discriminating ability of the test. Any test having AUC of <0.5 is generally considered as non-discriminating and not useful.

When choosing the diagnostic accuracy design, few important aspects should be kept in mind to avoid imprecise results. As the diagnostic performance of a new test is usually compared to the existing gold standard, appropriate gold standard/reference should be chosen for the particular disease. There should be a standard operational definition as to what is considered positive, negative and indeterminate test results. Since the test results depend on the spectrum and prevalence of the disease in the population, selection bias should be avoided and appropriate rater blinding should be applied to avoid overestimate or underestimate the diagnostic utility of the test. To avoid methodological flaws and deficiency, it is mandated at present that all the studies evaluating the diagnostic accuracy have to be conducted in a manner to fulfill the STARD (Standards for Reporting of Diagnostic Accuracy) and QUADAS (Quality Assessment of Diagnostic Accuracy Studies) criterion lists [13].

Appropriate consent with respect to subjecting the individual for the new diagnostic test or for collecting specimen for the new test should be taken. The protocol of the study should be submitted for the ethics committee review. If the diagnostic accuracy is studied form the collected and de-identified data, expedited review by the ethics committee may be requested [11].

Experimental/Interventional Study

The experimental/interventional studies include studies which aim at comparing the effect of a treatment or intervention between various groups. The study plan allows the researcher to have control over all factors that can affect the result. The experimental research approach is used when there is a temporal association, consistency in the causal relationship and when the magnitude of correlation is high with observational studies. The typical design has the experimental and the control group. Experimental group receives the independent variable, i.e, intervention, whereas control group does not. The dependent variable, i.e, outcome is compared between the two groups. Interventional studies can be classified as clinical or field trials [6].

Clinical trials are carried out in a hospital setting to study the various forms of treatment of a disease. Field trials are carried out in the community and evaluates if a particular agent or treatment reduces the risk of occurrence of a particular disease in disease-free individuals [6]. The classical example of an interventional trial is the Randomized Controlled Trial which will be discussed in detail in this chapter.

Randomized Controlled Trial

A randomized controlled trial (RCT) is defined as a study design which randomly assigns participants to either group, experimental or control arm [14]. The participants have equal chance of being allocated to either group by use of "randomization" and hence are not influenced by researcher or the participant thus reducing bias. The word "controlled" is often misinterpreted as presence of a control group, however, it indicates that the study design ensures that all steps in the study occur in a controlled manner. Randomized controlled trials can be classified further based on design or based on hypothesis.

Based on design, RCT can be classified as follows [14–16]:

- Parallel arm: Participants are assigned to either experiment or control group and receive and does not receive an intervention respectively. The participants remain in the same group as assigned throughout the study.
- Cross over study: the patients are allocated to two groups (experiment and control). After a wash out period, the patients switch the groups. The effect of intervention is analyzed both by self-control (patient acts as their own control) and independent controls. This design is powerful, but not always feasible. It's often used for assessing effects of drugs which have a faster wash-out period.
- Factorial: This design indicates presence of more than two parallel arms and each arm receives various permutations and combinations of intervention and control.

Based on the hypothesis, RCT can be classified as follows [14–16]:

- Superiority trials: One intervention is hypothesized to be superior to another or existing treatment. For example, in the study of Adapted Enhanced Recovery After Surgery (ERAS) pathway for perforated duodenal ulcer patients compared to the standard care to assess the effect of ERAS in the Length of Hospitalization (LOH) (primary end point), the ERAS path way is expected to reduce the LOH. Study design was superiority trial considering that the equal LOH or lon-

ger LOH than the standard care in ERAS group is not acceptable. The sample size also calculated as per the superiority design of the study [17]. Similarly, study evaluating the efficacy of sequential vs. concomitant eradication regimen for *H. pylori* where the sequential therapy is expected to have better eradication rate is designed as superiority trial [18].
- Non-inferiority trials: This is carried out to establish that the new modality is no-worse than the existing standard treatment.

The superiority of the RCTs is owing to its capability of reducing bias, which is determined primarily by randomization, blinding and attrition [19]. The study design should clearly explain how each of these processes is carried out for the conduct of the study. Randomization is the process by which the participants are randomized into either group. This can be done by various methods such as table of random numbers or computer generated random sequence. These are often coupled with allocation concealment measures to avoid the subjective bias in selecting participants.

The randomization can be simple, block or stratified. Simple randomization is used when the sample size is small and the study is expected to be completed with the calculated sample size. Block randomization allocates the samples into defined block sizes where in each block, equal number of control and intervention group population exist. The very advantage of block randomization is that even if the trial is stopped at some point of time due to any circumstances, the analysis can be done including the latest completed block as there will be equal number of study and control population. Block size is usually taken as the smallest units possible. For example in an RCT with two groups, block size is taken as 4 with the chance of two patients each in the case and control group. Blocks can be of varying sizes to avoid predicting the last patient in the block. For example, in a two-group open labeled RCT with the block size of 4, if already three patients have been recruited with two controls and one case, the investigator can predict or guess that the next or last patient in that block has to be the case [20]. A varying size of block in the said example with the block sizes of 4 and 6 arranged in random sequence prevents such guessing as the investigator will not know which block size (block size 4 or 6) he is recruiting the patients.

Stratification is done when one of the prognostic variables is known to affect the outcome of interest but may present in both the study and control population in unequal number [21]. The population is divided into strata based on the particular prognostic variable followed by permuted block randomization within each stratum. For example, the study involving high concentration oxygen during colorectal surgery, which is expected to reduce the postoperative surgical site infection (SSI), the presence of stoma, which is created in selected patients of colorectal surgery by itself, is known to increase the SSI. Hence to study the real effect of high concentration oxygen on SSI, the stoma should be equally distributed in both the groups. In the said study, the population will be stratified as having or not having stoma at first, followed by randomization into each stratified group separately so as to include equal number of cases and controls in stoma group and no stoma group.

The results can be made objective and bias can be further reduced in an RCT by blinding [14–16]. Blinding is the process by which patients, treating clinicians or the analysts are masked the group to which the patient belongs to. This will help in avoiding the bias such as patient who behaves differently or a treating clinician offering biased treatment based on personal preferences. Based on blinding, RCT can be single-blinded (only patient is blinded), double-blinded (patients and treating clinicians are blinded) or triple-blinded (patients, treating clinician and the observer are blinded). A triple-blinded randomized study is expected to provide the best-reliable results, however very rarely carried out. It is the double-blind study which is often done when feasible.

Allocation in an RCT can be open-label, where neither the patient nor the investigator is blinded. For example, when a surgical procedure is compared to the non-surgical treatment, where it is not possible to blind the investigator, surgeon and the patient. In cases of drug trial, blinding is possible by making a similar looking placebo. In both the scenarios, allocation concealment is very important to avoid selection bias [22]. The common method used for allocation concealment is serially numbered opaque sealed envelope technique (SNOSE). In this method, a note containing allocation to a particular group (Group A/B, Drug A/B) is kept inside an opaque envelope and sealed. The envelope should be opaque so that the note containing allocation of the group is not visible when held against light so as to reduce bias. The envelope is then numbered serially (as per the simple or block randomization) and provided to the third person who is not involved in the study to open only at the time of intervention. It is important to note that allocation concealment and blinding are not the same. Allocation concealment, as described above, occurs before randomization, whereas blinding occurs after randomization.

Randomized trials often have follow-up periods to study the effect of the treatment or intervention and hence there is a chance of attrition as the study progresses. This is a major source of bias, if not accounted for during analysis. It is ideal to carry out an Intention-to-treat (ITT) analysis [23]. This means that all participants are analyzed in the group to which they are originally assigned, all outcomes are analyzed and all events during follow-up are accounted. All patients who lose follow-up will be regarded as treatment failures while performing ITT analysis. However, in per-protocol analysis, patients who completed the original allocated intervention are only included in analysis, and hence has a potential for bias.

RCTs are considered as the most reliable tool in clinical research, but are slow and expensive to conduct [19]. It does not describe the cause-effect relationship, but rather effectively tests an intervention/experiment. Although it is a superior study design, it is not always better. The quality will be poor if it is not adequately sized, appropriately randomized or blinded and has many violations of the protocol. Hence, one must be cautious while accepting the conclusions from an RCT [24]. The reporting of a RCT should follow the CONSORT (CONsolidated Standards Of Reporting Trials) guidelines to ensure quality [16].

Any interventional trial are categorized as having more than minimal risk or high risk as per the ethical guidelines, and hence necessary measures should be taken such as submitting for the full ethical committee review, getting an informed written consent from the participants separately for cases and controls, compensation in case of research related unexpected adverse events, insurance coverage for the compensation, compensation for participating in the trial etc [11].

Non-Randomized Controlled Trials

Non-Randomized trials are chosen when for certain reasons the randomization is not possible or when randomization may lead to reduced compliance from the study participants. It is a type of quasi-experimental study where the allocation to case or control group is done in non-random method either as per the patient's preference or by the investigator's decision [25]. This type of study design is suitable when intervention and follow-up require significant patients' compliance which may be affected by their faith or preferences. This design can also be used when cost or logical factors make the RCT not feasible. Since the allocation is non-random, influence of confounding factors may affect the outcome of the study. A non-randomized trial can show the association or trend, however establishing the cause-effect relationship between the intervention and the outcome may not be possible due to confounding factors.

Meta-analysis

Individual RCT may be underpowered to answer the research question of interest in many instances. Meta-Analysis is done to obtain more definitive evidence by analyzing the pooled data form multiple RCT's so as to increase the statistical power to find the definitive answer to the research question [26]. However, when selecting the RCT for meta-analysis, few important aspects should be given due consideration. All the selected RCT's should be homogenous with respect to patient population, comparable case and control groups, defined intervention and outcome of interest. Any heterogeneity in the said criteria may lead to incorrect conclusion. QUOROM (Quality Of Reporting Of Meta-Analysis) guidelines have been made mandatory while reporting to ensure the adherence to defined criteria so as to improve the quality of meta-Analysis [27]. Details of meta-analysis is beyond the scope of this chapter.

How to Choose an Appropriate Study Design?

Selecting an appropriate study design is the most important step in the research process as the study design determines the methodology, the only part of the study which cannot be reversed once carried out. The understanding that a flawed methodology can affect the credibility of the results further emphasizes the importance of choosing study design. It can be the most daunting task for a researcher if a systematic approach is not followed. After formulating the research question, the first step is to assess the feasibility of the available resources. The next step is to design the study, the keystones in the decision-making process being "reducing bias" and "increasing efficiency" [28]. Assess if a triple blinded randomized trial can be designed as it is regarded as the gold standard; however, very often, it is not practical in clinical scenarios. Hence the order of preference for the study design should be in the order of potential for reducing bias. When a RCT is not a suitable design due to ethical/practical constraints, the same principle of "reducing bias" applies in selecting the most appropriate observational design as well. This approach to selecting the study design is shown in Fig. 3.

The decision about study design will also depend on other factors such as whether it is a common or uncommon exposure or outcome that is being studied, ethical issues and available resources [28]. As described earlier in the chapter, when it is an uncommon outcome or a rare disease that is being studied, a case-control study is appropriate. Although case-control studies are of retrospective nature, it should be carried out ideally with a prospectively maintained database. When it's an uncommon exposure, a cohort study is the best option to ensure including adequate number of patients with the exposure. In a resource-limited setting, carrying out a prospective cohort study with long follow-up may not be feasible, but a case-control or a retrospective cohort might suffice. Ethical issues play a major role in deciding the feasibility of RCTs. For instance, it will not be ethical to randomize patients into a placebo arm when some therapy is available as a standard of care. However, RCT can be conducted effectively, once the feasibility has been established for the research question being studied.

It is important for the researcher to understand that all the study designs are useful and contribute to the clinical knowledge. The best design is the one that answers

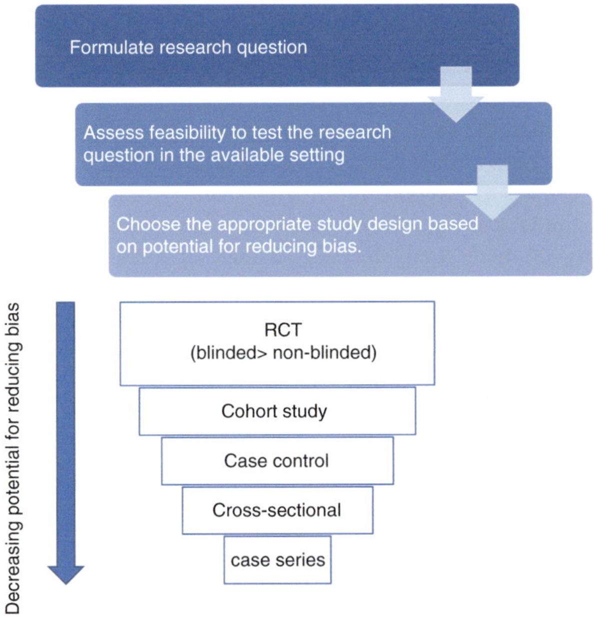

Fig. 3 Steps in choosing an appropriate study design. *RCT* randomized controlled dial

the research question most explicitly. Although a daunting task, choosing an appropriate design can be done with ease by systematically approaching the research question.

Case Scenarios

1. You want to study the association between Hepatitis B and development of liver cancer. Which is the suitable study design to address this?
   (a) Case-control
   (b) Prospective Cohort study
   (c) Single-blinded RCT
   (d) Cross-sectional study
2. You have designed a novel type of procedure for treating hernia. What type of study will you plan to test its efficacy?
   (a) Cohort study
   (b) Superiority randomized controlled trial
   (c) Case-control study.
   (d) Cross-sectional study

References

1. Jolles BM, Martin E. Study designs in orthopaedic clinical research. Clin Orthop Relat Res. 2011;469:909–13.
2. Altman D. Introduction to study design. 2014. http://www.equator-network.org.
3. Rohrig B, du Prel JB, Wachtlin D, Blettner M. Types of study in medical research: part 3 of a series on evaluation of scientific publications. DtschArzteblatt Int. 2009;106:262–8.
4. Sut N. Study designs in medicine. Balkan Med J. 2014;31:273–7.
5. Dawson B, Trapp RG. Basic and clinical biostatistics. New York: Lange Medical Books/McGraw-Hill; 2004.
6. Silva DS. Overview of study designs. In: Silva DS, editor. Cancer epidemiology: principles and methods. France: IARC Publications. http://www.iarc.fr/en/publications/pdfs-online/epi/cancerepi/.
7. Lewallen S, Courtright P. Epidemiology in practice: case-control studies. Commun Eye Health. 1998;11(28):57–8.
8. Szumilas M. Explaining odds ratios. J Can Acad Child Adolesc Psychiatry. 2010;19(3):227–9.
9. Song JW, Chung KC. Observational studies: cohort and case-control studies. Plast Reconstr Surg. 2010;126(6):2234–42.
10. Andrade C. Understanding relative risk, odds ratio, and related terms: as simple as it can get. J Clin Psychiatry. 2015;76(7):e857–61.
11. National Ethical Guidelines for Biomedical and Health Research Involving Human Participants. 2017. http://www.icmr.nic.in/guidelines/ICMR_Ethical_Guidelines_2017.pdf. Accessed 22 Nov 2017.
12. Šimundić A-M. Measures of diagnostic accuracy: basic definitions. EJIFCC. 2009;19(4):203–11.
13. Cook C, Cleland J, Huijbregts P. Creation and critique of studies of diagnostic accuracy: use of the STARD and QUADAS methodological quality assessment tools. J Man Manip Ther. 2007;15(2):93–102.
14. Kabisch M, Ruckes C, Seibert-Grafe M, Blettner M. Randomized controlled trials: part 17 of a series on evaluation of scientific publications. Deutsches Ärzteblatt Int. 2011;108(39):663–8.

15. Hopewell S, Dutton S, Yu LM, Chan AW, Altman DG. The quality of reports of randomised trials in 2000 and 2006: comparative study of articles indexed in Pub Med. BMJ. 2010;340:c723.
16. Iaggio G, Elbourne DR, Altman DG, Pocock SJ, Evans SJ, CONSORT Group. Reporting of non-inferiority and equivalence randomized trials: an extension of the CONSORT statement. JAMA. 2006;295(10):1152–60.
17. Mohsina S, Shanmugam D, Sureshkumar S, Kundra P, Mahalakshmy T, Kate V. Adapted ERAS pathway vs. standard care in patients with perforated duodenal ulcer-a randomized controlled trial. J Gastrointest Surg. 2018;22(1):107–16. https://doi.org/10.1007/s11605-017-3474-2. [Epub ahead of print]
18. Das R, Sureshkumar S, Sreenath GS, Kate V. Sequential versus concomitant therapy for eradication of *Helicobacter Pylori* in patients with perforated duodenal ulcer: a randomized trial. Saudi J Gastroenterol. 2016;22(4):309–15. https://doi.org/10.4103/1319-3767.187605.
19. Concato J, Shah N, Horwitz RI. Randomized, controlled trials, observational studies, and the hierarchy of research designs. N Engl J Med. 2000;342(25):1887–92.
20. Efird J. Blocked randomization with randomly selected block sizes. Int J Environ Res Public Health. 2011;8(1):15–20. https://doi.org/10.3390/ijerph8010015.
21. Zhao W. A better alternative to stratified permuted block design for subject randomization in clinical trials. Stat Med. 2014;33(30):5239–48. https://doi.org/10.1002/sim.6266.
22. Doig GS, Simpson F. Randomization and allocation concealment: a practical guide for researchers. J Crit Care. 2005;20(2):187–91.
23. Hollis S, Campbell F. What is meant by intention to treat analysis? Survey of published randomised controlled trials. Br Med J. 1999;319(7211):670–4.
24. Suresh K. An overview of randomization techniques: an unbiased assessment of outcome in clinical research. J Hum Reprod Sci. 2011;4(1):8–11. https://doi.org/10.4103/0974-1208.82352.
25. Philip S. What is a non-randomised controlled trial? BMJ. 2014;348:g4115.
26. Haidich AB. Meta-analysis in medical research. Hippokratia. 2010;14(Suppl 1):29–37.
27. Moher D, Cook DJ, Eastwood S, Olkin I, Rennie D, Stroup DF. Improving the quality of reports of meta-analyses of randomised controlled trials: the QUOROM statement. Quality of reporting of meta-analyses. Lancet. 1999;354(9193):1896–900.
28. Checkoway H, Pearce N, Kriebel D. Selecting appropriate study designs to address specific research questions in occupational epidemiology. Occup Environ Med. 2007;64(9):633–8.

Data Management in Clinical Research

Karthik Balachandran and Sadishkumar Kamalanathan

You can have data without information, but you cannot have information without data.—Daniel Keys Moran

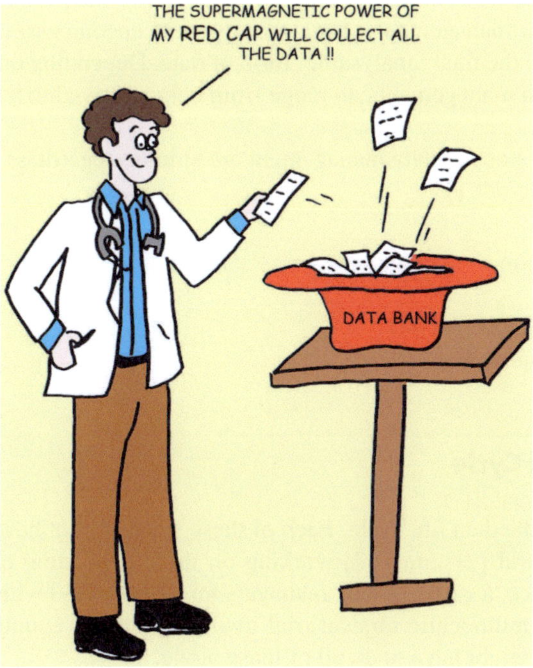

K. Balachandran
Assistant Professor, Department of Endocrinology, Sri Ramachandra Medical College and Research Institute, Chennai, India

S. Kamalanathan (✉)
Additional Professor and Head, Department of Endocrinology, Jawaharlal Institute of Post Graduate Medical Education and Research, Pondicherry, India

S. C. Parija, V. Kate (eds.), *Thesis Writing for Master's and Ph.D. Program*,
https://doi.org/10.1007/978-981-13-0890-1_9

Key Points

- Data management is an important part of clinical research.
- It involves planning, acquiring, processing, analyzing, preserving and publishing/sharing data.
- Each step needs to be documented for maximum reproducibility.
- Several software options exist to do the same—the choice of which depends on several factors.
- Using REDCap (or a similar software) takes care of each of these steps and is recommended for data management.

Everyone doing research has to contend with a singular problem—data management. The irony is that data management is rarely, if ever, taught to researchers. The thinking is perhaps, as long as the data that is output is in a format that can be analyzed, we don't need to worry about how it got there in the first place. Unfortunately, like much else in research, data management follows the GIGO rule—garbage in, garbage out. Thus we need to pay attention, not just to the product (data), but also the process (data management). Data management encompasses everything from data collection to the final 'analysable' form of data. Depending on the nature of the research, the data management can range from being a trivial to a remarkably complex task.

However, the steps of data management are similar, regardless of the size of the project. These include [1]

1. Data acquisition
2. Data entry
3. Data cleaning and analysis
4. Data archiving/backup

The Data Life Cycle

Figure 1 shows the data life cycle. Each of these stages might have several sub categories and several personnel [2] working on them depending on the size of the study. For instance, a group of data managers might be tasked with overseeing each stage in a large multicentre clinical trial involving several countries. In a student thesis, a student might have to do all of these alone.

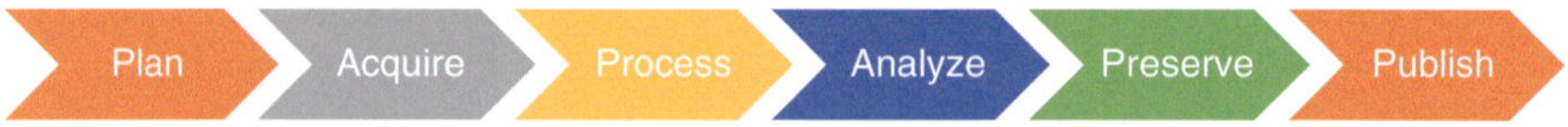

Fig. 1 Data life cycle

Data Acquisition

Before any data can be processed by the computer, it must be acquired, preferably in a useful format. This is the input part of the equation. The output critically depends on the input, as captured by the adage, "Garbage in, Garbage out" [3]. So the primary aim of the data acquisition is not only to collect data, but to collect it in the most appropriate manner possible. Designing the data collection instrument takes time and must be done in consultation with the domain expert and a statistical expert for maximum effectiveness.

Every database development has to go through a well-defined process, which has the following steps

1. Planning
2. Requirement gathering
3. Conceptual Design
4. Logical Design
5. Physical Design
6. Construction
7. Implementation
8. Support and Maintenance

The following considerations and best practices apply while collecting data

- Continuous vs categorical
  - Collect numbers whenever possible
  - Don't collapse continuous to categorical

e.g. The data on whether someone is overweight/obese can be collected as

Obese—yes/no
BMI
Height and Weight Separately.

The ideal option is C. One can derive BMI from Height and Weight, but not height and weight from BMI. Thus B is not a good option. Option a is the poorest option amongst these, as it gives very little information.

- Precision—Precision of measurement depends on the need and the available resources. For example, while acquiring the age of a person, one can ask for age or date of birth. For the purposes of research, being 60 years old and 60 years and 3 months old may not matter much. Thus adult physicians typically collect age as an integer variable. However for a pediatrician or neonatologist, this might mean a lot and thus they must collect the date of birth and subtract it from the current date—to get the desired precision in days, months or years.

- Feasibility—In the previous example, it might appear as though collecting maximum information is the best way forward. However this may not be always possible. For example, in a field research dealing with a lot of people who are illiterate, one may not be able to get the date of birth. Thus it is better to get an approximation using age instead of leaving the information out due to lack of feasibility.
- Construct—A construct is a difficult to measure entity. It is often abstract. For instance, if we want to measure drug compliance, it can be done in several different ways. Our goal is to use a validated method to measure what we intend to measure.
- Confounding and bias—These can adversely impact the quality of a study. Hence they should be taken into consideration even the stage of designing data collection instruments.
- Thoroughness—It is important to ensure that all the relevant data to be collected are anticipated in advance before making the case record form. While it may be possible to add some variables during the course of the study, this is not good practice. Even worse is trying to change the variables during the course of the study. This can lead to several problems in the later stages. The motto is—a case record form is open to growth, but closed to change.

The principles mentioned above must be used to guide the development of a data collection form. It is important to note that this is an iterative process, that takes input from various stakeholders and experts. The time invested in designing an appropriate data collection instrument pays off well in the later stages of data management.

The steps mentioned above involve planning, requirement gathering and conceptual design. It is important to note that no computer is needed for any of these stages.

The next stage is the implementation of our idea. This involves choosing a tool/software.

Thankfully, several tools exist for data management. Just like a surgeon wouldn't go to the operating room, thinking he would use 11 size blade and straight artery forceps alone, so too a researcher cannot say she would use only a particular tool. The research dictates the tool to be used and not vice versa. Thus a decent working knowledge of the various tools used to manage data is an asset.

Before we see the different tools which are used, it is useful to review the features of an ideal data management/collection tool.

These are

1. Easy to use—should not require extensive computer or programming skills
2. Free or open source (or low cost)
3. Secure
4. Platform independent—i.e.—it should work on most commonly used operating systems and devices
5. Limited system footprint—should be light on resources, as most researchers are unlikely to have advanced computers

6. Work online—this would enable easy creation of multisystem studies
7. Work offline—this would make it easier to collect data in the field

It is crucial to be clear about our requirements, as finding out midway that our choice of tools is inappropriate can be costly. Our choice of software depends partly on fulfilling these generic requirements and partly on project specific requirements. An example of project specific requirement is a multicentre study with researchers spread across several cities (or countries) all contributing data to a single repository. The relative importance of these requirements also varies from project to project, but ease of use, cost and security are sine qua non for most projects.

What Are the Options?

The data management options are summarized in Fig. 2. They include,

1. Spread sheet programs—Microsoft Excel, Apple Numbers, Libreoffice calc
2. Desktop relational databases—Microsoft Access
3. EpiData
4. EpiInfo
5. REDCap

There are several excellent internet resources for learning about proprietary software like MS Excel and open source tools like Epidata. The thrust of this chapter, however, is on using REDCap.

What Is REDCap?

REDCap is an acronym that stands for research electronic data capture. It is a web-based tool for data management. Unlike the other software mentioned in the list, REDCap is a software that is not installed on your computer. It is a robust web

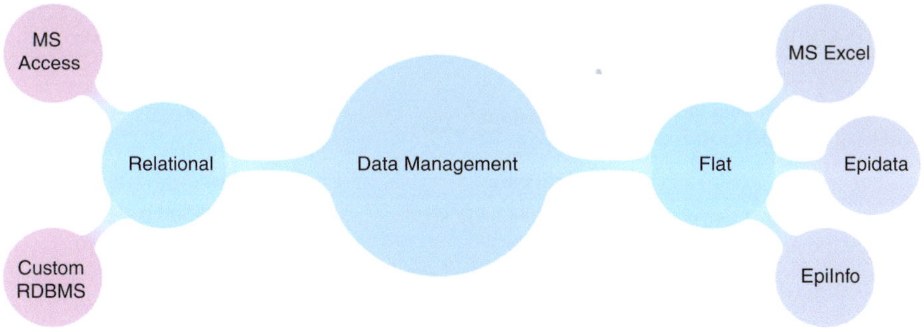

Fig. 2 Data management options

application that is installed on a webserver and can only be licensed to institutes (free of cost). It was built by Vanderbilt University in the early 2000s and has already been adopted by over 300 institutions. JIPMER for instance has made REDCap available to all its students, residents and faculty members.

If your college/university does not have REDCap at present, requesting the IT department for REDCap installation in the server is the first step. REDCap is easy on system resources and can be installed by a system administrator. It is a web application that uses PHP and MySQL, common web technologies that drive many websites.

Advantages of REDCap:

- Ease of data entry
- Avoidance of data entry errors
- Ability to collect longitudinal data
- Automatic statistics/graphs
- Secure—automatic data backups
- Device and operating system independent
- Ability to do surveys
- Ability to store images/pdfs/videos
- Export to common file formats of statistical software

How Does It Compare with Microsoft Excel?

Table 1 shows the differences between REDCap and Microsoft Excel, with respect to data collection.

Data Entry

Data entry in REDCap is much easier than data entry in other tools. This is because

1. Data of only one record can be modified at a time. Because of this there is no chance of parallax errors.
2. Data is stored on a server which is continually backed up. So even if the researcher's computer is destroyed/stolen/crashed, there is no chance of data loss.

Table 1 Comparison of REDCap and Microsoft Excel

Feature	REDCap	Excel
User	Multiple	Single
Secure	Yes	No
Data entry error	Very likely	Common
Survey	Yes	No
Secure data sharing	Yes	No
Automatic graphs/statistics	Yes	No
Store images and Pdfs	Yes	No
Suited for longitudinal data	Yes	No

3. It is optimized for longitudinal data collection, circumventing the problems of a flat file format like MS Excel.
4. Data can be entered by collaborators in various institutions at the same time
5. Data can be collected for regulatory trials—since the software is 21 CFR part 11 and HIPAA compliant

Even so, minimizing data entry errors and maximizing data entry efficiency is the goal during this stage. The following methods should be followed to minimize errors

- Use the paper form of the data collection instrument to collect data. Data entry errors are least common in this method. Data collection proforma can be printed out from REDCap for maximum fidelity between the paper and the screen and this can potentially improve the accuracy and speed of data entry.
- Before data entry, ensure data type validation—e.g. Only numbers should be allowed in a data entry field asking about age.
- Before data entry, ensure range checks—e.g. In a study involving adults, only age >18 should be allowed (and preferably an upper limit such as 90 years)
- Plan for double data entry—double data entry means same data as entered by two people in the same database format. By comparing the two data, one can identify the discrepancies, presumably random errors and errors due to illegibility in the paper forms [4]. All errors that are picked up must be tagged and then verified with the source document and errors must be resolved.
- After data entry, implement data quality rules—these rules give an additional layer of protection, especially when soft data validation was done. For example, one can create a rule to list the names and IDs of individuals whose age is >90 years. This is also helpful in detecting outliers.

Each of these methods can be done very easily using REDCap.

Data Cleaning, Storage and Analysis

It is said that 90% of time for data analysis is spent in data cleaning. If the rules for entering clean data are followed, data cleaning does not consume time. The trick is to have a quality assured data entry process (using REDCap or Epidata makes it easier to do so).

Data can be exported in several different formats in most of the tools mentioned above. While one may use a proprietary format for exporting and analysis of data, for data storage it is better to use a non-proprietary format that can be read in any device (csv—comma separated values is one such format).

The important rule during this phase of data management is

"Document everything. Work on a copy of the data, not the original data."

The following best practices are recommended during this stage

1. Keep a log book—to keep a log of all things that are done with the data. For larger studies, this helps in maintaining the audit trail.
2. Keep a codebook—to understand what the variable names and values mean.
3. Develop a naming convention for files and folders and stick with it.
4. Back up the data (and code files).
5. Develop separate coding files for data modification and derived variables.

If you use REDCap, it automatically does steps 1, 2, 3 and 4. Step 5 will depend on which software is being used for analysis. The role of REDCap in data management is depicted in Fig. 3. In general, software which rely only on a graphical user interface to do the analysis are harder to document and keep a trail of. If however, scripts are written for data analysis, this becomes relatively simple.

Data Backup and Archival

Backing up data is very important and should preferably be done on a separate computer. If you are not using REDCap, consider using any of the cloud storage services for this purpose. Backup and archiving, though might seem similar, have different aims. Data back up is a daily process, where we protect against data loss by storing a copy of the data. It is like an insurance for data.

On the other hand, we archive the data, when are sure that all we want to do with the data is done and we are preserving it for posterity. In both cases, the security of the data is paramount. It is important to ensure that identifiable personal information is not leaked inadvertently. REDCap for example, does this automatically.

For clinical trials, the study closeout is also marked by database lock, beyond which the researcher cannot access the data. At this stage too, the data is archived.

Conclusions

Data management is an important part of clinical research. Students require specific training for data management, preferably in an easy to use software. This software at its core should make the right thing easier to do and the wrong thing harder to do. REDCap is one such software and is particularly recommended for research of any scale. If however, the reader's institution doesn't have access to REDCap, then EpiData can be used. Regardless of the software used, the principles mentioned in the chapter should help the reader develop good data management practices.

Case Scenarios

1. A gastroenterologist is doing a study on using endoscopy videos to teach post-graduate students about various gastric lesions. He collects data about student

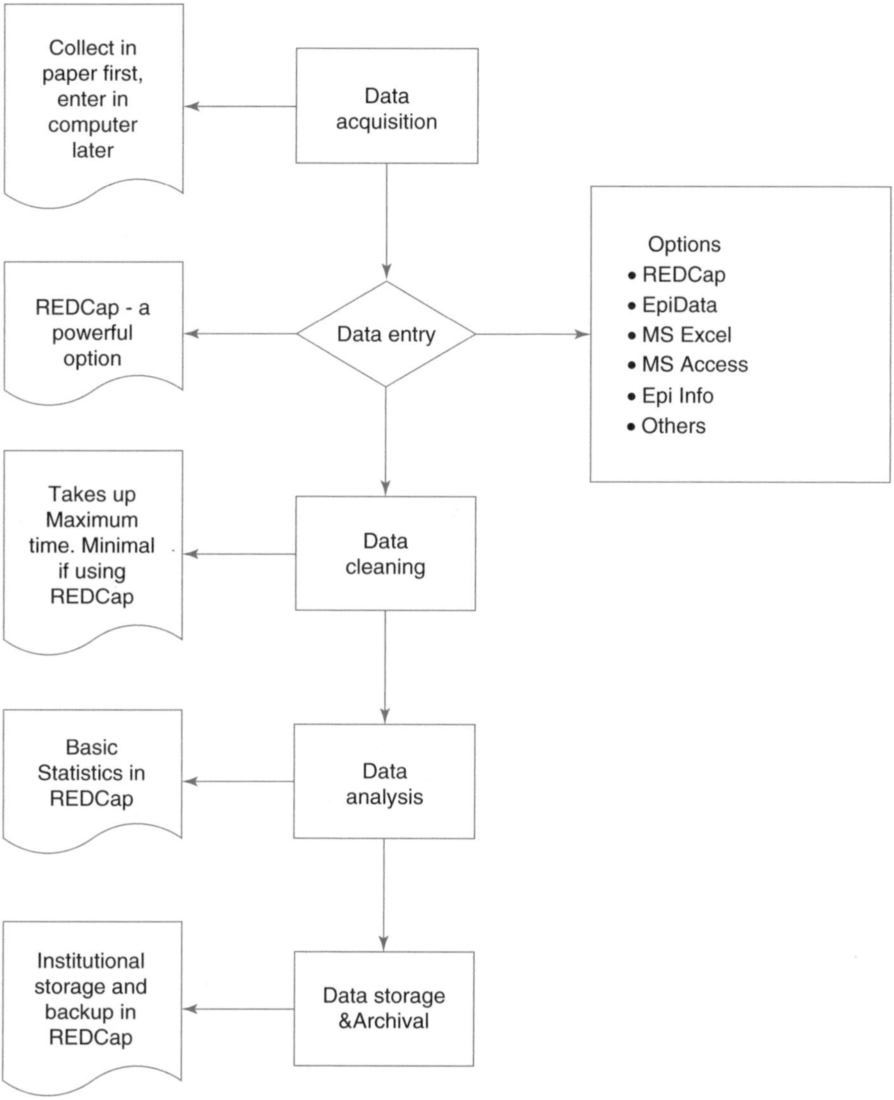

Fig. 3 Data management and REDCap

comprehension pre and post-viewing of the videos. He has ten videos in total. He is wondering if there's an efficient way to store 'complex' objects like videos in a spreadsheet. What would you advise him?

2. An endocrinologist is creating a registry of a rare disease called Acromegaly. She wants to keep the neurosurgeon, the radiologist and the radiation oncologist in the loop so that they can also enter their data into the same database. How can this be achieved?

References

1. Krishnankutty B, Bellary S, Kumar NBR, Moodahadu LS. Data management in clinical research, an overview. Indian J Pharmacol. 2012;44:168–72.
2. Perrier L, Blondal E, Ayala AP, et al. Research data management in academic institutions, a scoping review. PLoS One. 2017;12:e0178261.
3. Williams M, Bagwell J, Nahm Zozus M. Data management plans, the missing perspective. J Biomed Inform. 2017;71:130–42.
4. Juul S. Take good care of your data. Aarhus: Aarhus University, Department of Public Health; 2006.

Preparing and Decoding the Master Chart

Meenakshi Girish and Senthil Amudhan

Organising is what you do before you do something, so that when you do, you do not get it mixed up—AA Milne

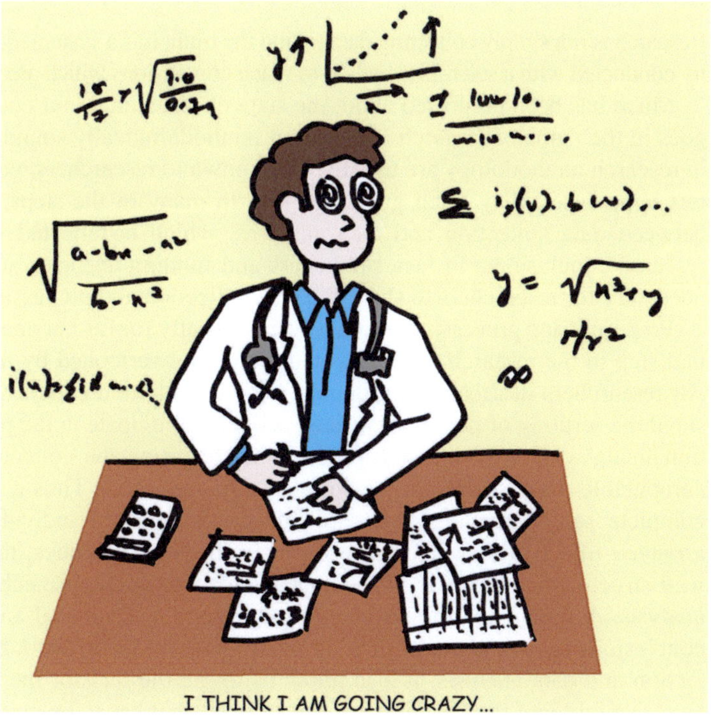

M. Girish (✉)
Associate Professor, Department of Pediatrics, NKP Salve Institute of Medical Sciences, Nagpur, India

S. Amudhan
Associate Professor, Department of Epidemiology, National Institute of Mental Health and Neuro Sciences, Bangalore, India

S. C. Parija, V. Kate (eds.), *Thesis Writing for Master's and Ph.D. Program*,
https://doi.org/10.1007/978-981-13-0890-1_10

Key Points

This chapter discusses the key processes involved in preparing the data for analysis (i.e., Preparation and decoding of Mater Chart) and will be helpful especially for those readers who have limited skills and access to advanced computer software for data management and have limited resources to acquire one. The key points covered in this chapter are as follows:

- Importance of data handling in research
- The processes involved in making a Master Chart
- How to handle errors in data compilation
- Decoding of Master Chart - Classification and Tabulation

Introduction

Research is not simply collecting data to find the truth; it is a systematic, sequential activity conducted with a scientific method to reach conclusions which are valid and reliable.

Much has been published about the state of research in our country where what goes in the name of research is often not methodologically sound [1, 2]. The steps in research methodology are usually well known to researchers, yet in their haste to test hypotheses, they often give a go—by to many of the steps, especially those between data collection and data analyses, which is reflected in the quality of research conclusions. In fact, publishers and funding agencies are now making it necessary for researchers to share the data collection and processing details [3].

Preparing and processing the data systematically for further analysis is an important step in the research processes that are often overlooked by many researchers. All researchers desirous of producing reliable and valid conclusions which could stand the scrutiny of peer review must actively participate in the process of 'operationalising' data, which is the process of converting the collected raw data into computable data, usually in the form of a master chart. Thus a master chart is a complete set of raw research data (all the answers of individual respondents) arranged in a sequence and represented in the form of codes, thereby forming a well-structured and formatted data matrix/database of the research to facilitate data analysis. A well-made master chart would simplify statistical analyses and make conclusions easy to arrive at. It is an intermediary stage of work between data collection and data analysis. It also allow us to get the feel for the data and provide better insight into the feasibility of the analysis that has to be performed as well as the resources that are required.

Preparing a master chart requires the following steps:

1. Data screening
2. Data coding
3. Data entry
4. Data cleaning
5. Data organisation (Classification and tabulation)

Data Screening

Errors in recorded data are not unusual, the values may be recorded with incorrect units of measurement, they may be entered in the wrong cell, or response may be recorded illegibly, and so immediately after data collection, the researcher should carefully screen for three 'i's—inconsistencies, inaccuracies, incompleteness. This can be done either manually or electronically. When raw data are collected electronically through computerized assessment instruments, potential inconsistencies between the responses are minimised. For large scale studies, electronic data collection has been shown to be more economical when one considers the savings in staff time spent on data screening and data entry [4, 5].

When errors are detected during screening, there are basically three approaches to rectify them:

(a) Go back to the case/respondent/questionnaire for clarification. This approach is adopted for variables which are of considerable importance to the research objectives. If it is not feasible to revisit the case, then the value may be coded as 'no answer' and such edited values should be highlighted with distinctive colors.
(b) Infer from other responses: If there is a missing entry, for example, missing response to the question 'previous experience with breastfeeding', we look for any other variable for a clue. For example, we may note that the respondent is a primigravida ("primigravida" refers to first pregnancy and hence cannot have 'previous experience with breastfeeding') which explains the missing data and by inference we can enter 'not applicable' in the cell in question. Such a change should only be made when a definite clue exists or there are multiple evidences to infer.
(c) Discard responses altogether: A decision to exclude data should be considered carefully as it may affect the validity of the study. If a question elicits ambiguous or vague answers from all respondents, then the whole question should be excluded from further analysis. Such omissions must be accounted for and mentioned in the final report.

Data Coding

Data screening will be followed by data coding. The process of converting the collected data into a format which is usable for computer-based data analyses is called coding. In other words, data coding is a systematic way to condense large quantities of recorded data into a form that can be more easily handled, especially by computer programs. Coding involves converting raw data into numbers or letters of the alphabet. Each piece of information collected is known as a variable and the options under that variable are called categories (Fig. 1), coding is done for each category and the variable is given a name (discussed later). While assigning codes the following properties should be kept in mind:

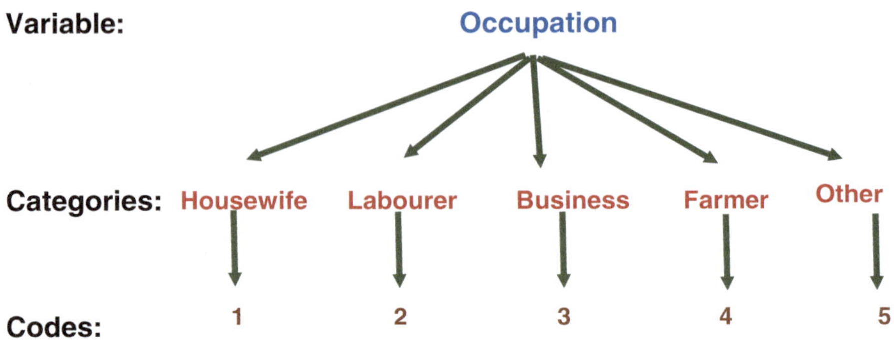

Fig. 1 An example of a variable with its corresponding categories and assigned codes

1. Exhaustive: there should be a code for all potential categories of the variable
2. Mutually exclusive: Codes given for one category should not be applicable to any other category
3. Consistent: Code values should be consistent across all variables

When to Code

1. Coding can be decided in advance and placed on the case record form (CRF) or the questionnaire itself by providing space while constructing the instrument.
2. Coding in qualitative studies: Where there are descriptive responses, codes are generated after examination of the textual data, which includes identification of themes and categories from the descriptive responses (grounded theory approach). Response categories may also be determined in advance and coded while framing the questions (inductive categorisation approach) [6]. There are computer programmes which can categorise data directly from the respondents or the CRF, thereby bypassing the need for detailed study of the responses for the purpose of giving them codes. Transcription software HyperTRANSCRIBE or Computer Assisted Qualitative Data Analysis Software (CAQDAS) are few examples [7].

Coding Tips

Type of data often determines the coding style [8, 9].

1. For Nominal data, codes are usually arbitrary but remain mutually exclusive and exhaustive. For example, 'Occupation' is a variable which contains nominal data and in creating codes, a separate code number is given for each category under this variable (Fig. 1). If a special category 'other' is created to capture all responses which are not covered in the original list of options, a unique code is assigned to this category. For example, if the categories are housewife, labourer, business, farmer, then the codes assigned are 1, 2, 3 and 4. The 'other' category is a way to

ensure that the code frame is exhaustive, to deal with information the researcher did not anticipate and given a code, say, 5. These code numbers remain mutually exclusive; meaning housewife always gets a code 1, never 2 or 3.

2. For ordinal data, numerical codes may be assigned in rank order to denote the hierarchy of responses in ascending order. So for a variable like APGAR score, a category of 0–3 is given a code of 1, category 4–7 would be code 2 and 8–10 a code of 3. Code 3 here will always represent a higher category than code 1.
3. For continuous data, even a zero is a meaningful number and the values are directly used as codes. Sometimes, continuous variables can be categorised. Decisions concerning how to categorize continuous data can be made after they have been collected. For example, for the variable 'age', we may decide to have two age groups: 40 and above, and age below 40 or we may also want to have three categories: 20–29, 30–39, and 40 upwards (categories are decided based on their pragmatic utility, plausibility or from previous literature). Codes are then assigned as for ordinal data.
4. For variables with binary responses, codes zero and one are used. Example, first-born is the variable in which firstborn is coded 1 and others 0. In gender, male may be coded 0 and female 1. (Kindly note that code "0" is also used for "Not Applicable" category. So the category corresponding to code "0" has to be mentioned explicitly in codebook)
5. Codes for open-ended questions (in questionnaires) are usually done after examining a sample of (say 20) questionnaires. Similar types of responses are grouped into single categories (so as to limit their number to at the most 6 or 7) and then given code numbers. 'Others' category may be included, to capture remaining responses but they should be as small as possible, preferably containing fewer than 5% of the total answers.
6. Common responses should have the same code in each question, as this minimises mistakes by coders [10]. For example:
   Yes (or positive response) code—Y or 1
   No (or negative response) code—N or 2
   Don't know code—D or 8
   No response/unknown code—U or 9

Figure 2 is an example of how a properly coded data should appear.

Codebook

The codes as shown in Fig. 2 make no sense to anyone other than the individual who assigned the codes. Thus explanatory details must be recorded somewhere for ready reference during analysis. Such a record is known as the codebook. A codebook specifies the question number on the questionnaire from which the data is taken, the variable name, the operational definition of the variable, scale of measurement, unit of measurement of the variable, the coding options, (Boxes 1 and 2) and any other information as required [9]. Codebooks also contain documentation about when and how the data was created. A good codebook helps in communicating the research data clearly and ensures that data is understood and interpreted properly. Codebooks are often created manually; however, it is possible to generate a codebook from an existing spreadsheet using statistical software like SPSS. Given below are examples of a codebook formed for different types of questionnaire (Boxes 1 and 2)

S no	Job	SE status	Fam_Type	Mat HB	Parity	Amen_dur	Del mode	Resusc	rest time	Past exp
01	1	1	0	9	0	1	0	0	2	0
02	1	0	1	1	0	1	1	0	2	0
03	1	1	1	1	1	1	0	0	2	1
04	1	1	0	1	1	1	0	0	1	1
05	1	1	0	1	0	1	1	0	2	0
06	1	1	1	1	0	1	0	1	2	0
07	1	1	1	1	0	1	0	0	2	0
08	1	1	0	1	0	1	1	0	2	0
09	1	0	0	0	1	1	1	0	2	1
10	1	1	1	0	1	1	1	0	2	1
11	1	0	0	0	0	1	1	0	2	0
12	1	0	0	0	1	0	1	0	2	1
13	1	1	0	1	1	1	1	0	2	1
14	1	1	0	1	0	1	0	0	0	0
15	1	1	0	1	0	1	2	0	2	0
16	1	0	1	1	1	1	0	0	2	1
17	1	1	1	1	1	0	0	0	0	1
18	1	1	1	1	1	0	1	0	2	0
19	1	1	0	1	1	1	1	0	0	1
20	1	0	0	0	0	1	1	0	2	0
21	1	0	0	0	1	1	1	0	2	1
22	1	0	1	1	1	1	1	0	2	1
23	1	1	0	0	0	1	0	0	2	0
24	1	0	0	1	0	1	0	0	2	0
25	1	1	1	1	0	1	0	0	2	0
26	1	0	1	0	1	0	1	0	2	1
27	1	1	0	1	0	1	1	0	0	9

Fig. 2 A master chart with coded data in spreadsheet

Box 1: Codebook Sample

Case Record Form

Q1. NAME __________ Q2. AGE ____ Q3. SEX____

Q4. OCCUPATION:

Professional
Skilled
Semiskilled
Unskilled
Unemployed

Codebook

Q. no.	Variable no.	Variable name	Response	Scale of measurement	Codes
1	1	Name	Name of the respondent	Nominal	ID number can be created and linked
2	2	Age	Age of the respondent	Continuous	1 for 0–39 2 for 40 and above
3	3	Gender	Male Female	Nominal	1—Male 2—Female
4	4	Occupn	Professional Skilled Semiskilled Unskilled Unemployed	Ordinal	5—Professional 4—Skilled 3—Semiskilled 2—Unskilled 1—Unemployed

Box 2: Coding of Matrix Question (Multiple Questions with Identical Options)

Q.5. NATURE OF JOB:

Employer	Permanent	Temporary
Government		
Private		

CODE BOOK—SAMPLE I

The matrix questions can be coded by considering each row as one variable.

Q. no.	Variable no,	Variable name	Response	Scale of measurement	Codes
5	5	JOB_GOVT	Permanent Temporary	Nominal	1—Permanent 2—Temporary 0—Otherwise
	6	JOB_PVT	Permanent Temporary	Nominal	1—Permanent 2—Temporary 0—Otherwise

CODE BOOK—SAMPLE II

The matrix questions can be coded by considering each cell as response to one variable (depending on the objective of the study)

Q. no.	Variable no.	Variable name	Response	Scale of measurement	Codes
5	5	JOB_ NATURE	Govt-Permanent Govt-Temporary Pvt-Permanent Pvt-Temporary	Nominal	1—Govt-Permanent 2—Govt-Temporary 3—Pvt-Permanent 4—Pvt-Temporary 0—Otherwise

How to Name Variables in the Codebook

While naming the variable, certain general rules have to be followed especially if the spreadsheet is to be exported to statistical software (like SPSS) for analysis [11]. The variable names are usually short and often cannot exceed eight characters; numbers can be used but the name should always start with a letter, preferably lower case, as a computer may not register 'male' as equal to 'Male' or 'MALE'. Spaces, punctuations and special characters should be avoided (@.#,$,- etc.,). Underscore

Box 3: Giving Names to Variables

Preferred	Avoid
AGE	1AGE
DUR_AMEN	DUR-AMEN
NEWVAR	NEW,VAR
JOB_SAT	JOB SAT
OCCUPN	?OCCUPN
FAMTYPE	FAM@TYPE
ADAR_ID, ADARID	ADAR ID, #ADARID, ADAR$ID

Table 1 Coding missing data

	Variable coding		
Missing data type	Single digit	Double digit	Triple digit
Not applicable	0	00	000
Refused to answer	7	97	997
Dont know	8	98	998
Truly missing	9	99	999

(_) can be used. Certain variable names like COMPUTE, SUM, TEST, NOT, OR, ALL etc should be avoided as sometimes the software would not be able to distinguish between a command and a variable (Box 3). Each variable name must be unique and duplication should be avoided.

How to Handle Missing Data

For proper data analysis, coding 'missing data' is as important as creating codes for existing data. In fact no cell in the datasheet should be left blank. When coding missing data, care should be taken to choose a value beyond the maximum valid value for the variable [12]; if it is numeric then the code for missing value should also be numeric and the value may be '9' or '99' or '999' depending on the number of characters used for coding other categories of the variable. For variables which are not applicable (NA) for some respondents, special coding should be done to distinguish from codes for missing data. For instance, a respondent may have marked 'primiparous' for question on parity and the next question is on previous experience with breastfeeding, if the respondent leaves this space blank, it will be coded as for NA and not as missing data. Codes traditionally assigned to different categories of missing data are given in Table 1 [13]:

Data Entry

Coding of data is followed by entering the data into a spreadsheet using the codebook. This data entry results in a well-structured format called Master Chart that contains raw data of all the individual respondents of the study in a particular sequence using pre-determined codes. A Master Chart also serves as a storage format from which it can be read by any software application for statistical analysis. Spreadsheets like MS Excel are commonly used to create a Master Chart. Computerised database programs (e.g., EPINFO) can also be used for data entry.

The steps of data coding and data entry can be addressed in a single operation as in a quantitative study or for multiple choice type of questions in the qualitative study, but for open-ended question responses, coding is done separately prior to data entry into the computer.

General guidelines for data entry [14]

- Each respondent should be given a unique, sequential number (ID) and entered in the first column on the left.
- Details of each respondent should be entered on a single row (each row for single ID)
- Letters, words, and symbols should be converted to plausible numbers. E.g., Y/Yes/✓—1, N/No/X—0
- Do not leave blanks and do not enter "?", "*", or "NA" for missing data because this becomes a string variable that cannot be used for any arithmetic computation.
- Do not combine variables in one column and do not enter any units (Box 4). The units like days, years, months, mm Hg, gm, Kg etc., can be documented in the codebook or included in the variable name for reference.
- Use 0/1 for 2 groups with 0 as a reference group
- Colors are used to delineate or highlight the variables (e.g., outliers, homogeneity, related variables etc.).
- When data are collected multiple times for the same variable, a horizontal format is preferred for simplicity (Box 5). Some software can convert longitudinal format to horizontal format.
- Enter ordinal variables into one column if they are mutually exclusive (Box 6)

Box 4: Data Entry for Combination of Variables

Incorrect	Correct	
BP	SBP	DBP
120/80 mm Hg	120	80
110/60 mm Hg	110	60
130/70 mm Hg	130	70

Box 5: Data entry for single variable collected multiple times

Longitudinal format			Horizontal format						
Date	ID	SYSBP	ID	DATE1	SYSBP1	DATE 2	SYSBP2	DATE 3	SYSBP3
2/2/2017	1	120	1	2/2/2017	120	2/4/2017	110	2/6/2017	100
2/4/2017	1	110	2	4/3/2017	130	4/4/2017	120	4/6/2017	NO RECORDING
2/6/2017	1	100							
4/3/2017	2	130							
4/4/2017	2	120							
4/6/ 2017	2	NO RECORDING							

Box 6: Data entry for ordinal variables

Incorrect

ID	Education			
	Primary	Secondary	Higher secondary	College
1	0	0	0	1
2	1	0	0	0
3	0	1	0	0

Correct

ID	EDU
1	4
2	1
3	2

Footnote: 1 is code for primary, 2 is code for secondary, 3 for higher secondary and 4 for college

A	B	C	D	E	F	G	H	I	J	K
Sr.NO.	Occupation W/H	S/E Status	Jt/Nuclear Family	Mat HB	Parity	Duration of Ammenor	Mode od Del.	Need for Resuse	sleepless Int before deliv	Prev .exp breast fd
1	Stud/ Property Deler	Middle	Jt Family	-	Primi	38w+5	Normal	No	NO	NO
2	House wife /Labour	Lower	Nu- family	10.6 gm	Primi	40week	L.S.C.S.	No	NO	NO
3	House wife /Labour	Middle	Nu- family	10gml	Para2Previoss	40+2	Vaginal	no	No	Yes
4	House wife / Farmar	Middle	Jt-Family	10.2	3	38 week	Vaginal	NO	Yes	Yes
5	House wife /P.Worker	Middle	Jt-Family	10gml	Primi	39 weeks1day	L.S.C.S.	No	NO	NO
6	H0use wife/Labour	Middle	Nuclear	10.4gml	Primi	40week2days	Vaginal	Yes	No	No
7	House wife/Chemist	Middle	Nuclear	11.3gml	Primi	39weeks 1day	Normal	No	NO	NO
8	House wife/Labour	Middle	Jt-Family	10.6gml	Primy	38+5	L S C S	No	No	No
9	Housewife/Farmar	Lower	Jt-Family	9.2gml	Para2	9month	L.S.C.S.	No	No	YES
10	House wife /P.Worker	Middle	Nu- family	9.7gml	Para 2	40+2week	L.S.C.S.	No	NO	Yes
11	House Wife/P.Worker	Lower	Jt-Family	8gm	Primi	37Weeks	L.S.C.S.	No	NO	NO
12	House Wife/P.Worker	Lower	Jt-Family	8.40gml	Para2	36 Weeks	L.S.C.S.	No	NO	Yes
13	HouseWife/Survice	Middle	Jt-Family	10.8gml	Para2	39Week6day	L.S.C.S.	No	No	Yes
14	HouseWife/ShopKeepar	Middle	Jt-Family		Primi	39Week	Normal	No	7hour	NO
15	HouseWife/Driver	Middle	Jt-Family	10gml	Primi	39weeks 1day	Forcep	No	24 hour	NO
16	Housewifw/Labour	Lower	N-Family		para2	39weeks 1day	Normal	No	12hour	Yes
17	Housewife/ Tailor	Middle	N-Family	10.4gml	para2	36week 4day	Normal	No	8 hrs	Yes
18	Housewife/Chemist	Middle	N-Family	12.20gml	Para2	36week3day	L.S.C.S.	No	12hrs	NO
19	HouseWife/ Farmar	Middle	Jt-Famali	11.8gml	Para 2	38+1	L.S.C.S.	No	8hour	Yes
20	House Wife/ Labour	Lower	Jt-Famali	9.8gml	Primi	37+1	L.S.C.S.	No	12 hour	No
21	House Wife /Labour	Lower	Jt-Famali	6.8gml	Para3	38.2day	L.S.C.S.	No		Yes
22	Housewife/ Labour	Lower	Nt- Famali	11.6gml	Para2	39+3 day	L.S.C.S.	No	12hour	Yes
23	HouseWife/ Driver	Middle	Jt-Family	9.3gml	Primi	37+4days	Normal	No	12hour	no
24	HouseWife/P. Worker	Lower	Jt- Family	10.6gml	Primi	39+5day	Normal	No	24hour	No
25	House Wife/P.Worker	Middle	N-Family	11.6gml	Primi	39week	Normal	No	12hour	NO
26	House Wife/ Labour	Lower	N-Family	9.39gml	Para2	36+4day	L.S.C.S.	No	10hour	Yes
27	House Wife/ Shopkeepar	Middle	Jt-Family	10gml	Primy	40weeks	L.S.C.S.	No	2hour	

Fig. 3 Example of poor data entry in master chart

An example of a master chart with faulty data entry procedure is given below to highlight the importance of proper data entry (Fig. 3). The highlighted cells are empty, column B has combined two categories in one cell, column D is named inappropriately, unit of measurement is inconsistent in columns E and G, column H has ambiguous categories and in the remaining columns there is inconsistency in using capital letters.

This data is entered by a novice who believes that a spreadsheet is nothing but a simple table with rows for entering results and columns for giving headings. Such a master chart will not be suitable for analysis by any statistical package.

Entry of Derived Variables

Sometimes two variables may be used to construct another variable (e.g. BMI using height and weight). Information about such a variable and its computation should be entered in a codebook. These derived variables can be computed easily in a spreadsheet using simple arithmetic operations. At this point, the possibility of missing value codes altering the derived variable should be kept in mind. In such cases, appropriate missing value codes (0 etc.,) should be identified before derived variables are constructed [15].

Spreadsheet programmes like the Microsoft Excel do not replace statistical packages for analysing data. But they will save the data and provide an output in the form of a plain text or ASCII file, which can then be exported to software packages (SAS, SPSS, or STATA) for analysis. So it becomes important to integrate codebook with the master chart for better communication and understanding for further data analysis.

Data Cleaning

The most important aspect of any research process is the control of data quality. Sometimes errors can be missed during the initial data screening (especially logical and arithmetic relations). Similar to data screening that is done immediately after data collection, data is checked for the three 'i's immediately after complete data coding and entry (or during data entry). Needless to emphasise, this step determines the validity of the conclusions and hence should be performed with due diligence.

Data cleaning can be done by visually scanning the entire datasheet if the sample is small or a small portion (say 10–15%) of the sample can be scanned by one researcher or multiple researchers when it is a large study. There are computer programmes which interact with researchers through pop-up windows, when their inbuilt mathematically modelled programme detects data items that appear suspicious. A more detailed description of computerised quality control can be found elsewhere [16], but some examples of automated ways of checking for inconsistencies, incompleteness and inaccuracies are given below:

- Admissible range checks carried out by inputting minimum and maximum values in the software used for data entry. This can be used to check single variables.
- Use of Arithmetic relations between variables: Multiple variables are taken together for this function. For example, if variable A refers to maternal Hb and B for packed cell volume then a set of ranges can be put in place using variable B to check accuracy or inconsistency in variable A.
- Logical relations: Multiple variables are taken together to calculate a logical response to the variable in question. If for example, column X contains the variable 'total members in family', then it can be computed logically that column Y with variable 'number of children in the family' could never have values greater than those in variable X. Such logical relations are based on criteria specifically defined by the researcher using "if—then" or "if and only if" functions.

- Special consideration can be given to dates, outliers and derived variables while cleaning/checking the data. All the dates should be within reasonable time span, valid (e.g 30 February not possible) and correctly sequenced (e.g, birth, surgery and death dates). Usually continuous variables reveal some outlying values that are incompatible with rest of the data. Such suspicious values should be checked carefully. If there is no evidence of mistake and the value is plausible, then it should not be altered. Awareness about outliers will be highly helpful while analysing the data.

Data Organisation (Classification and Tabulation)

Classification

So far we have discussed all the steps required for preparing a master chart, namely, data screening, data coding, data entry and data cleaning. Data in the master chart are still in raw form or ungrouped and need to be organised and presented in a meaningful and understandable form to facilitate further statistical analysis. The process of grouping raw data into different classes according to some common characteristics/attributes is known as classification [17, 18]. By classifying data, unnecessary details are eliminated which helps in drawing meaningful inferences for further statistical treatment. The classified data are then arranged systematically and presented through the process of tabulation. Thus classification is the first step in the process of decoding master chart into tabulation [19].

Broadly there are four types of classifications: geographical, chronological, qualitative and quantitative nature [18, 19] and they are illustrated in Tables 2, 3, 4 and 5.

In general, class intervals should be mutually exclusive. Number of class intervals should be neither too large not too small. They should have equal width for easy comparison and computation. Sturges has given a formula to determine the number of classes (k), i.e., $k = 1 + 3.322 \log N$ (N = total number of observations) [20]. In practice, the number of classes as well as class intervals is determined based on previous literature or based on plausible utility and justification.

Classes can be called exclusive when upper limit of one class is lower limit of next class and the upper limit is not included in the class and inclusive when both the upper and lower limits of the class are included within the same class itself (Table 6)

When number of observations are distributed across the different classes, frequency distribution is formed which are usually represented using simple tables (Table 5).

Table 2 Geographical classification (according to geographical region or place)

Place of residence	Panchayat A	Panchayat B	Panchayat C	Panchayat D
Birth rate	20	16	18	22

Table 3 Chronological classification (according to order of time expressed in years, months, weeks, etc., The data is generally classified in ascending order of time)

Year	2014	2015	2016	2017
Birth rate	26	24	23	21

Table 4 Qualitative classification (data are classified on the basis of same quality/attributes like sex, education, religion, etc. that cannot be measured along with a scale)

Simple/dichotomous (based on one attribute)				
Group	Male	Female		
Number of people	10	16		

Manifold (based on more than one attribute)				
Group	Male employed	Female employed	Male unemployed	Female unemployed
Number of people	20	6	8	12

Table 5 Quantitative classification (classification of data according to some characteristics that can be measured such as height, weight, etc., on the basis of class intervals)

Height (in cm)	Frequency
110–120	5
120–130	20
130–140	26
140–150	30
150–160	19
Total	100

Table 6 Exclusive and Inclusive type of class intervals

Exclusive type	Inclusive type
60–70 (60 and above but <70)	60–69 (60 and above but ≤ 69)
70–80 (70 and above but <80)	70–79 (70 and above but ≤ 79)
80–90 (80 and above but <90)	80–89 (80 and above but ≤ 89)
90–100 (90 and above but <100)	90–99 (90 and above but ≤ 99)

Tabulation

Tabulation is the process of summarizing classified or grouped data in a detailed and orderly form. A table is a systematic arrangement of classified data in columns and row.

Classification and Tabulation are not two distinct processes and therefore are carried out concurrently. For tabulation, data are classified and then displayed under different columns and rows of a table. Classification sorts the data for further analysis while tabulation emphasizes on the presentation of sorted data [19].

Tabulation of data helps in several ways, as given below:

- It helps the process of data cleaning
- Data can be presented in a compact form to show relations and make comparisons.
- It facilitates organisation of data to align different variables in accordance with the objectives or hypothesis of the study
- It provides a basis for further statistical computations, especially when manual analysis is attempted in quantitative data.
- It simplifies complex data and present facts in minimum space

Table 7 Components of table
(**Table number**) -----------(**Table Title**)---

Row heading	Column heading		Total
	Column sub-heading	Column sub-heading	
Row designations	Body of the table		
Total			

Preparing a Table

The purpose of tabulation and utility of its information has to be kept in mind while preparing a table. An ideal table has the following components (Table 7):

- **Table number**
- **Table title**
- **Column headings or Captions** (usually relatively less important or shorter classification are tabulated in columns)
- **Row designations or Stub** (usually a relatively more important classification or variable with a large number of classes are tabulated in rows).
- The arrangements of rows and columns should be in a logical and systematic order. This arrangement may be alphabetical, chronological or according to size.
- **Body of the table** (all the cells except those on the top row and first column)
- **Totals** (The totals of rows should be given at the right of the table and that of columns at the bottom of the table. Totals for every sub-class too should be mentioned.)
- **Footnote** (for explaining or providing further details about the data, that have not been covered in title, column and row headings)
- **Sources of data** (source from where information has been taken are given at the bottom of the table for readers to check the figures and gather additional information)

Other Requirements of Good Table

1. Column headings and row headings should be clear and brief with units of measurement specified at appropriate places.
2. The columns and rows should be clearly separated with dark lines
3. Comparable data should be put side by side.
4. The figures in percentage should be approximated before tabulation.
5. Explanatory footnotes concerning the table should be placed at appropriate places.

Types of Tables

Based on purpose

General tables (used for common purpose and not with reference to specific objectives. E.g., socio-demographic table) or,

Specific tables (represents data relating to specific objectives).

Based on originality

Primary table (containing data in the form in which they are originally collected) or, Derived tables (presents totals, averages etc., derived from original data).

Based on number of characteristics

Simple (data on only one characteristic) or,
Complex table (data on more than one characteristic).

Developing table based on number of characteristics has more practical utility and are explained in Tables 8, 9 and 10.

Table 8 Simple or one-way table (contains data of one characteristic only)

Table no. x: Reported cases of dengue by age in city Y, 2017	
Age in years	**No. of cases**
<20	12
20–40	16
40 and above	15
Total	43

Table 9 Two-way table (contains data of two variables) (This table is the most commonly used in most research studies)

Table no. x: Reported cases of dengue by age and sex in city Y, 2017			
Age in years	No. of cases		Total
	Male	Female	
<20	8	4	12
20–40	10	6	16
40 and above	9	6	15
Total	27	16	43

Table 10 Manifold table (contains data of more than two variables)

Table no. x: Reported cases of dengue by age, sex and working status in city Y, 2017							
Age group in years	No. of cases						Total
	Male			Female			
	W	NW	Total	W	NW	Total	
<20	5	3	8	3	1	4	12
20–40	8	2	10	4	2	6	16
Above 40	6	3	9	5	1	6	15
Total	19	8	27	12	4	16	43

Footnote: W stands for working and NW stands for not working

Table 11 Sociodemographic profile

Characteristics	Number	Percent
Total cases	43	100
Sex		
Male	27	63
Female	16	37
Age		
<20	12	28
20–40	16	37
Above 40	15	35
Smoking		
Smoker	23	53
Non-smoker	20	47

Composite Table

To conserve space in a report or manuscript, several tables are sometimes combined into one (Table 11) [21]. It is important to realize that this type of table should not be interpreted as for a three-way table (manifold table). It does not indicate the interrelationship of the included variables (sex, age, smoking), merely, several one variable tables have been concatenated for space conservation.

When the data set is small, it could be classified and tabulated manually using manual sorting and tally counting [10]. However, with the availability of the statistical softwares, decoding Master Chart into classification and tabulation as the initial step in routine data analysis is now being done by the computers. Figure 4 shows a summary of preparing and decoding a master chart.

Final Thoughts

To generate or test any hypothesis, a good data collected through a well-conducted research study is essential. But it is only one part of the whole story. To make the huge mass of data meaningful and amenable to proper analysis and for drawing valid and reliable inferences, it is equally important to process and assemble the data properly. Construction of a Master Chart is a sine qua non of this process. Unfortunately, most researchers are woefully ignorant of the various steps involved in the preparation of Master Chart. This chapter takes the reader through the various steps of this process and hopefully will fill the void in the published literature on this topic.

Case Scenario

1. A study was conducted among 150 healthy individuals and 100 cases to assess the sex and blood group distribution. Following data were observed,
   (a) 50% of healthy individuals and 55% of cases were males.

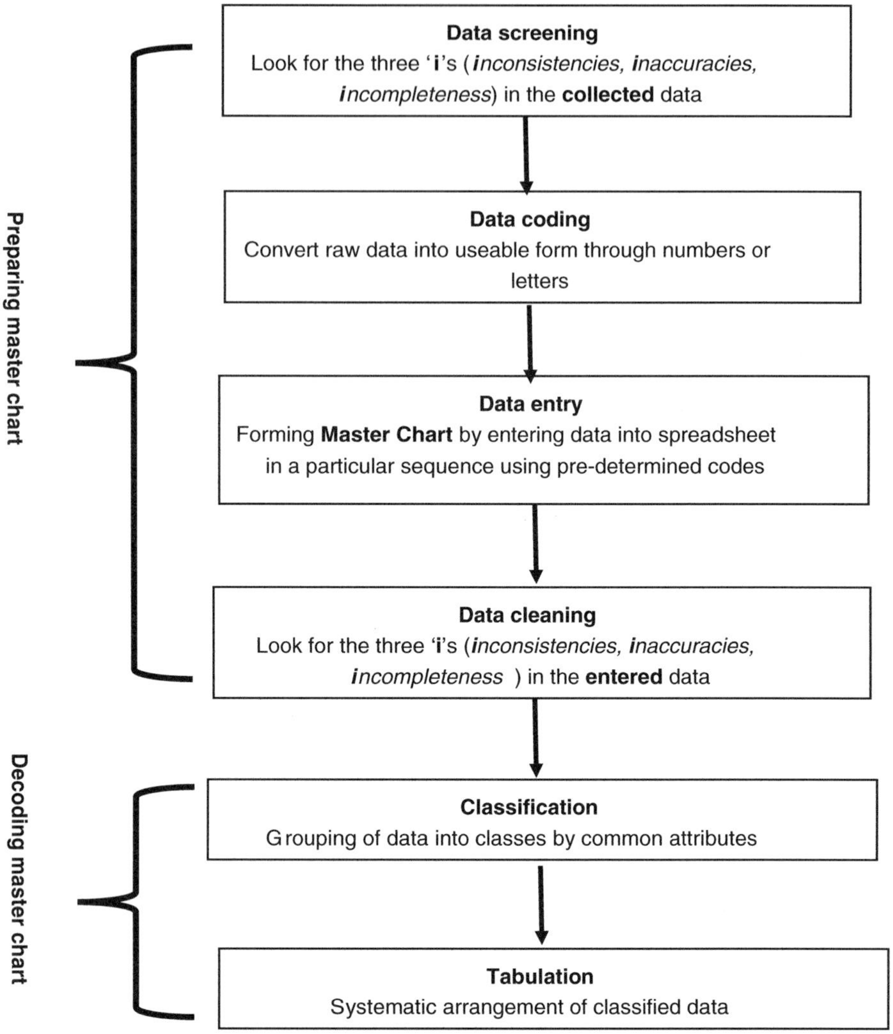

Fig. 4 Preparing and decoding the Master Chart: Summary

(b) 30% of healthy individuals and 40% of cases had blood group "A"
(c) 20% of male healthy individuals and 40% of male cases had blood group "A"

- Tabulate the distribution according to sex and disease status
- Tabulate the distribution according to blood group and disease status
- Tabulate the distribution according to sex, blood group and disease status

2. Prepare a masterchart in a excel sheet along with codebook from the following hypothetical information on ten individuals who attended the medicine outpatient department.

Male	10 years	Primary School	Not applicable	Not applicable	Dengue positive	120/80 mm Hg	2.5 lakh platelet/μl
Female	12 years	Primary School	Not applicable	Not applicable	Dengue negative	110/70 mm Hg	3.5 lakh platelet/μl
Male	22 years	Middle School	Private job	Unmarried	Dengue negative	120/70 mm Hg	1.84 lakh platelet/μl
Male	32 years	Graduate	Private job	Divorced	Dengue negative	114/78 mm Hg	4.5 lakh platelet/μl
Male	44 years	High School	Govt job	Married	Dengue negative	124/82 mm Hg	1.96 lakh platelet/μl
Male	56 years	Illiterate	Govt job	Married	Dengue positive	100/78 mm Hg	0.5 lakh platelet/μl
Male	67 years	Graduate	Govt job	Married	Dengue positive	90/60 mm Hg	2.34 lakh platelet/μl
Female	34 years	Higher secondary School	Private job	Widow	Dengue negative	118/76 mm Hg	3.1 lakh platelet/μl
Female	36 years	Illiterate	Private job	Divorced	Dengue positive	128/98 mm Hg	1.2 lakh platelet/μl
Female	12 years	Higher secondary School	Private job	Married	Dengue negative	122/92 mm Hg	2.3 lakh platelet/μl

References

1. Sharma DC. Poor research output from India's medical schools. Lancet. 2016;387(10034):e28.
2. Tullu MS, Karande S. Quality research in Indian medical colleges and teaching institutions: the need of the hour. J Postgrad Med. 2016;62(4):213–5.
3. Surkis A, Read K. Research data management. J Med Libr Assoc. 2015;103(3):154–6.
4. Nahm ML, Pieper CF, Cunningham MM. Quantifying data quality for clinical trials using electronic data capture. PLoS One. 2008;3(8):e3049.
5. Newgard CD, Zive D, Jui J, Weathers C, Daya M. Electronic versus manual data processing: evaluating the use of electronic health records in out-of-hospital clinical research. Acad Emerg Med Off J Soc Acad Emerg Med. 2012;19(2):217–27.
6. Epstein L, Martin A. Coding variables. In: Kempf-Leonard K, editor. Encyclopedia of social measurement, vol. 1. New York: Academic press; 2005. p. 321–7.
7. Gibbs GR, Friese S, Mangabeira WC. The use of new technology in qualitative research. Introduction to issue 3(2) of FQS. Forum Qual Soc Res. 2002;3(2):8.
8. Sarvela PD, McDermott RJ. Health education evaluation and measurement: a practitioner's perspective. Madison, WI: Brown & Benchmark; 1993. p. 334.
9. Schleicher A, Saito M. Data preparation and management. In: Ross KN, editor. Quantitative research methods in educational planning: IIEP training modules, No010. Paris. International Institute for Educational Planning & UNESCO: France; 2005. p. 78.
10. Varkevisser CM, Brownlee AT, Pathmanathan I. Designing and conducting health systems research projects: proposal development and fieldwork. Vol. 1. Amsterdam: KIT Publishers and the International Development Research Centre (IDRC); 2003. p. 357.
11. Collier J. Using SPSS Syntax: a beginner's guide. New Delhi: SAGE Publications India Pvt Ltd; 2009. p. 35–6.
12. Inter-university Consortium for Political and Social Research. Guide to social science data preparation and archiving: best practice through the data life cycle. 5th ed. Ann Arbor, MI: ICPSR, Institute for Social Research, University of Michigan; 2009.

13. Bourque LB. Coding. In: Lewis-Beck MS, Bryman A, Liao TF, editors. The SAGE encyclopedia of social science research methods. Thousand Oaks: SAGE Publications, Inc.; 2004. p. 132–6.
14. Muraya PI, Coe RI, Garlick CSSC. Research data management, vol. 123. Nairobi, Kenya: World Agroforestry Centre; 2002.
15. Altman DG. Preparing to analyse data. In: Practical statistics for medical research. 1st ed. London: Chapman and Hall; 1991. p. 122–32.
16. Casley DJ, Lury DA. Data collection in developing countries. 2nd ed. Oxford, NY: Oxford University Press; 1987. p. 240.
17. Anderson TW, Sclove SL. Introduction to the statistical analysis of data, vol. 704. Boston: Houghton Mifflin; 1978.
18. Elhance DN. Fundamentals of statistics, vol. 4. 32nd ed. Allahabad: Kitab Mahal Agencies; 1986. p. 1–4.30.
19. Pillai RSN, Bagavathi V. Statistics (theory & practice). 7th ed. New Delhi: S. Chand & Company LTD; 2008. p. 50–79.
20. Sturges HA. The choice of a class interval. J Am Stat Assoc. 1926;21(153):65–6.
21. Centers for Disease Control and Prevention (CDC). Displaying public health data. In: Principles of epidemiology in public health practice: an introduction to applied epidemiology and biostatistics. 3rd ed. Atlanta: Office of Workforce and Career Development, CDC; 2006. p. 511.

Statistical Analysis: Data Presentation and Statistical Tests

Mahalakshmy Thulasingam and
Kariyarath Cheriyath Premarajan

Statistics without science is incomplete, science without statistics is imperfect.—KV Mardia

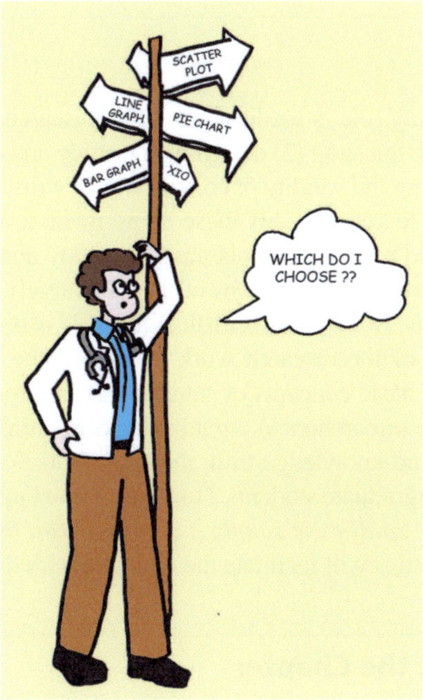

M. Thulasingam (✉)
Associate Professor, Department of Preventive and Social Medicine, Jawaharlal Institute of Postgraduate Medical Education and Research, Pondicherry, India

K. C. Premarajan
Professor and Head, Department of Preventive and Social Medicine, Jawaharlal Institute of Postgraduate Medical Education and Research, Pondicherry, India

S. C. Parija, V. Kate (eds.), *Thesis Writing for Master's and Ph.D. Program*,
https://doi.org/10.1007/978-981-13-0890-1_11

Key Points

- Data analysis should be planned in line with objectives of the study. Quality assured data entry, data cleaning and construction of dummy tables are essential steps before data analysis.
- Descriptive statistics summarize the data obtained from the study subjects. The measures could be rate, proportion, odds ratio, relative risk, mean, median, mean difference, etc.
- Inferential statistics make inference about the population using the data from the study sample. In inferential statistics, 95% confidence interval and p-value are calculated.
- In comparison with p-value, 95% confidence interval gives information on the magnitude of effect in addition to statistical significance. Clinical significance is important than statistical significance.
- Choice of statistical test of significance depends on the type of data (numerical, categorical) and its distribution (normal or non-normal).

Introduction

Statistics play a key role in medical research. Research has six logical steps:(1) formulating the research question (2) designing the study and data collection (3) interpretation of results (4) testing the validity of conclusion (5) writing the research work (6) contemplation of the research [1]. All these steps involve reasoning and critical thinking. Researchers spend a lot of time planning the study and in collecting valid and reliable data. Making correct interpretations of the data largely relies on the use of appropriate statistical methods. Sometimes statistical analysis is done by a trained statistician who may not be part of the research work. However, the researcher should have a good understanding of basic concepts of statistics and interpretation of the statistical results. Statistics help the researchers to organize the data, think critically, and derive meaningful information and knowledge from the data. Statistics is often feared by both undergraduate and postgraduate students. However, Steve Gull, a modern Bayesian, physicist, comments "*Data analysis is simply a dialogue with the data*" [2]. Understanding the essentials of statistics will facilitate the dialogue with the data to find the truth.

Objectives of the Chapter

This chapter primarily focuses on statistical analysis of quantitative data. The chapter

1. gives an overview of the approach to a dataset
2. briefly explains how to choose commonly used statistical tools for a given data set and to make interpretations from it
3. explains descriptive and inferential statistics and its interpretation
4. describes the uses of figures and graphs for data presentation

This chapter does not explain qualitative research analysis, detail theory behind the statistical tests, multivariate analysis and uncommon or exceptional scenarios which require a thorough understanding of the statistical concepts. This chapter summarises the common thumb rules in data analysis. However, there are exceptions to these thumb rules and approach to the data may vary on a case to case basis.

Basic Terms Used in Data Analysis

Types of Variables

Choosing appropriate statistical test or presentation of data largely depends on the type of variable. The two major divisions of variables are (i) Categorical Variable (ii) Numerical variable [3]. Categorical variable are non-numerical variables and the data in these variables fall into finite number of categories. Binary variables (has only two possible values) and ordered categorical variables (they have a natural order) are special types of categorical variable. Examples of categorical variables are presence or absence of hypertension (binary variable), socio-economic status and Body Mass Index (BMI) classified as overweight, obese, morbid obesity (ordered categorical variable). Numerical variables could be discrete or continuous. Discrete variables take whole numbers such as the number of patients attending the OPD, heart rate. Continuous variables are measured on a continuous scale and include decimal numbers. Examples are haemoglobin, weight.

Types of Distribution

For numerical variables choosing the right statistical tool depends on the type of distribution of the data—normal or non-normal distribution. Central Limit Theorem which forms the backbone for the inferential statistics is based on the normal distribution. The key characteristics of a normally distributed data are: (1) mean = median = mode and (2) 68% of the values in the data set lie between mean ± 1 SD, 95% of the values lie between mean ± 1.96 SD and 99.7% of the data lie between mean ± 3 SD. One of the key steps while proceeding with the statistical analysis, is to find if the data follows a normal distribution? (Box 1) The normality of data may be further tested by exploring the dataset using various statistical packages [4].

Box 1: Thumb Rule to Identify If a Data Set Is Normally Distributed
In most situations data follow normal distribution when

1. mean ≈ median ≈ mode and
2. SD is <50% of mean or
3. Co-efficient of variance (SD/Mean × 100) is less than 50% of mean

Linking Data Analysis with Objective

To do a sound statistical analysis, the researcher should have clear objectives. He should link the analysis with the objectives. Broadly, objectives of studies are either descriptive or analytical. In a descriptive study, the researcher wants to estimate a proportion or mean and does not have a comparison group. The objective 'to estimate the incidence of Tuberculosis among PG residents working in a tertiary care hospital' is an example of descriptive studies [5]. In analytical studies, the researcher wants to establish a relationship between two variables by having a comparison group. The study would either find an association between risk factor and disease or treatment and outcome. An example for objective in analytical study design is 'to compare two antibiotic regimens for treatment of neonatal sepsis' [6].

Descriptive Statistics and Inferential Statistics

The data analysis usually has two parts: (1) descriptive statistics and (2) inferential statistics. In descriptive statistics, the researcher describes and summarises the data in terms of measures of central tendency, dispersion. Descriptive statistics also explores the distribution of data and identifies patterns. The researcher proposes to make inference or assumptions about the population based on the data collected from a sample. This is done through inferential statistics, which includes estimation of 95% of Confidence Intervals (95% CI) and calculation of p-value. As a logical sequence descriptive statistics is followed by inferential statistics.

Precursors of Data Analysis

1. **Dummy tables** or planned tables are empty tables which outlines how the results will be represented [7]. It is ideal to make dummy tables while writing the protocol as this would guide the development of data collection tool. It is a good practice to follow the various reporting guidelines such as CONSORT, STROBE while making the dummy tables [8]. Even if dummy table is not made in the protocol it is essential to make it before analysing the data. The dummy tables are filled as the data analysis is done. It helps in organizing the analysis at each step and gives clarity during the analysis [9].
2. **Quality-assured data entry**: Adequate emphasis has to be given to quality-assured data entry which is described as the 'Cinderella' of medical research. Double data entry and validation is considered as the definitive gold standard of good clinical practice. Therefore, wherever possible double data entry and validation should be done. During the data entry and before starting the analysis the researcher should make sure that the variable are labelled appropriately [10, 11].
3. **Data cleaning** is an essential step which is done before the researcher starts analysing the data. In this step we look for any errors or inconsistencies. Here

we remove or verify data points which are obviously disconnected or erroneous. A few examples are (1) haemoglobin entered as 101 instead of 10.1, (2) a pregnant male (3) a person working as professional and educated up to fifth class. In this step we also look for outliers, to identify wrongly entered numerical data, any logical connections such as gender and pregnancy, education and occupation. Overlooking data cleaning may lead to wrong interpretations or identifying the mistake towards the end of the analysis leading to waste of resources.

Approach to Statistical Analysis [12, 13]

Studies Without Comparison Groups (Descriptive Study)

Descriptive statistics: As described earlier, we start the analysis with descriptive statistics. Descriptive statistics depend on the type of variables. If the variable is categorical, then we calculate either **proportions or rates** [14]. A few examples of proportion (formula 1, Box 2) are: percentage of patients reporting to the emergency ward with snake bite, the percentage of low birth weight babies having neonatal sepsis. Incidence rates (formula 2, Box 2) [15] are the appropriate descriptive statistics in follow up studies (longitudinal studies) where the patient is followed for a defined period of time. A few examples of rates: the rate of ventilator acquired pneumonia in the first month of artificial ventilation, the rate of surgical site infection during the first post-operative week. Formulae for proportion and incidence rate are given below:

For a numerical variable, the descriptive statistics are measures of central tendency and dispersion. **Measures of central tendency** are mean, median, mode. These summary measures attempt to describe the data-set with a representative or central value. Arithmetic mean equals sum of all the values divided by the number of values in the data set. Arithmetic mean is commonly used in medical research, for example: average haemoglobin of pregnant mothers at delivery, average BMI of a patient presenting with gall stones. Mean is highly influenced by outliers, and does not depict central tendency in case of non-normal distribution. In situations, where the numerical data is not distributed normally, median is the better measure of central tendency, for example: duration of hospital stay for emergency appendicectomy (usually duration of hospital stay follow non-normal distribution), number of per vaginal examinations done during active labour. Median is the middle value in the data set.

Measures of dispersion are standard deviation, variance, range and inter-quartile range. Measures of dispersion capture the degree of spread/variability of the data. As a thumb rule when mean is used as measure of central tendency, standard deviation is used as a measure of dispersion; in case of median, we use inter-quartile range (IQR). Formula for standard deviation is given in Box 2 (formula 3). Interquartile range is the range between the first and third quartile. When the data are arranged in ascending order, quartile are the three points which divide the data set into four equal parts. In terms of percentile, first quartile (Q1) is 25th percentile, second quartile (Q2) is 50th percentile (median), third quartile (Q3) is 75th percentile. First quartile (Q1) divides the lowest 25% of the data and the highest 75% of the data (formula 4). Median and IQR are more robust and not affected by extremes of data.

Inferential Statistics

After the descriptive statistics, we try to estimate the true population value. Sampling errors occur while estimating the true population value from the sample statistics. Hence, there is uncertainty associated with making inference about population with the values from the sample. Therefore, we report a range in inferential statistics, which is called as the confidence interval. Usually, we report 95% confidence interval (Box 3, formula 5).

The 95% confidence interval (95% CI) is interpreted as 'there is 95% chance that the mean population value will be between the confidence interval range. However

Box 2: List of Formulas Used in Descriptive Statistics

$$\textbf{\textit{Formula}}\,\mathbf{1}: Proportion = \frac{\begin{array}{c}number\ of\ partcipants\\ with\, a\ given\ characteristics\end{array}}{\begin{array}{c}total\ number\ of\\ participants\ in\ the\ group\end{array}} \times 100$$

$$\textbf{\textit{Formula}}\,\mathbf{2}: Incidence\ rate = \frac{\begin{array}{c}number\ of\ new\, cases\ of\ disease\\ during\ specified\ time\ interval\end{array}}{\begin{array}{c}summed\ person-time\\ of\ observation\end{array}} \times 100$$

$$\textbf{\textit{Formula}}\,\mathbf{3}: Standard\ deviation = \sqrt{\frac{\Sigma(x-\overline{x})^2}{n-1}}$$

x indicates data
$\overline{x}$ indicates sample mean
n indicates sample size

$$\textbf{\textit{Formula}}\,\mathbf{4}: Interquartile\ range = Q3 - Q1,$$

$$Q3 = value\ that\ divides\ the\ lowest\, 75\%\ of\ the\ data\, from\ highest\, 25\%$$

$$Q1 = value\ that\ divides\ the\ lowest\, 25\%\ of\ the\ data\, from\ highest\, 75\%$$

there is 5% chance that the confidence interval will not include the mean population value. For example, if mean haemoglobin of the 200 study participants is 11 gm% (95% CI: 9–13). It means that there is 95% chance that the mean population haemoglobin will be between 9 and 13. However, there is 5% chance that the population value would be <9 and >13. Another example with proportion, if prevalence (proportion) of tuberculosis is 10% among a sample of subjects with HIV and 95% CI is 5–15%. It implies that the descriptive statistics is 10% and there is 95% chance that the population (representing the sample)prevalence will be between 5 and 15%. Confidence interval is calculated based on Central Limit Theorem and normal distribution, hence not usually calculated in case of non-normal distribution. The analysis of descriptive studies is summarised in Fig. 1.

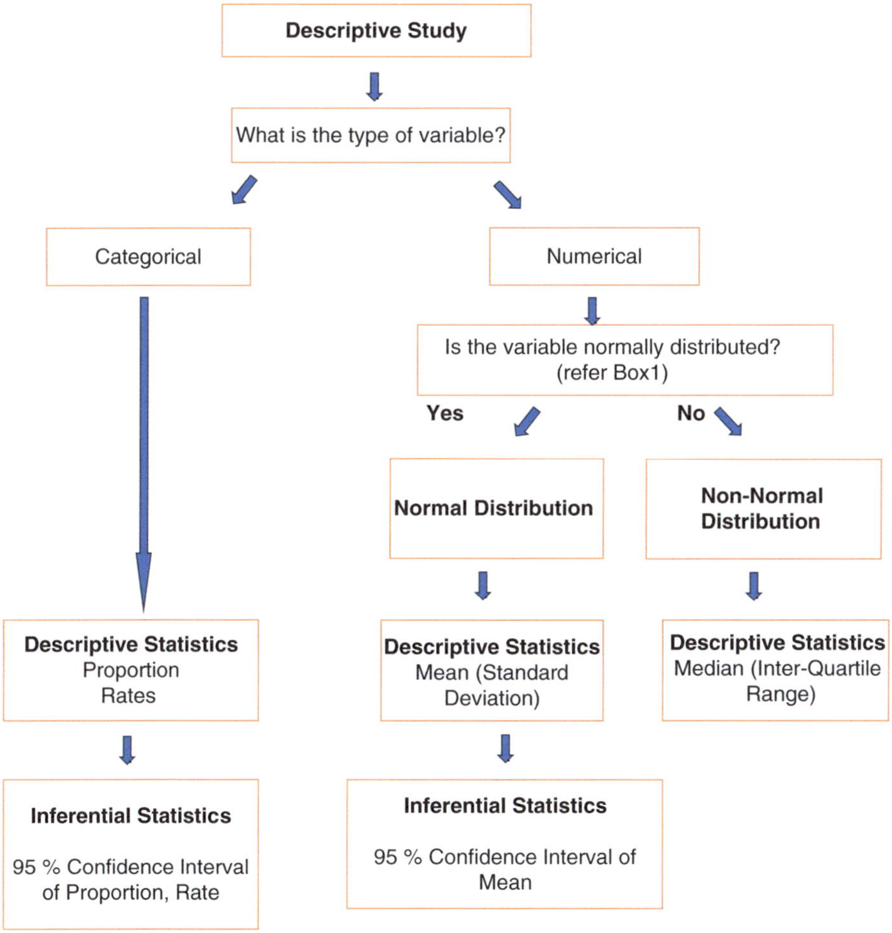

Fig. 1 Approach to statistical analysis for descriptive studies

Studies with Comparison Group (Analytical Study)

Null Hypothesis and p-Value

Before proceeding further, it is important to understand the concept of null hypothesis and p-value. In science, it is usually impractical to 'prove' a hypothesis as you cannot account for all possible objections. Hence, we either 'reject' or 'fail to reject' a hypothesis. Routinely, we start with the assertion that "there is no difference between groups or there is no association between the exposure and outcome". This is the Null Hypothesis. If the collected data shows that the observed variations cannot be due to mere statistical randomness or 'chance' then we reject the null hypothesis and conclude that there is an association. On the contrary, we may 'fail to reject' the null hypothesis, indicating that the data is not sufficient to accept the alternative hypothesis [16]. However, when the researcher accepts the null hypothesis it should be ensured that power of the study is at least 80%.

The p-value indicates the probability that any observed difference between groups is due to chance when the null hypothesis is true. For example, p-value<0.05 means the probability that the observed difference between the two groups due to chance is <5%. If the p-value is <0.05 then we 'reject' the null hypothesis and it is conventionally mentioned as a statistically significant difference/association. If the p-value is ≥0.05 then we 'fail to reject' the null hypothesis. Generally, p-values is rounded up to two decimal places or up to one significant digit. For example, p-value = 0.0434 is mentioned as 0.04, p-value = 0.00532 is mentioned as 0.005. If p-value is less than 0.001 it should be written as <0.001. For example 0.000031 is mentioned as <0.001 [17].

Analytical studies usually aim to find association between exposure and outcome. Analysis starts with descriptive statistics and is followed by inferential statistics. The inferential statistics of measuring association has two components: (1) 95% Confidence Interval of the measure of association (2) calculation of p-value. The interpretation of 95% confidence interval is similar to that explained earlier. Selection of statistical test for calculation of p-value largely depends on the type of the exposure and outcome variable. Exposure variable could be risk factor or a treatment modality. Outcome could be a disease or event or treatment outcomes. The exposure and outcome variables of a research studies could be:

1. exposure and outcome are categorical, example: two antibiotic regimens for treatment of neonatal sepsis (exposure) and survival of the child (outcome)
2. exposure categorical and outcome numerical, example: two treatment regimens for treatment of severe anaemia (exposure) and improvement in Haemoglobin (outcome)
3. exposure and outcome are numerical example: weight (exposure) with systolic blood pressure (outcome)

The approach to statistical of the above three scenarios are given in Figs. 2, 3 and 4.

Box 3: List of Formulas Used in Inferential Statistics

$$\textbf{Formula 5}: 95\%\ \textit{confidence interval}(\textit{numerical data}) = \textit{mean} \pm 1.96(\textit{standard error of mean})$$

$$95\%\ \textit{confidence interval}(\textit{categorial data}) = \textit{proportion} \pm 1.96(\textit{standard error of proportion})$$

$$\textit{Standard error of mean} = \frac{\textit{standard deviation}}{\sqrt{n}}$$

$$\textit{Standard error of proportion} = \sqrt{\frac{p(1-p)}{n}}$$

p indicates proportion
n indicates sample size

Two by two table when both exposure and outcome are categorical

Exposure		Outcome	
		Present	Absent
	Present	a	b
	Absent	c	d

$$\textbf{Forumla 6}: \textit{Relative risk} = \frac{\textit{incidence of event among exposed subjects}}{\textit{incidence of event among non-exposed subjects}}$$

$$\textbf{Formula 7}: \textit{Odds ratio} = \frac{ad}{bc}$$

$$\textbf{Formula 8}: \textit{Prevalence ratio} = \frac{\textit{prevalence of event among exposed subjects}}{\textit{prevalence of event among nonexposed subjects}}$$

Data Analysis in Scenarios When Exposure and Outcome Are Categorical

To measure association, between categorical exposure and categorical outcome we use relative risk or prevalence ratio or odds ratio (descriptive statistics) depending on the types of study (Fig. 2). While we calculate these measures of association, it is essential to pay attention to the construction of two by two table (Box 3). In cohort studies, we calculate incidence rates in the exposure groups and calculate relative risk (RR) (Box 3, formula 6). Generally odds ratio (OR) is the measures of association for

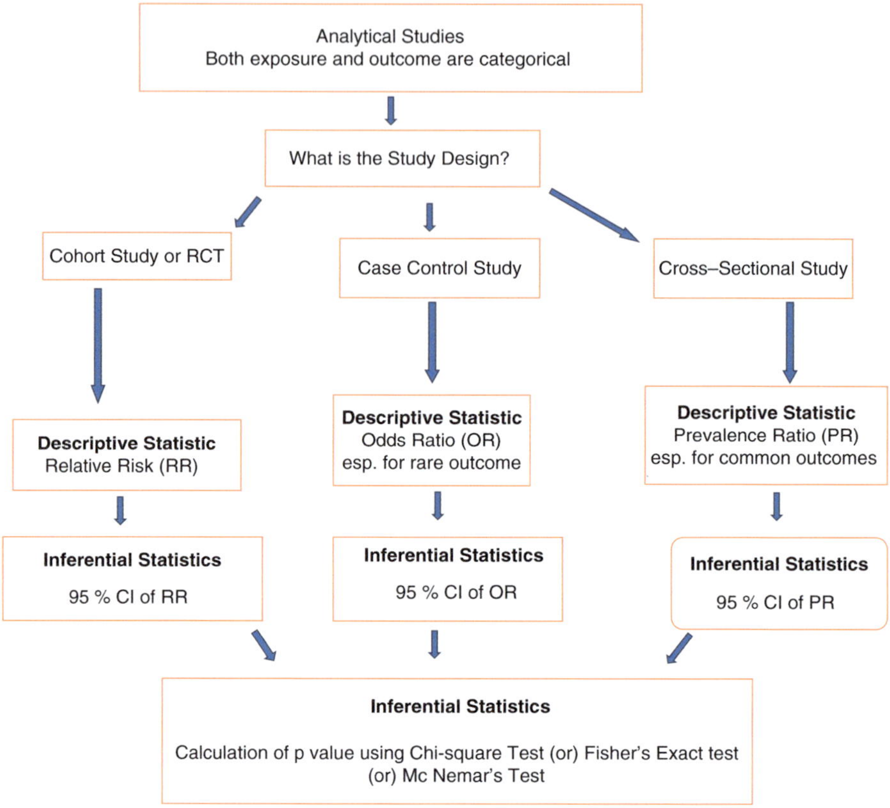

Fig. 2 Approach to statistical analysis for analytical studies where both exposure and outcome are categorical

case-control study. However, the measure of association in case-control study depends on case and control selection methodology [18, 19]. Odds ratio (Box 3, formula 7) is approximately equal to relative risk when the outcome is rare (<5%). In cross-sectional studies prevalence ratio (PR) is a better measure of association especially when the outcome is common (Box 3, formula 8) [20]. The interpretation of OR, RR, PR are given in Table 1. Most statistical software calculates 95% CI for RR, OR and PR. In addition, p-value is calculated using chi-square test in most scenarios. Chi-square test is a robust test and are used even when there are more than two rows or columns. Fisher's exact test is better than chi-square when one or more cells have expected cell count less than 5. In case of paired or matched data, paired analysis should be done in which the table construction, calculation of measures of association and test of significance are different from that used for unpaired data.

Data Analysis in Scenarios Where Exposure Is Categorical and Outcome Is Numerical

In situations where exposure is categorical and outcome is numerical descriptive statistics of the outcome in each of the exposure categories is calculated. These descriptive statistics is considered as the effect size. For example, mean

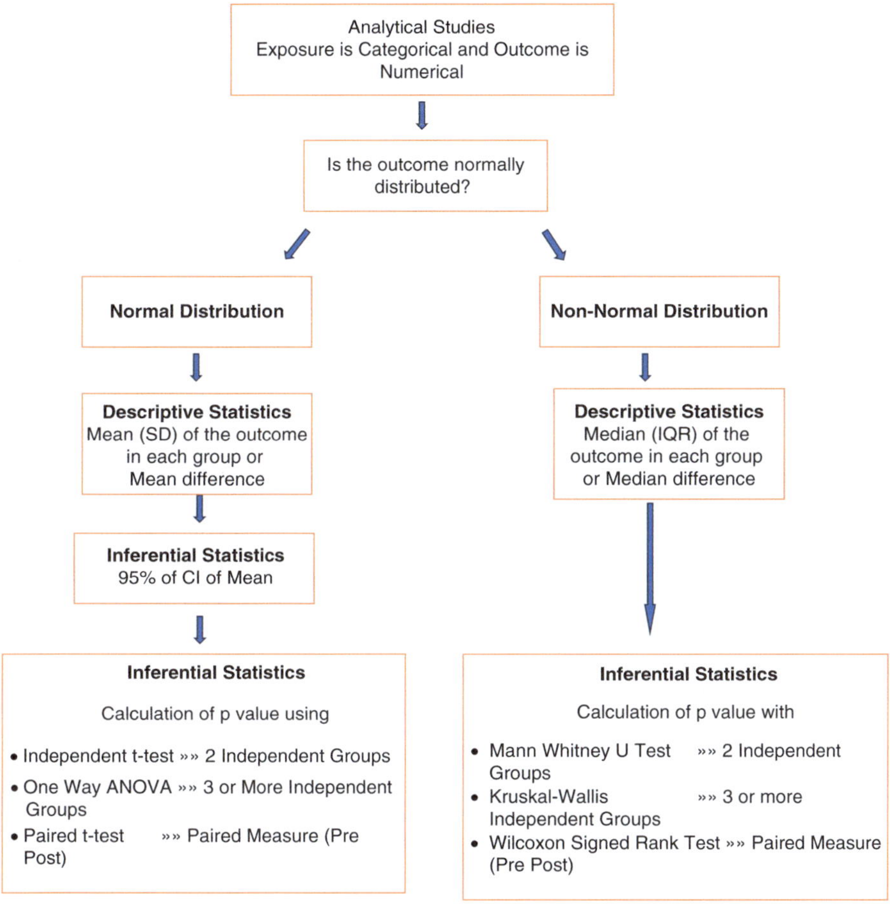

Fig. 3 Approach to statistical analysis for analytical studies where exposure is categorical and outcome is numerical

haemoglobin in group 1 is 13 gm% and in group 2 is 9 gm%, it is interpreted as 'in the sample, the haemoglobin of group 1 is higher than that in group 2'. Next step is calculation of confidence interval for the means. For example, in group 1, 95% CI of haemoglobin is 12–14 gm%, 95% CI of group 2 is 7–11 gm%. Third step is calculation of p-value. A guide to the choice of the test is given in Fig. 3.

Data Analysis in Scenarios Where Both Exposure and Outcome Are Numerical

In this scenario, the measure of association is correlation coefficient (r). It is obtained using Pearson's correlation when both the exposure and outcome are distributed normally. We use Spearman's correlation when either exposure or outcome or both does not follow a normal distribution. The correlation coefficient (r) value ranges from −1 to +1. This test also give 95% CI and p-value (Fig. 4).

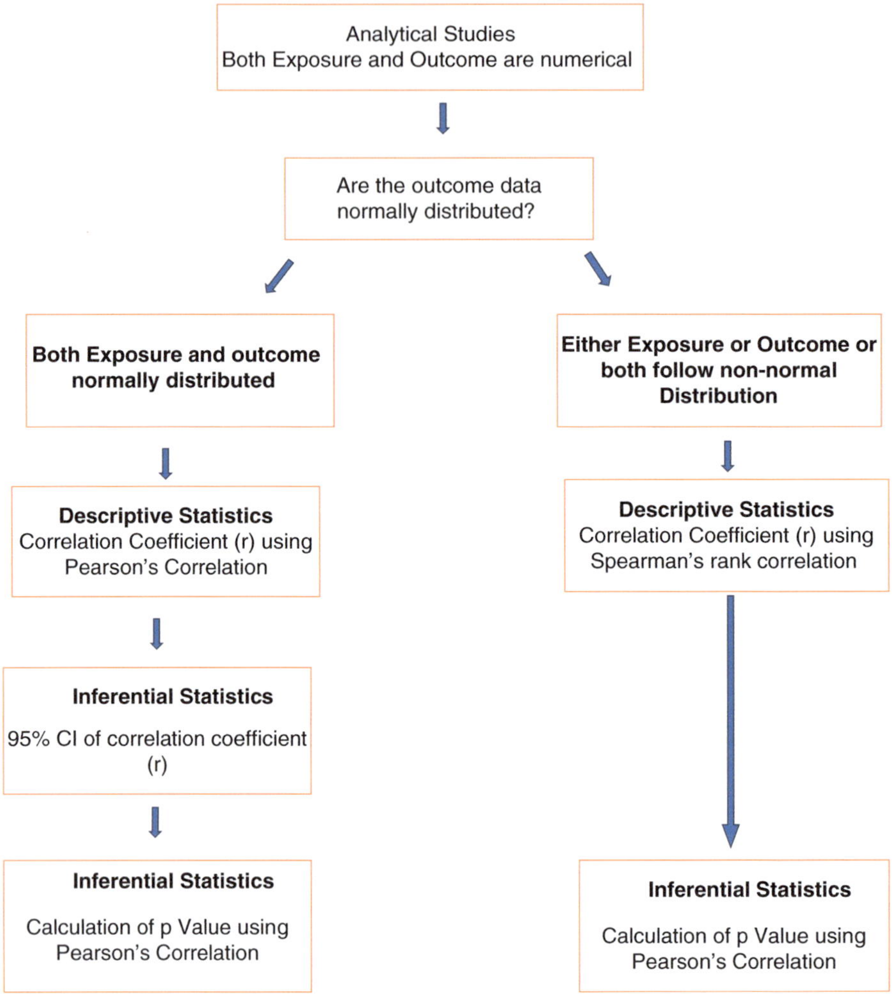

Fig. 4 Approach to statistical analysis for analytical studies where both exposure and outcome are numerical

Evaluation of a Diagnostic or Screening Tool/Test

Sometimes, medical research evaluates a diagnostic or screening tool. The statistical analysis in this situation includes calculation of sensitivity, specificity, positive predictive value, negative predictive value and likelihood ratios along with 95% CI [13]. Receiver Operating Curve (ROC) is also plotted. ROC is used for identifying an appropriate cut-off for a test, considering the clinically apt sensitivity and specificity. Area under the curve of ROC is used to discriminate and identify a clinically relevant test [21]. Gold Standard Test should be selected carefully, as most of the above indicators rely largely on the gold standard test.

Table 1 Interpretation of relative risk, odds ratio and prevalence ratio

Measure of association	Interpretation
Relative risk, odds ratio, prevalence ratio >1	The exposure is a risk factor for the outcome
Relative risk, odds ratio, prevalence ratio <1	The exposure is protective factor for the outcome
Relative risk, odds ratio, prevalence ratio = 1	The exposure has no impact on the outcome
Examples	
Relative risk = 2	The ***incidence*** of the outcome is two times more likely among exposed as compared to unexposed
Odds ratio = 2	The ***odds of exposure*** among cases are two times higher than the odds of exposure among controls. It is approximately equal to relative risk when the disease is rare.
Prevalence ratio = 2	The ***prevalence*** of disease among exposed is two times higher than the prevalence of disease among unexposed
Relative risk = 0.8	The incidence of outcome is 20% [(1 − rr) × 100] less in the exposed as compared to the unexposed
Relative risk = 2 (95% CI: 1.5–3)	RR of the sample in the study is 2 and there is 95% chance that the true population value of RR will be between 1.5 and 3.

95% Confidence Interval and p Value [22]

As already mentioned 95% confidence interval and hypothesis testing (p-value calculation) are inferential statistics. 95% CI are usually given by the statistical software or is calculated using the formula 5, Box 2. The p-value is calculated using the various test of significance such as chi-square test, Fischer's Exact test, t test, ANOVA etc. In most situations, when the 95% CI includes the null value then the p-value is ≥0.05. For relative risk, odds ratio and prevalence ratio the null value is 1 (Table 2). For numerical variables, when the 95% CI of mean of the two groups overlap then the p-value would mostly be ≥0.05 (statistically not significant). It is often commented that 'Statistical significance is the least interesting thing about the results'. The 95% CI indicates the magnitude of the impact and predicts the population value [23].

Clinical Significance vs Statistical Significance

Statistical significance does not always imply clinical significance. The magnitude of association is more important than statistical significance. Even a small difference may be statistically significant because of larger sample size and a big difference may not statistically significant because of less sample size and less power. 95% CI also gives information about the precision of the results. While choosing a treatment option the researcher/clinician looks into many factors such as magnitude of benefit, side-effects, cost involved, convenience of use and patient preferences [24].

Table 2 Scenarios explaining the relation between 95% Confidence Interval and p Value

Scenario	95% Confidence interval (CI)	Visual depiction of the measures of association and 95% CI ● Depicts null value —— depicts 95% CI	Comment	Statistical significance
Association between Smoking and COPD	95% CI of Relative risk 1.5–3	● 1.5 —— 3	95% CI does not include the null value*	Statistically significant
Association between treatment success and two interventions	95% CI of Relative risk 0.8–2	0.8 ——●—— 2	95% CI includes the null value*	Statistically not significant
Compare two drug formulations in improving haemglobin	95% CI of Mean Hb of group 1 12–14 gm% 95% CI of Mean Hb of group 2 7–11 gm%	7 —— 11 12 —— 14	95% CI of the two means does not overlap	Statistically significant
Compare two drugs in improving haemglobin	95% CI of Mean Hb of group 1 10–13 gm% 95% CI of Mean Hb of group 2 9–11 gm%	10 —— 13 9 —— 11 Overlap	95% CI of the two means overlaps	Statistically not significant

*for Relative risk null value is 1

Multivariate Analysis

When we note an association in analytical studies, the next question which needs to be addressed is, if the association could be due to confounding. To identify the influence of confounding, we either use stratified analysis or multivariate analysis. For multivariate analysis either linear regression or logistic regression is used based on the type of outcome variable.

Choosing Figures and Charts

Charts/figures are the visual representation of a data. Charts facilitate understanding and highlight the important patterns. Charts are chosen based on the message that needs to be highlighted (Fig. 5) [25]. Charts are not apt when the observations are very few or numerous or when there is little variation.

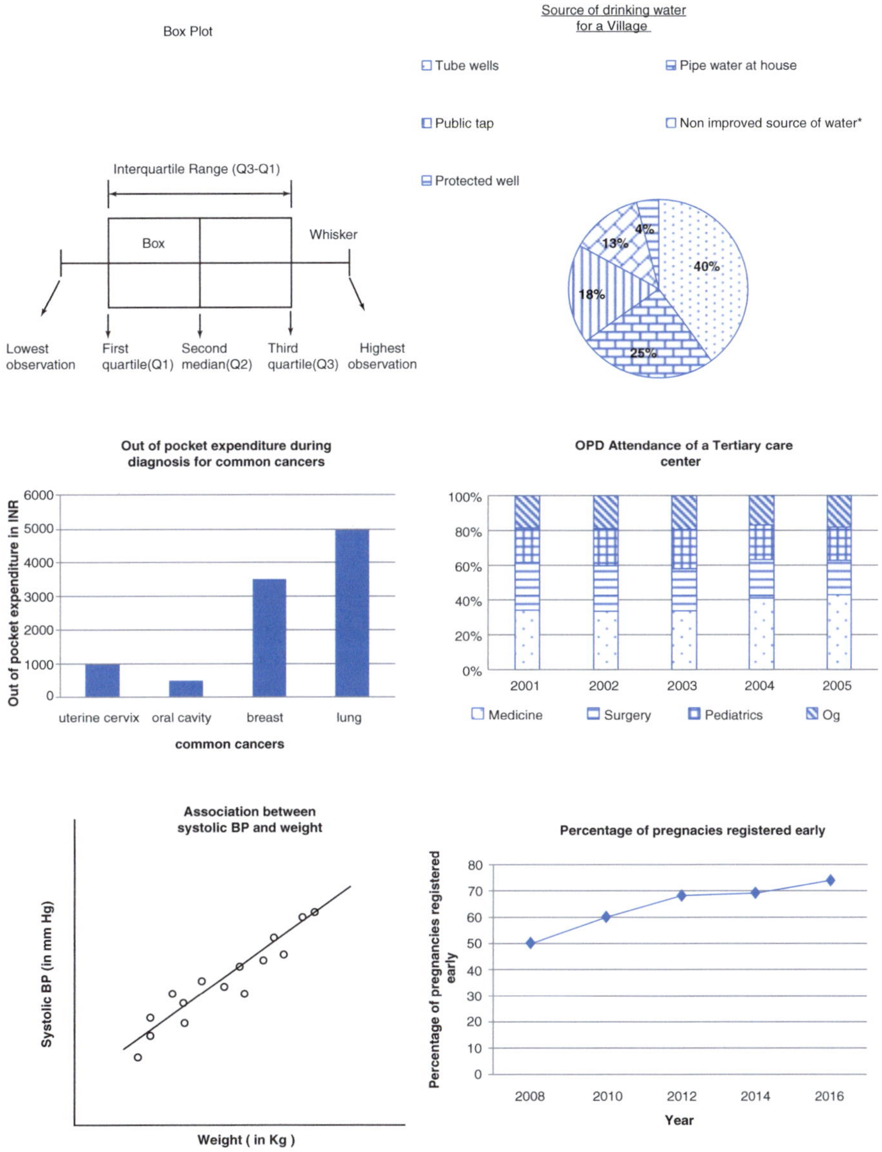

Fig. 5 Various types of charts and figures used to present data. (**a**) Box plot which shows the distribution of data. (**b**) Pie chart showing source of drinking water of a village. (**c**) Simple bar chart showing out-of-pocket expenditure during diagnosis for common cancers. (**d**) Component bar chart which depicts the OPD attendance at various departments of a tertiary care centre. (**e**) Scatter plot showing the association between systolic BP and weight. (**f**) Line diagram showing the changing trend in early registration of pregnancy since 2008 to 2016

Conclusion

Statistical analysis helps in summarising, organizing the data (descriptive statistics). Following descriptive analysis, 95% confidence interval is calculated to predict the true population value. In case of analytical studies, p value is calculated to identify if the association would be by chance. The choice of the statistical tool used depends on the type of variable and the research question. Though statistical analysis is an essential component of research, the researcher should not blindly go with only the statistical analysis. The researcher needs to look at the validity and reliability of the data collection method, biases involved in the study and more importantly the clinical significance of the result.

Case Scenarios

1. Prevalence of anaemia was around 60% in a community. The researcher did a cross sectional study to study the association between anaemia and type of diet. He reported an odds ratio (OR) of 65 with 95% CI as 30–130. Comment on the measure on association.
2. A research article reports a study with objection of studying the association between diabetes mellitus and intake of excessive saturated fat. They calculated prevalence ratio and 95% CI. Prevalence ratio was 1.1 (95% CI = 0.9–1.2). The p value was calculated using chi-square test and was reported p value as <0.05. Comment of the observation.

Acknowledgement The authors thank Dr Tanveer Rehman, Junior Resident and Dr Gunjan Kumar, Senior Resident, Department of PSM for critically reviewing the manuscript

References

1. Dutton WA. Reasoning in research. Can Med Assoc J. 1959;81(6):489–93. http://www.ncbi.nlm.nih.gov/pubmed/13818921. Accessed 28 July 2017
2. Sivia DS. Data analysis- a dialogue with the data. 2005. http://bayes.wustl.edu/sivia/lisbon05.pdf. Accessed 28 July 2017.
3. Kirkwood BR, Sterne JAC, Kirkwood BR. Essential medical statistics. Victoria, Australia: Blackwell Science; 2003.
4. Sarkar. Understanding data for medical statistics. Int J Adv Med Heal Res. 2014;1(1):30. https://doi.org/10.4103/2349-4220.134449.
5. Rao SA, Kadhiravan T, Swaminathan RP, Mahadevan S. Occupational exposure and tuberculosis among medical residents in a high-burden setting: an open-cohort study. Int J Tuberc Lung Dis. 2016;20(9):1162–7. https://doi.org/10.5588/ijtld.15.0638.
6. Ramasamy S, Biswal N, Bethou A, Mathai B. Comparison of two empiric antibiotic regimen in late onset neonatal sepsis—a randomized controlled trial. J Trop Pediatr. 2014;60(1):83–6. https://doi.org/10.1093/tropej/fmt080.
7. Paul Vogt W, editor. Dummy table. In: Dictionary of statistics & methodology. Thousand Oaks, CA: SAGE Publications, Inc. https://doi.org/10.4135/9781412983907.n596.
8. Schulz KF, Altman DG, Moher D, for the CONSORT Group. CONSORT. Statement: updated guidelines for reporting parallel group randomised trails. BMJ Med. 2010;340:c332.

9. Developing a quantitative data analysis plan for observational studies developing a quantitative data analysis plan 2013. http://nceph.anu.edu.au/files/Data_Analysis_Plan_Guide_20131125.pdf. Accessed 13 Aug 2017.
10. Kumar AMV, Naik B, Guddemane DK, et al. Efficient, quality-assured data capture in operational research through innovative use of open-access technology. Public Heal Action. 2013;3(1):60–2. https://doi.org/10.5588/pha.13.0004.
11. Ohmann C, Kuchinke W, Canham S, et al. Standard requirements for GCP-compliant data management in multinational clinical trials. Trials. 2011;12:85. https://doi.org/10.1186/1745-6215-12-85.
12. Gravetter FJ, Wallnau LB. Essentials of statistics for the behavioral sciences. Baltimore: Wadsworth Cengage Learning; 2014.
13. Gordis L. Epidemiology. Philadelphia: Elsevier; 2013.
14. Gerstman B. Epidemiology kept simple. 3rd ed. Oxford: John Wiley & Sons; 2013. http://www.sjsu.edu/faculty/gerstman/eks/. Accessed 1 Sep 2017
15. Epidemiology kept simple. http://www.sjsu.edu/faculty/gerstman/eks/formula_sheet.pdf. Accessed 13 August 2017.
16. Dahiru T. P-value, a true test of statistical significance? A cautionary note. Ann Ibadan Postgrad Med. 2008;6(1):21–6. http://www.ncbi.nlm.nih.gov/pubmed/25161440. Accessed 15 Aug 2017
17. The UNION. Course material of UNION SORT-IT operational research workshop.
18. Knol MJ, Vandenbroucke JP, Scott P, Egger M. Practice of epidemiology what do case-control studies estimate? Survey of methods and assumptions in published case-control research. Am J Epidemiol. 2008;168(9):1073–81. https://doi.org/10.1093/aje/kwn217.
19. Vandenbroucke JP, Pearce N. Case-control studies: basic concepts. Int J Epidemiol. 2012;41(5):1480–9. https://doi.org/10.1093/ije/dys147.
20. Thompson ML, Myers JE, Kriebel D. Prevalence odds ratio or prevalence ratio in the analysis of cross sectional data: what is to be done? https://www.ncbi.nlm.nih.gov/pmc/articles/PMC1757577/pdf/v055p00272.pdf. Accessed 31 Aug 2017.
21. Park SH, Goo JM, Jo C-H. Receiver operating characteristic (ROC) curve: practical review for radiologists. Korean J Radiol. 2004;5(1):11–8. https://doi.org/10.3348/kjr.2004.5.1.11.
22. Ajay Kumar M. Confidence intervals and test of significance. Indian J Community Med. 2006;31(1):46. https://doi.org/10.4103/0970-0218.54942.
23. Coe R. It's the effect size, stupid: what effect size is and why it is important. September 2002. https://www.leeds.ac.uk/educol/documents/00002182.htm. Accessed 25 Aug 2017.
24. Mariani AW, Pêgo-Fernandes PM, Mariani AW, Pêgo-Fernandes PM. Statistical significance and clinical significance. Sao Paulo Med J. 2014;132(2):71–2. https://doi.org/10.1590/1516-3180.2014.1322817.
25. Government of Canada SC. Statistics: power from data! Using graphs. http://www.statcan.gc.ca/edu/power-pouvoir/ch9/using-utilisation/5214829-eng.htm. Accessed 15 Aug 2017.

Part III

Structuring the Material and Writing the Thesis

Preparing a Title Page, Abstract and Table of Contents Page

Kiruthika Sivasubramanian, Rajive Mathew Jose, and Stuart Enoch

A stunning first impression was not the same thing as love at first sight. But surely it was an invitation to consider the matter.—Lois McMaster Bujold

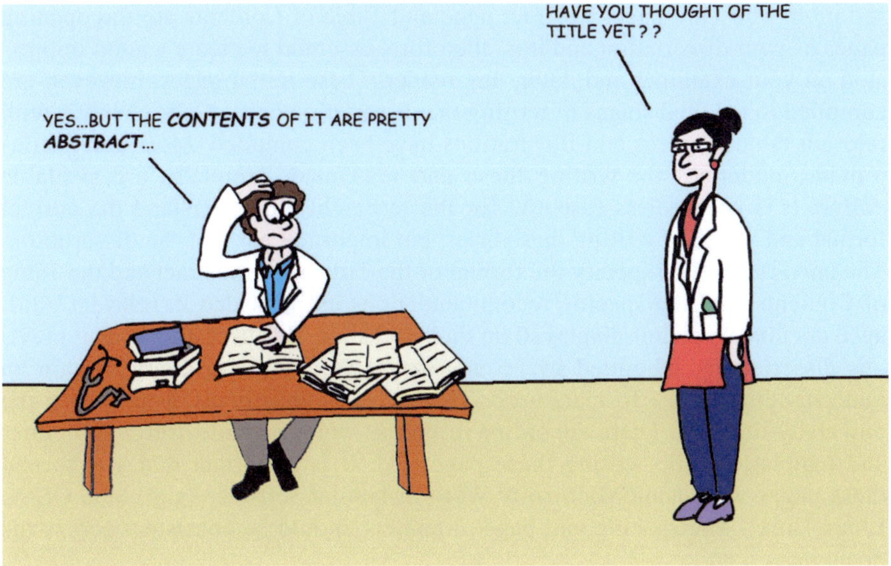

K. Sivasubramanian
Consultant in Child and Adolescent Psychiatry, Black Country Foundation Trust, West Bromwich, UK

R. M. Jose (✉)
Consultant in Plastic Surgery, University Hospital Birmingham, Birmingham, UK

S. Enoch
Director of Education and Research, Doctors Academy Group (Intl), Cardiff, UK

S. C. Parija, V. Kate (eds.), *Thesis Writing for Master's and Ph.D. Program*,
https://doi.org/10.1007/978-981-13-0890-1_12

Key Points

- The Title page, Abstract page and Table of Contents are the opening pages of a dissertation and therefore, essential to create a good impression on the reader.
- The first page of a dissertation should succinctly summarise your work.
- The abstract also called as the 'executive summary', follows the Title page and Declaration Statement and should encapsulate the essence of the dissertation.
- The Table of Contents lists the contents contained within the dissertation with pagination helping the examiners and readers to find the information easily.

Introduction

Writing and submitting a dissertation frequently involves months, if not years, of work that involves commitment, perseverance, and hard work. The initial pages should reflect the great effort that would have gone into writing the dissertation. The Title page, Abstract page and Table of Contents are the opening pages of your dissertation and it is, therefore, essential to create a good impression on your examiner and, later, any reader. These initial pages, however, are compiled in the final stages of writing the dissertation once all the chapters with relevant tables, figures and illustrations have been compiled. Most universities provide guidelines for writing these and readymade templates are available online. It is nonetheless essential for the researcher to understand the correct format and styles of writing these brief, but important parts of the dissertation. The universities also specify the format of the Title page, Abstract and the Table of Contents, and the specific recommendations are provided in relevant guidance documents and/or displayed on their websites. It is useful to look at previous dissertations submitted by researchers at the same university to gain an understanding of the formats used. These copies are usually available in the university libraries. There are online resources which provide useful guidelines and templates while writing these pages [1]. It is important that you format these pages well using Microsoft® Word or similar software (e.g., Mac OS X, Linux/Unix). The spacing and page alignment should be consistent across the documents.

Title Page

This is the first page of your dissertation and should succinctly summarise your work. It is considered to be the first page of the document though the page number does not appear on this page. There are sample templates of Title pages available online [2].

The title page should contain the following information:

1. The Title of the dissertation. The title should remain the same on all the documents. It should ideally be in typescript or black ink and in block letters.
2. Name of the author. This should include the first name, middle name and surname. This should match the name you have provided in the university records.
3. Previous academic credentials (qualifications) of the author. These are written in descending chronological order and each qualification is written in a single line. An example is shown below:
   M.S (General Surgery), Pondicherry University, 2007
   MBBS (Pondicherry University), 2003

However, in some universities, only the name of the candidate without academic qualifications is put on the title page.

4. The degree award title for which the dissertation is presented. This should be written in the form of a statement which reads as "…in partial fulfillment of… (write the name of the course or degree)
   For example:
   Dissertation submitted in partial fulfillment of the requirements for the Doctorate of Philosophy
5. The Institution or Department in which the work was carried out.
6. The month and year during which it is submitted for examination (or re-presentation in the case of a dissertation that is to be re-examined).
7. If there is more than one volume that is submitted, then the Title page should state the total number of volumes and the particular volume.
8. A Copyright Statement that should include your name, year and name of the university
   For example:
   © *Dr Arvind Gupta, 2010, Pondicherry University*

However, this is not mandatory in all the university guidelines.

9. Reuse Statement. This clarifies the terms of reproducing the work. The copyright usually rests with the author or the Department in which the work is carried out.
10. A Declaration Statement is usually placed in the page following Title page that outlines a statement signed by the candidate that states, "Except where indicated by specific reference within the dissertation, the work submitted for examination is the result of the candidate's own investigation and the views expressed are those of the candidate".
11. The Declaration Statement should also include a signed statement by the candidate that states, "No portion of the work presented in this dissertation has been submitted in substance for any other degree or award at this university or any other university, nor is being submitted concomitantly in candidature for any degree or other award".

Abstract Page

The abstract follows the Title page (and Declaration Statement) and should encapsulate the essence of the dissertation. It is also called 'executive summary'. Although it might appear to be a small part of the overall dissertation write-up, it is nonetheless a vital section as it gives the examiner and the reader an overview of the work. Examiners are often provided a copy of the abstract by the university prior to inviting them as formal examiners. If the abstract is not compiled in a proficient manner the examiners may choose not to examine a candidate. In a Ph.D. thesis, a brief summary of the thesis called as "Synopsis" is sent to the prospective examiners so as to get their concurrence for evaluation of the thesis.

It is important that you make the abstract concise and include all the salient features of your research. There is usually a word restriction for abstracts and it ranges between 300 and 500 words depending on the type of work. While writing Masters or Ph.D. dissertations, you presume background knowledge of the subject for the reader and it is not necessary to explain terminologies or scientific terms. Tables, images, illustrations and references are not included in the abstract. The verb tense should be in the past tense as you are describing what was done. The only section where you might use a future tense is when you outline the scope for further research or what this research might lead to. It is important to use the same structure as the main dissertation for the abstract and should include all the elements albeit in a condensed form. It is a common mistake to not dedicate enough space for the results in the abstract. At least half of your abstract should be about what you found and interpreting the results [3].

The key points to cover in the abstract include:

- What is the background to your research?
- What body of evidence already exists in the area studied?
- What was the question you were trying to answer?
- Was there a hypothesis and, if so, were you testing the null or alternative hypothesis?
- How was the research carried out, i.e., materials and methodologies?
- What were the results?
- How did you ascertain that your results were significant?
- What statistical tests did you use to come to a conclusion?
- How have the results of your research contributed to the area of the study?
- What are the future research prospects in this area?

The abstract is usually written at the end of writing the dissertation since it is a summary of the work. Summarising the dissertation in an abstract form adhering to the word count can be a challenge and frequently a number of drafts are required before the perfect, final version can be produced. It might be useful to look at other dissertations and their abstracts to get an idea. The information in the abstract should only be what is contained in the rest of the dissertation and no new information should be introduced. The abstract frequently form the first page of the dissertation but the page number is written in lowercase Roman numeral. Likewise, the pagination for the information listed in the Table of Contents is also in lowercase Roman numerals. The pagination in Western-Arabic (also known as Hindu-Arabic) numeral will start only from the first chapter of the dissertation. Figure 1 shows how to prepare an abstract.

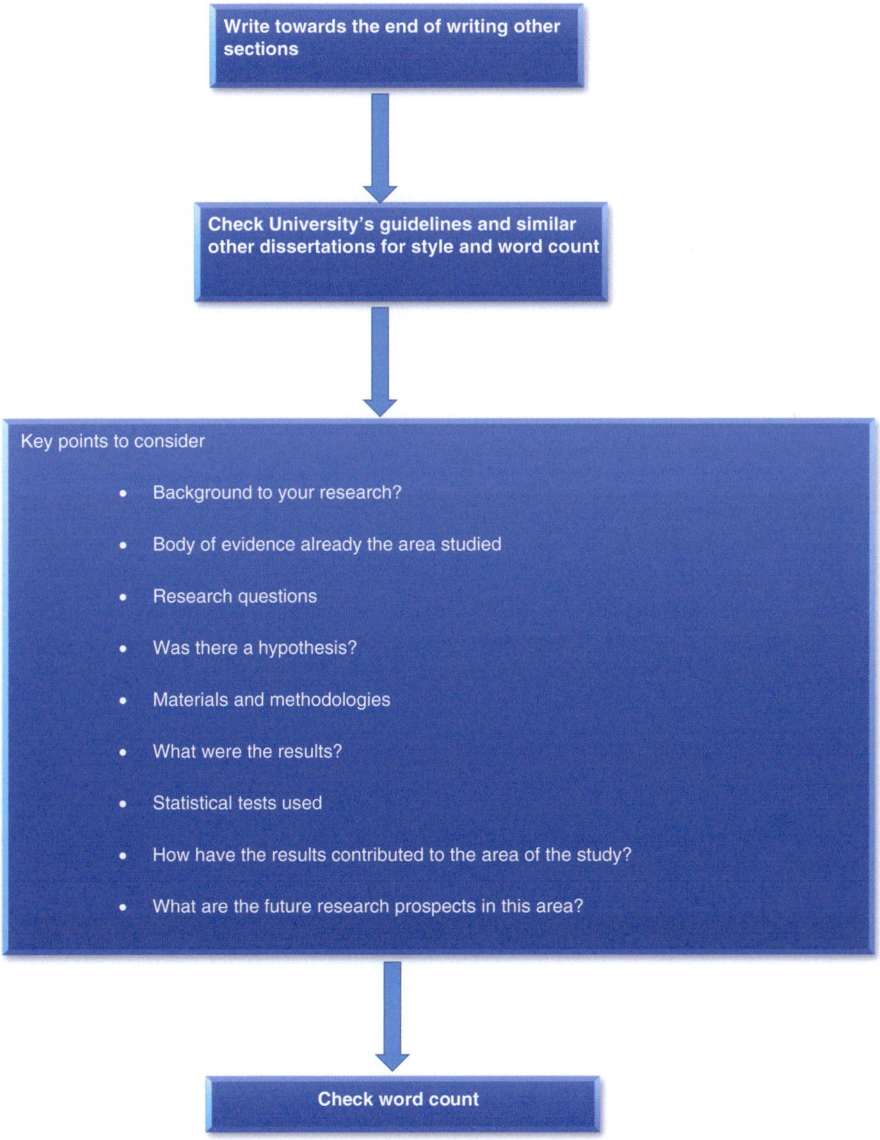

Fig. 1 Flow chart showing how to prepare an abstract

Table of Contents

The Table of Contents lists the contents contained within the dissertation with pagination. It helps the examiners and readers to find the information easily. There are several templates for these available from online resources. It can also be formatted in Microsoft® word, Mac OS X or Linux/Unix using one of the available standard templates. The Table of Contents page frequently follows the Abstract page and Acknowledgements. As such, the pagination for the Table of Contents will start at lowercase Roman numeral 'ii' or 'iii'.

The usual sequence for the Table of Contents page is as follows:

1. Abstract (page i)
2. Personal Statement and Acknowledgements (page ii)
3. List of Contents (All subsections of the dissertation including chapter titles and sections) (pages iii—any relevant number)
   (a) Chapter 1 and subsections listed as 1.1., 1.1.1, 1.1.2 etc
   (b) Chapter 2 and subsections listed as 2.1., 2.1.1, 2.1.2 etc
   (c) Chapter 3 and subsections listed as 3.1., 3.1.1, 3.1.2 etc
   (d) Chapter 4 and subsections listed as 4.1., 4.1.1, 4.1.2 etc
   (e) Chapter 5 and subsections listed as 5.1., 5.1.1, 5.1.2 etc
   (f) Chapter 6 and subsections listed as 6.1., 6.1.1, 6.1.2 etc
   (g) Any further chapters as relevant
4. List of Tables
5. List of Figures
6. List of Illustrations
7. List of Videos
8. List of any other Accompanying Material
9. Abbreviations
10. Appendices
11. Bibliography
12. Index

This sequence is only a guide and can vary between different universities. If there are no specific guidelines the candidates may discuss with their supervisor for advice.

If the dissertation has more than one volume, then the Table of Contents are written separately for each volume although pagination is continuous for all the volumes. The Title page is the first page of the dissertation but the page number is not listed. The pagination, therefore, starts from the abstract page as described earlier.

In summary, these three sections, which form the initial part of the dissertation, are important as they create the first impression on the reader. It is important to be aware of the formatting guidelines of individual universities while preparing these.

Case Scenarios

1. You are writing the Title page for your dissertation. Which amongst the following will you not include in the Title page?
   (a) Your surname
   (b) Your academic credentials
   (c) Your membership with professional bodies
   (d) The Institution in which the work was carried out
   (e) The month and year during which it is submitted for examination
2. You are preparing an abstract for your Ph.D. dissertation. Which of the following sections will you not include in the abstract?
   (a) Background of your research
   (b) Research question
   (c) Methodology
   (d) Results
   (e) Key References

References

1. https://learn.solent.ac.uk/mod/book/view.php?id=2744&chapterid=1272
2. http://www.graduateschool.colostate.edu/documents/Dissertation-Title-Page.pdf
3. https://www.sfu.ca/~jcnesbit/HowToWriteAbstract.htm

Methods and Materials in a Thesis

Sanjay Gupta

The real purpose of scientific method is to make sure nature hasn't misled you into thinking you know something you actually don't know.—Robert M. Pirsig

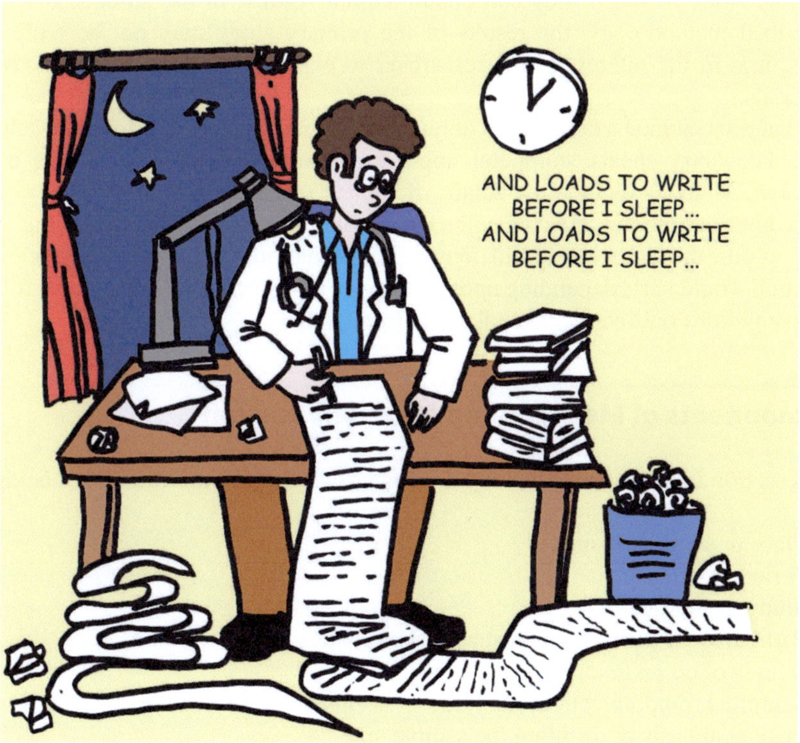

S. Gupta
Director Professor and Head, Department of Surgery, University College of Medical Sciences, New Delhi, India

S. C. Parija, V. Kate (eds.), *Thesis Writing for Master's and Ph.D. Program*,
https://doi.org/10.1007/978-981-13-0890-1_13

Key Points

- Clearly written methods and materials is the first step to good scientific research.
- Enough details should be provided about the cases, controls and methods to permit replication of study by other researchers.
- Adherence to ethical guidelines must be ensured in the proposed research.
- The basis of calculating the sample size and proposed analysis of results should be valid and clearly defined.

Introduction

A fundamental essential of all scientific research is that it is transparent and its results are independently verifiable. A study may claim path-breaking results, but if the methodology used to achieve those results is vague in its details, the scientific community would not readily accept it. As is usually the case with any scientific research, especially the ones that claim different outcome, peers attempt to duplicate the study to see if they can obtain similar results. In the absence of clearly described methodology, the results of the primary study may not be replicated. Thus, it is in the interest of the researcher to explain all aspects of methods and materials.

Materials include a description of human or animal subjects, instruments, chemicals, data entry sheets, computer applications and other similar aspects of the research. Methods include the details of subject selection, the tests/investigations/procedures carried out, the data collection techniques and statistical handling of the data. While the exact details of materials and methods section of any scientific research would vary, depending upon the type of study being carried out, the following paragraphs outline the general guidelines.

Components of Methods and Materials Section

This section includes the following details, usually in the order described below:

- Place or setting of study
- Period of study
- Study design
- Particulars of the subjects/materials in the study
- Details of comparison group, if any
- Sampling, randomization, allotment concealment and blinding
- Statistical basis of deciding the sample size
- Consent and ethical committee approval
- Details of intervention/procedure done
- Outcome measures
- Data management and statistical analysis

Place or Setting of Study

When writing a thesis, it is customary to mention the name and place of the institution where the research was conducted. However, when writing for a journal, the guidelines prescribed by the journal need to be followed. Some journals discourage naming the institution in this section [1], though this policy is debatable. Identifying the place of study lends credibility to the research, especially if the work has been carried out in an institution with good standing for scientific research. Naming the setting of the study also gives an idea about the likely ethnic and socio-demographic profile of the subjects, which is important when the peers wish to duplicate the research.

Period of Study

The materials and methods section should include the starting and ending dates, especially for clinical studies. The reader can interpret the results in the context of the period of study. As an example, a study done for the efficacy and side effects of a new drug soon after it has become available, may have a different outcome from a study done much later, when the drug has become established in its therapeutic use. This difference may occur because dosing and indications for the drug may change over time. Similarly, the duration is an important parameter in follow-up studies. For instance, the result of a study for efficacy of a newly introduced surgical technique for hernia repair, conducted over a period of 18 months, is likely to be viewed with skepticism. This is because the recurrences following hernia repair may occur much later in the postoperative period. The same study, when conducted over 10 years, is likely to be much more credible.

Study Design

Choosing an appropriate study design, to address a research question most effectively, is of utmost importance. However, when writing the study design in the materials and methods section, the details to be included depend upon the publication. For most journal articles, naming the study design is sufficient. For more exhaustive research publication, such as a thesis, the justification for choosing a particular study design is often included. Table 1 shows a summary of study designs and their indications.

Details of Subjects/Material Included in the Study [3]

Inclusion criteria are those characteristics which a potential subject must possess for recruitment into the study. The aim of writing the inclusion criteria is to define the study population and ensure uniformity of the subjects recruited. The subjects could

Table 1 Study designs [2]

Broad category	Characteristics	Types of study	Most suitable to
Experimental study	• Researcher manipulates exposure • Comparison group present	• RCT • Non-RCT	• Describe association • Determine causality
Observational - Analytical	• Researcher only measures exposure • Comparison group present	Cross-sectional	• Measure disease prevalence
		Case-control	• Identify multiple exposures • Describe association
		Cohort study	• Measure disease incidence • Identify multiple exposures • Identify multiple outcomes • Describe association • Determine causality
Observational - Descriptive	• Researcher only measures exposure • No comparison group	• Case reports • Case series • Surveys	• Give idea about a disease or its prevalence

be human, animal, body fluid or tissue. In human studies, the details should include age, gender, ethnicity, the population from which the subjects are selected (hospital/community-based) and the disease being studied.

It is important to define the disease condition. For instance, only mentioning 'wound infection' or 'peritonitis' as inclusion criteria are not sufficient. Wound infection could range from inflammation of wound edges to frankly purulent wound discharge. Similarly, 'peritonitis' could be interpreted differently by two clinicians. The issue is best resolved by adhering to the standard definition of diseases. If there is no unanimity in the literature regarding the precise definition of a disease condition, then the definition chosen by the researcher should be spelt out, preferably with supporting references.

Exclusion characteristics apply to those subjects who meet the criteria for inclusion. These features, if present, either interfere with the result of the research or expose the prospective subject to the likelihood of harm. For instance, subjects younger or older than a defined age may be excluded from a drug trial because of a greater risk of toxicity in these individuals. Similarly, people suffering from renal or hepatic dysfunction may be excluded from drug trials. Inability to give a valid consent may be yet another criterion for exclusion from a study. The investigator must be ready to provide a rationale for the inclusion or exclusion criteria chosen for the research.

A common mistake in listing the exclusion criteria is to name those characteristics which would have prevented the subject from being considered for inclusion in the first place. Thus, 'obesity' would not be exclusion criteria in a study of nutritional supplements in 'underweight children.' However, the presence of 'milk intolerance' could be valid exclusion criteria in this study.

Table 2 Correct and wrong grouping of inclusion criteria

Correct order	Illogical order
1. Stage I breast cancer	1. Total serum albumin ≥2.5 g/dL
2. Karnofsky performance scale = 90	2. Age ≥ 21 years
3. Age ≥ 21 years	3. Karnofsky performance scale = 90
4. Total serum bilirubin ≤1.2 mg/dL	4. Stage I breast cancer
5. Total serum albumin ≥2.5 g/dL	5. Total serum bilirubin ≤1.2 mg/dL

It is preferable to write inclusion criteria as positive statements. For instance, if the research is planned in nonpregnant women, it is advisable to write 'pregnancy' as exclusion criteria rather than writing 'non-pregnant' as inclusion criteria. When writing the inclusion criteria, the order should be logical and similar parameters should be listed together (Table 2).

Comparison Group

A control group is present in experimental studies, where it is treated differently from the intervention group. While the intervention group receives the treatment under study, the control group receives one of the following: no treatment, placebo, different dose, or different treatment. Except for this, the comparison group should match the intervention group in all the other aspects.

In observational analytical studies such as the case-control study, the control group comprises of the individuals who have had similar exposure to risk factors but do not have the disease. For example, while studying the risk factors for developing urinary bladder cancer in workers in the chemical industry, controls could be those employees who have worked for a similar period but are free from the disease.

Unlike the experimental studies, where the controls are randomly chosen from the group of individuals suffering from the disease, selecting controls for the case-control studies is more challenging and needs greater care. While population-based controls are ideal, there are logistic problems in choosing them. Instead, controls are selected from hospitalized individuals, family members or volunteers. Care is needed, when hospitalized people are taken as controls, to ensure that the concurrent condition, for which the control is hospitalized, does not confound the study. As far as possible, the control group should match the intervention group regarding age, gender, ethnicity and sociodemographic profile. The size of control and intervention groups should match.

Sampling, Randomization, Allotment Concealment and Blinding

In an ideal situation, all the subjects of the population should be included in the study to get the most accurate result. However, as this is not practical, a sample is chosen from the population for the conduct of the research. The study sample is selected from the population by different sampling methods. The sampling method could be random or non-random. In random sampling, each subject in the study population has an equal chance of getting selected. Such a sampling could be done using random number tables. Random sampling methods are suitable for community-based research, where the study population is present in a defined area at a given time. On the other hand, for most of the hospital-based clinical studies non-random sampling methods are more suitable, as all the subjects are not available at the same time. They are recruited over a period, as and when they present themselves to the hospital for treatment. Table 3 gives the features of these two sampling methods and their subtypes.

An experimental study, such as a drug trial, randomizes the subjects into treatment and control groups. This randomization could be done using a random number table or a randomizer application. The entire study population could be randomized at once (simple randomization) or could be divided into smaller blocks (block randomization). Thus, the cases and controls at any point in time are relatively equal in number. This method is especially useful if the condition is uncommon, the study population is small, or the study is prematurely terminated.

While randomization of subjects into intervention and control groups is essential, it is equally important to conceal from the researcher, the study group allocated to a subject. This may be done using opaque and sealed envelopes, or allocation by a person independent from the study. In the absence of allocation concealment, the researcher may knowingly or otherwise influence the selection of subjects into intervention or control group.

Just as randomization and allocation concealment minimize the bias at the time of treatment allocation, blinding reduces the bias while recording the results and

Table 3 Sampling methods [2]

Broad category	Sub-types	Features
Random (probability) sampling	Simple	• Subjects are selected one at a time, using draw of lots or random number table
	Systematic	• Sampling technique is devised in a way that all the subjects are randomly selected at one go
	Cluster	• The population is divided into homogeneous groups. The study population is selected from any one group using simple or systematic sampling technique
	Stratified	• The study population is stratified based on characteristics such as age, gender or severity of the disease. Subjects are randomly selected from each stratum
Non-random (non-probability) sampling	Convenience	• Subjects selected according to researcher's convenience • No specific selection criteria
	Purposive	• Subjects selected according to researcher's convenience • Selection based on a list of selection criteria
	Quota	• Sampling stops once a certain number of subjects are recruited • Sampling done in a non-random fashion

evaluating the outcome. Depending upon the feasibility, the subjects could be unaware of their study group (single blinding) or both the subject and the researcher may be unaware whether the subject is allocated intervention or control group (double blinding). It is imperative to mention the details of the techniques of sampling, randomization, allocation concealment and blinding, when applicable.

Deciding the Sample Size

The outcome of a research study and its extrapolation to the general population is predominantly based on statistical methods. In a well-done study, the results are fairly representative and applicable to the larger population. The materials and methods section should define the basis for arriving at a given sample size for the proposed study.

The prior information needed to calculate the sample size includes the study design, nature of variable under evaluation, an estimate of the expected outcome and the desired level of precision. There are computer applications available which calculate the sample size, once the required values are put in the program. The sample size needs to be an adjustment for dropouts or covariates. Some of this information is based on previous similar studies, which should be cited at this stage. For pilot studies, which are novel and for which no prior data is available, sample size calculation is not necessary [2, 4–6].

Since most of the theses for a postgraduate medical course are completed within a limited timeframe, it may not be feasible to recruit the calculated number of subjects during the available time. Under such circumstances, the researcher must first calculate the sample size and then explain why a lesser number of subjects are proposed to be included in the study. It should be understood that the outcome of such a study is not valid and generalizable.

Ethical Considerations and Informed Consent

It is mandatory for all human and animal research to conform to guidelines issued by the regulatory bodies. Templates for informed consent are available at the World Health Organization web page [7]. Indian Council of Medical Research has published a document which describes the ethical considerations relating to human research [8].

In the materials and methods section, it only needs a mention that the subjects gave informed consent to participate in the study and the institutional committee has cleared the research proposal. Some journals compulsorily require registration of the research project with the clinical trial registry. For clinical trials in India, the plan requires registration at the website of Clinical Trials Registry—India (CTRI). [www.ctri.nic.in/] The consent certificate, patient information sheet, and institutional ethics committee certificate should be included in the annexures.

The consent form suggested by the WHO has two parts: participant information sheet and consent document. The patient information sheet broadly consists of the following details:

- Name, contact information and institutional affiliation of the principal investigator.
- Details about the research proposal in language easily understood by the participant.
- The reason for selecting the participant.
- Possible risks, benefits, and compensation for the participant.
- Permission to use and share results without breaching confidentiality.
- The option of withdrawing from the study at any point.

Some of the general principles in biomedical research include:

- The need to conduct human clinical trial is essential as there is no other option.
- The participants should have given a voluntary informed consent.
- There is non-exploitation of the participants due to any reason.
- Ensuring the privacy and confidentiality of the participants at all times.
- Due care and precaution must be maintained at all times to minimize the risks to the participant.
- Preserving and dissemination the records relating to the research in the public domain, for the benefit of all.
- The researcher must take full responsibility for the conduct of the study according to the guidelines.

Details of the Intervention/Procedure Done

After having described the subjects, the next step is to give details of the data collection, intervention and follow-up, if any. The data collected could be in the form of demographic details, clinical history and examination, questionnaire, laboratory investigations, radiological tests, molecular biology techniques and others. For using a standard data collection procedure, giving reference to the source of information is sufficient. However, a modification of a technique or a new method should be described in detail, to enable the readers to duplicate it.

In experimental studies, the exact particulars of the intervention should be described. The units of measurement, evaluation scales, laboratory kits and instruments used should be mentioned. In follow up studies, the frequency of follow up and data collection should be described. This information is often best given in the form of a flowchart. At times, it may be advisable to provide the details of the procedure as an annexure.

Outcome Measures

All medical research starts with a research question and a hypothesis. The study is designed in a way to answer the research question most effectively. Depending upon the objective of the study, the research question may be about the efficacy of a treatment modality, risk factors or causation of a disease, sensitivity, and specificity of a diagnostic modality or prevalence or incidence of a disease condition.

The researcher must identify at the outset, the one result of the study which will answer the research question. For instance, in a study of the effectiveness of a new antibiotic in surgical prophylaxis, the incidence of postoperative wound infection would be the primary outcome measure. Similarly, in a case-control study of the association of pesticide exposure to breast cancer, serum levels of pesticide in cases and controls would be the primary outcome measure.

A study may aim to explore more than one parameter. For example, in the previously mentioned study of the effectiveness of a new antibiotic for surgical prophylaxis, the researcher may also plan to explore the cost and the safety of the medicine. The latter goals of the study are called secondary outcome measures. Identification of the primary outcome measure is necessary because it is used for calculation of the sample size. While a study may have many secondary outcomes, it is preferable to have a single primary outcome.

Data Management and Statistical Analysis

The researcher must describe the type of data expected at the end of the study period. The proposed statistical tests to be applied and the possible computer application to be used for the statistical analysis must also be mentioned at this stage. It is possible that the data obtained at the end of the study period may turn out to be different from the one expected at the beginning. For instance, the distribution of the data may be skewed, while the tests were proposed for normally distributed data. Under such circumstances, the researcher may apply the appropriate statistical tests, which may be different from those planned at the start of the study. The reason for such a change must be explained, especially in a research thesis. Figure 1 shows a plan for the research methodology.

General Guidelines for Writing the Materials and Methods Section

Following are the broad guidelines to be followed while writing this section:

- This section is written in future tense at the proposal stage. On completion, at the time of reporting, either as a journal article or as a thesis, past tense is used.
- Enough details should be provided, preferably with references, to enable other researchers to replicate the study.
- All the data proposed to be collected in this section should be presented in the results section. It is important that the results must not give data for which there is no proposal in the materials and methods section. Similarly, it is to be ensured that no data proposed in materials and methods are missing from the results

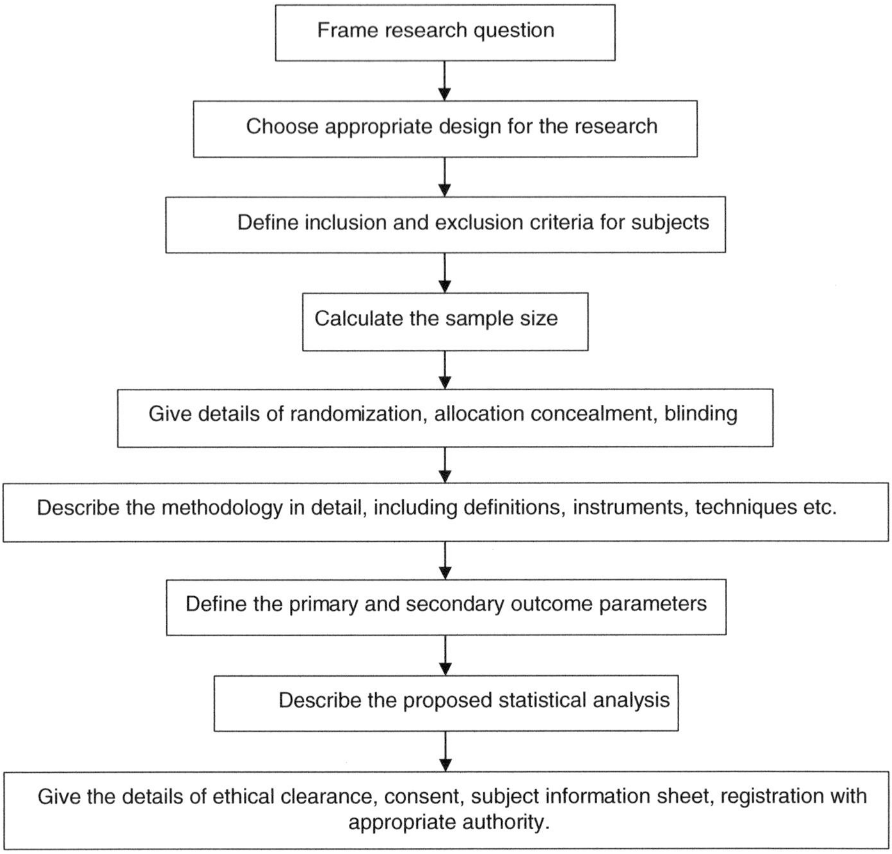

Fig. 1 Flowchart for research methodology

section. It may occasionally happen that the researcher may not be able to carry out all the components of proposed study due to unforeseen events, such as non-availability of some equipment or laboratory test. Under these circumstances, the reason for deviation from the proposal must be explained.

In conclusion, materials and methods section lays down the framework for conduct of research, not only for the peers but also for the researcher as well. Precisely written methodology ensures reproducible results and valid outcome.

Case Scenarios

1. What is wrong with the following inclusion and exclusion criteria?
   "The inclusion criteria were patients with painless hematuria, histologically proven grade 1 transitional cell carcinoma of urinary bladder and normal renal functions. Patients with painful hematuria, grade 2 and 3 transitional cell carcinoma and deranged renal function were excluded from the study."

2. Which of the following study designs needs the smallest sample size?
   (a) Descriptive study.
   (b) Experimental study with crossover design.
   (c) Experimental design with a control group.
   (d) Experimental study in a single group with pre and post type of design.

References

1. Erdemir F. How to write a materials and methods section of a scientific article? Turk J Urol. 2013;39(Suppl 1):10–5.
2. Ab Rahman J. Brief guidelines for methods and statistics in medical research. Singapore: Springer; 2015. p. 7–10.
3. Gupta P, Singh N. How to write the thesis and thesis protocol A primer for medical, dental and nursing courses. New Delhi: Jaypee Brothers; 2014. p. 75–82.
4. Chow SC, Wang H, Shao J. Sample size calculations in clinical research. New York: CRC Press; 2007. p. 6–21.
5. Biggam J. Succeeding with your master's dissertation: a step-by-step handbook. London: McGraw-Hill Education (UK); 2015. p. 88–91.
6. Patra P. Sample size in clinical research, the number we need. Int J Med Sci Public Health. 2012;1(1):5–9.
7. World Health Organization Informed Consent Form Template for Clinical Studies. Available from: http://www.who.int/rpc/research_ethics/informed_consent/en/.
8. Ganguly NK, Geeta J, Roli M, Valiathan MS. Ethical guidelines for biomedical research on human participants. New Delhi: ICMR; 2006. p. 2–7.

Writing the Review of Literature in a Thesis

A. M. Quraishi

If I have seen further than others, it is by standing upon the shoulders of giants.—Isaac Newton

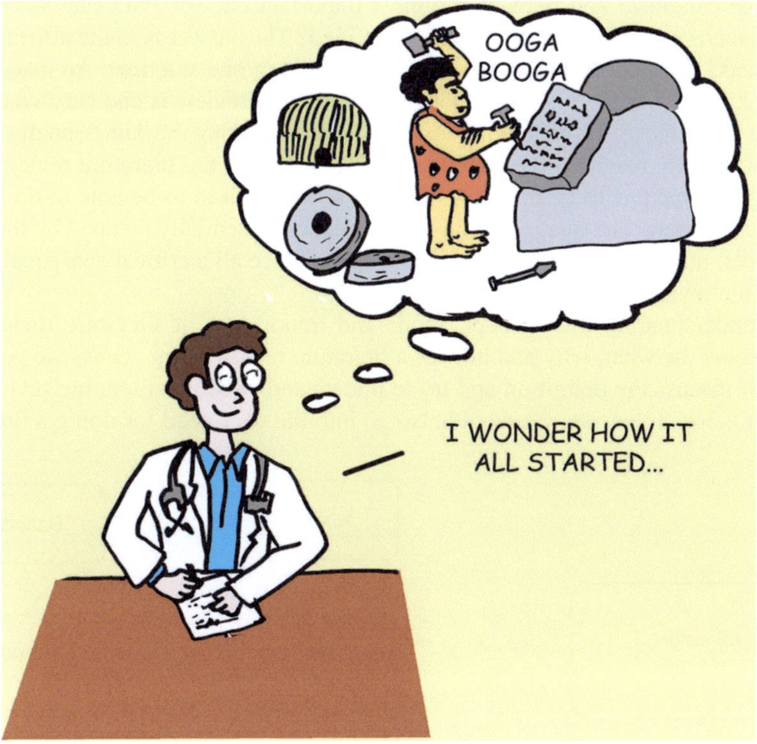

A. M. Quraishi
Professor, Department of Surgery, Government Medical College, Nagpur, India

S. C. Parija, V. Kate (eds.), *Thesis Writing for Master's and Ph.D. Program*,
https://doi.org/10.1007/978-981-13-0890-1_14

Key Points

- Literature review is the search and critical appraisal of existing literature on a topic.
- It helps in formulating a research question after finding a knowledge gap.
- The research topic provides the roadmap to literature search.
- Literature search sources are scanned with the help of search tools.
- The retrieved data is put through the sieve of PICO format to shortlist articles.
- The literature is critically appraised analysed and synthesised.
- The results are compared and contrasted.
- The literature review is organised and written systematically.
- The knowledge gaps are highlighted and scope for future research brought out.

Introduction

Thesis writing is a daunting task. It is one of the greatest challenges for a postgraduate candidate and perhaps the most important one for PhD candidates. The question is, can the whole exercise be simplified? The answer is in the affirmative if one breaks it into different parts and deals with them one at a time. An insight into the making of a thesis makes the job easy. Literature review is one very vital component of the thesis. From picking up the topic to collecting the data to analysing the result to finally reaching the conclusions one has to do the literature review again and again. One has to be diligent, focussed and organised to be able to do a good literature review. The quality of the final product is essentially decided by the reading skills, note-taking, organised approach and above all a critical analytical thinking of the reviewer.

In understanding the concept, scope and importance of literature review one must know the what, why and how of a literature review? (Fig. 1). As we go along we will discuss the definition and try to understand what is a literature review and what it is not. Likewise, we would also go into the very need for doing a literature

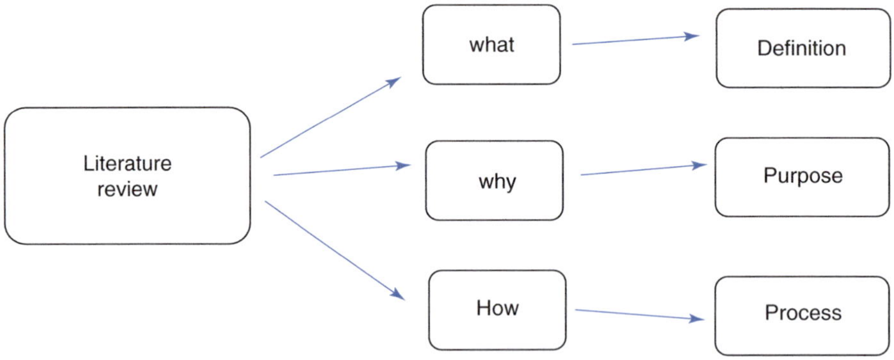

Fig. 1 What, why and how of literature review

review. Last but most importantly we will see how a literature review has to be actually done. This would include literature search strategies, analysis of the relevant literature, synthesis of the findings and organisation of the literature review. In the later section, we would also discuss the pitfalls and how they should be avoided.

What Is a Literature Review?

A literature review is an objective, thorough summary and critical analysis of the relevant available research and non-research literature on the topic being studied [1]. This analysis finally leads to what is known on the said topic and identifies what is not known. It thus finds the knowledge gap and brings forth areas where research can be done. This is how one finds a research question. The answer to the question is sought by analysing the literature in the light of the new insights from our own study. It thus opens a window of opportunity for original contribution to the existing knowledge.

A good literature review compares and contrasts existing knowledge about a topic. One must understand that it is not just a summary of literature or an annotated bibliography. It is a more encompassing concept which includes selection of topic, collection of data and summarising of the gathered data. But most importantly it is the critical appraisal of the collected literature.

Depending on the approach to the collection of data, its analysis and presentation we have different types of literature reviews. These include the traditional or narrative literature review and the more detailed systematic review. Meta-analysis and meta-synthesis involve complexities of statistics and are thought to be research in their own right.

What Are the Different Types of Literature Reviews?

There are many different types of literature reviews. Many different names are used to describe literature reviews but in actuality there is an overlap of all types which means they are not mutually exclusive. It is necessary to understand the elements of various types of reviews to be able to critically analyse published literature. If a review is described as a systematic type of review one must know what parameters make it so. If the review, which is, claiming to be a systematic review fails to come up to those parameters, the same can be criticised on that account. It is also important, while you are conducting a review, to know the requirements of various types of reviews. Thus, we must know the features of each one of them.

Essentially all types of literature reviews entail collecting, evaluating and presenting of data. The difference lies between the structured approach to a topic with a range from least structured to the most structured reviews. Although they are described by different names which are loosely applied, there is a lack of consistency in definition [2]. There is no 'ideal' type of literature review and appropriate methodology has to be employed depending on the focus of the study.

Traditional Review

Traditional review is also known as narrative or descriptive review. Its aim is to identify, analyse and interpret literature on a topic. It does not follow a rigorous methodology. However, in the age of evidence-based practice some basic standards of methodology have to be followed. Such reviews are sometimes labelled as 'systematic'. It only means that there has been some attempt to follow a methodology of search and analysis but it is nowhere near an actual systematic review which follows rigorous protocols of search and analysis.

Narrative reviews are often done for thesis and dissertation to justify the choice of topic or as a part of proposals for funding where it is used to find knowledge gaps. It can also be a part of a chapter of a book to describe the state of existing data on a topic. By and large these reviews are less specific as compared to the systematic review.

Systematic Review

The practice of evidence-based medicine has made it mandatory for systematic reviews to be conducted for evidence-based practice guidelines. The knowledge boom brought about by the information on the internet has made it all the more imperative that the relevant literature be reviewed critically and systematically to come out with evidence-based solutions for clinical issues.

The Systematic review is different from other types of reviews in the fact that it follows a rigorous protocol methodology and is precise and transparent. A clear policy of inclusion and exclusion is made before embarking on the review. This not only helps in retrieving relevant data but also reduces the selection bias leading to more credible evidence on the topic. Generally systematic review includes randomised control trials (RCT) as they are considered to be on the highest level in the hierarchy of evidence. However, in certain clinical situations RCTs are difficult to conduct and may even be unethical. Thus, reviews may include studies other than RCTs [3].

Meta-analysis

Meta-analysis is the statistical analysis of the results of the pooled data of individual studies. For undertaking meta-analysis, the studies must have methodology, populations and outcome which are homogenous [4]. Meta-analysis gives strength of evidence to effectiveness of an intervention. Meta-analysis also resolves the controversies arising out of conflicting claims and results from individual studies [5].

What Is the Purpose of Doing a Literature Review?

There are multiple purposes of doing a literature review. They are as follows:

1. To evaluate the contribution of various works to the understanding of the topic.
2. To bring forth the relation of one work to that of others on the topic.
3. To identify what has already been said on a topic.
4. To identify gaps in the existing research.
5. To identify conflicts and contradictions in previous studies.
6. To contextualise your own work in the existing literature.
7. To find areas of future research on the topic.

Steps in Literature review

Although it is depicted as though the literature review follows a linear step by step pattern one must understand that this perception is far from true. This means although the focussed literature search on a topic starts after the topic is selected, the topic selection itself entails a fair amount of literature search. One would realize that more than anything else it boils down to good reading ability and critical thinking on a focussed topic (Fig. 2).

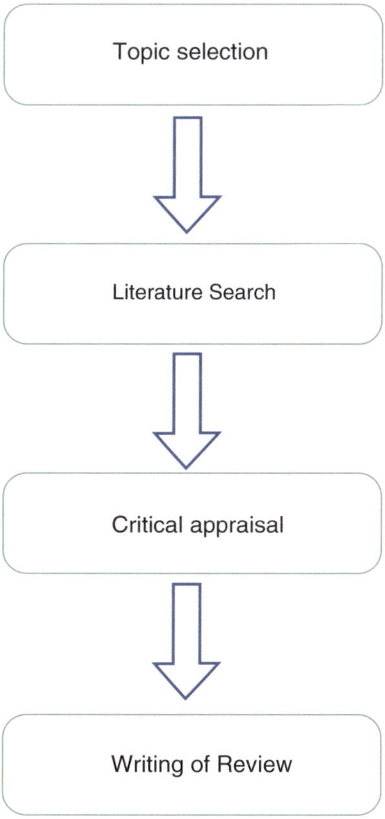

Fig. 2 Steps of literature of review

Topic Selection

A literature review has to be approached systematically. Usually the search starts with the selection of the topic of research and framing of a research question. The following aspects need to be considered while selecting a topic.

1. It should be of interest to you
2. It should be of clinical relevance
3. It should be focussed

For a post-graduate student in surgery this may start with search on laparoscopic groin hernia repair. One of the laparoscopic approaches to groin hernia is Trans-Abdominal Pre-peritoneal (TAPP) repair. The guide may ask the student to find something relevant and important to work on this topic. During the preliminary search, the student is likely to come across various studies covering various aspects of laparoscopic groin hernia repair. These studies may be on open versus laparoscopic groin hernia or they may be on comparisons of the two different laparoscopic techniques trans-abdominal pre-peritoneal repair (TAPP) versus total extra-peritoneal repair (TEP) of groin hernia. He will also find that the two most important outcome measures are recurrence of hernia and chronic groin pain. This would lead him to the topic of fixation of prosthetic mesh versus non-fixation. A related topic could be tacking of mesh versus use of fibrin glue. Thus, a focussed research question would be "*Does use of fibrin glue for fixation of mesh reduce chronic groin pain after TAPP repair for groin hernia*". A secondary question would be does the use of fibrin glue have any adverse effects. Thus, selection of topic would depend on the interest of the guide, availability of trained staff and availability of reasonable number of patients for the proposed study and its clinical relevance. The research question is the roadmap to literature search. The research question can be formulated using the PICO format (Fig. 3).

P—Population being studied
I—Intervention done during the study
C—Comparison
O—Outcome measures

Literature Search

Sarah Gash has defined literature search as '*a systematic and thorough search of all types of published literature in order to identify as many items as possible that are relevant to a particular topic*' [6].

The literature review provides an in-depth view of a topic. For this purpose, literature search and data collection are crucial. The literature search must have inclusion and exclusion criteria so that only relevant data is collected. The number of years should also be defined. For example, one may collect data of past five years. Although this does not prevent one from quoting important seminal work of the past

Fig. 3 Formulation of a research question

Primary Question

Does mesh fixation with fibrin glue reduce chronic pain in TAPP repair for groin hernia?

⇩

Secondary Question

What are the adverse effects of fibrin glue fixation of mesh?

⇩

The search elements (PICO)

Population- Adult patients of groin hernia

Intervention- Laparoscopic TAPP repair

Comparison - Fibrin glue versus tacking

Outcome- Chronic groin pain/recurrence/ other adverse events

in the review. Literature search helps in finding areas of consensus as well as disagreement. It also leads the researcher to gaps in literature leading to potential of adding a new perspective to the topic. The reviewer should take down notes regarding the methodology which has been followed for the search. The databases and keywords used should be noted. This is essential for replicating the search and also for understanding as to how the search was done.

There are many databases which can be used to do a literature search like Medline, Cochrane library, and Embase. As a first step Medline can be used through the search engine of PubMed or Ovid. Other databases are Cochrane Database of Abstracts of Reviews of Effectiveness (DARE), PsychINFO and Cumulative Index of Nursing and Allied Health Literature (CINAHL) [7].

There are many tools for literature searching. One has to employ a suitable search strategy for one's own study. An attempt has to be made to balance between a sensitive and a specific approach. This means all relevant data has to be included by an exhaustive search but at the same time irrelevant data has to be kept to a minimum by a focussed approach. A smart use of available tools helps us to fulfil this objective.

One of the most common methods employed is the use of keywords. Keywords should be spelt properly and alternative keywords should be tried for literature search. Synonyms can be found on the thesaurus. The Cochrane database and the Medline use thesauri known as MeSH (Medical Search Headings). Many databases use "Boolean operators" like AND, OR and NOT. Boolean operators are used for expanding, excluding or joining keywords. This system was described by Graham Boole (1815–1864), the English mathematician and computer pioneer [8].

Thus, if one is performing literature search on the topic of "Mesh fixation in Groin hernia with glue", one would get about 3899 references on the PubMed as a response to the keywords, "groin hernia". If these keywords are appended by "AND mesh fixation", one would retrieve 298 references which fairly narrows the search. Similarly, one can modify the search by adding, "AND glue" to get 121 references, out of which the relevant ones can be selected. There are broadly two types of glues which are used viz. fibrin glue and cyanoacrylate glue. Since the literature has references for both, a search with the keyword as "glue" would retrieve references of both. If one wants to narrow the search with only fibrin glue, one can add "NOT cyanoacrylate. This reduces the number of references to 84. Likewise, if the guide feels fibrin glue is expensive and wants to look for the feasibility of a similar study with the cheaper cyanoacrylate glue, one can add "NOT Fibrin glue". This further reduces the number to 34. Similarly, if one wants to search literature on pressure sores one can put the keyword, "pressure sore". One would retrieve 44,025 references. If the search is to broaden one may put "OR decubitus ulcer". This reveals 44,752 references. If the guide wants the student to study on, "Role of Negative Pressure Wound Therapy (NPWT) in pressure sores", then, one can narrow the search by adding, "AND NPWT". This would give 156 references. Thus, one may have to use suitable Boolean operators with different combinations to make the search broad or narrow as desired.

Typically, literature search is conducted in a phased manner as follows:

1. Brainstorming phase—In this phase a search for all possible data is done. The search usually begins with searching on the internet databases like PubMed/ Google Scholar or Open access journals. The reviewer may find it easy to zero in on a few important journal articles and pick up relevant articles from the references of these articles. This is described as snow balling [9].
2. Evaluation phase—This phase entails refinement of literature search by accessing additional sources, contacting experts, and searching specific theme based journals for recent articles and revising search strategy. It's a good policy to consult the guide at this stage to get a feedback on the adequacy of the search done. Contacting lead players in the field through mail may be very fruitful though the yield of these efforts is often uncertain.
3. Documentation of the search process. This should be preferably in a tabular form with author, source and date format. This step helps in making the search transparent and reproducible.

Organising the Collected Literature

After the literature search, one is usually left with overwhelming amount of literature. Remaining organised is very important to deal with this situation. The first step is scanning of literature to find articles relevant to the research question. This process is usually done in a staged manner by sifting the data through various sieves. This starts by excluding articles after going through the titles; this would reduce the number of articles considerably. This is followed by reading the abstract and removing irrelevant articles. After this stage, the remaining articles are read in full and assessed for exclusion or inclusion. As the amount of data gets trimmed an inverted pyramid is formed with a vast amount of irrelevant data having been excluded (Fig. 4). The strategy of shortlisting has to be mentioned so that reasons for exclusion are known. One method to assess the studies for relevance is to gauge them on the above- mentioned PICO format. It is a good practice to save excluded material in a separate file so that if any article is required at a later date it can be retrieved.

The finalised list of articles has to be arranged preferably with the help of software like citation manager or reference manager. The articles then should be gone through thoroughly. This reading must be done systematically and a simultaneous

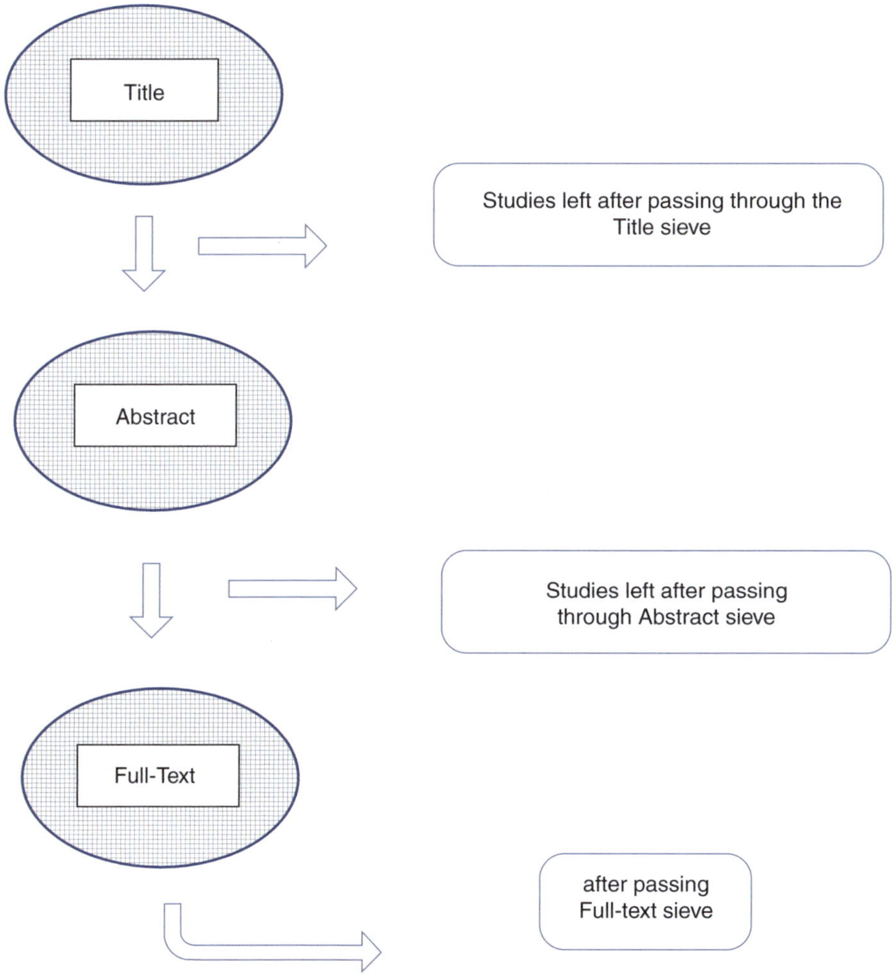

Fig. 4 Exclusion of data by staged sieving

notes-taking must be done. If one is not diligent enough on this issue one is lost with the huge amount of data and searching something again is frustrating. So, it's a good idea to have pegs to hang your clothes, so that you can find them easily.

Critical Appraisal of Literature

The next step is to group articles according to the themes and segregate them in subheadings. The articles are evaluated on the methodology and outcomes and are compared and contrasted. The review of literature should include alternative views and should try to bring forth reasons for differing outcomes of different studies. After the analysis, one may find the reason for this difference in the sample size, methodology or some other identifiable issue.

Once the studies are organised thematically they are critically appraised. The process of appraisal systematically assesses the evidence for its validity, results and relevance [9]. This is done to find the robustness and strength of the study. The limitations of the study are also identified. The limitations of the study should be minor for it to be robust. Robustness is decided on methodology and internal and external validity of a study. Internal validity means the results are true in the study setting. External validity is dependent on generalizability of the results. This means the results should also be true outside the study setting.

A detail appraisal starts from the aim of the study and goes on to evaluate different parts of the study systematically including methodology, results, appropriateness of method and data analysis employed, discussion and referencing. Each of these areas are scrutinised in all the relevant studies. The results are compared and contrasted. A data extraction table is made, to put, the type of study, the methodology employed and outcomes of all the relevant studies [10].

There are various tools for critical appraisal. These are in the form of checklists. Existing checklist from the guidelines for quality assessment can be used or a tailor-made checklist can be made. One may have to use more than one checklist when studies of different types of research designs are to be reviewed [11].

The commonly used checklists in the health field are:

CASP—Critical Appraisal Skills Programme

SIGN—Scottish Intercollegiate Guidelines Network

CEBM—Centre for Evidence Based Medicine

Cardiff University—Critical Appraisal Checklists

PRISMA—Preferred Reporting Items for Systematic Reviews and Meta-analyses

CONSORT—Consolidated Standards Of Reporting Trials. The CONSORT Statement describes minimum requirements for reporting Randomised Control Trials

STROBE—STrengthening the Reporting of OBservational studies in Epidemiology [4]

The Equator Network provides guidelines for improving reporting standards for health research.

Writing the Review of Literature

Writing of the literature review has to be done systematically and in an organised manner. It is usually done in a phased way. A rough initial draft is made and revised many times before a final draft is made. It's a good idea to have deadlines for various parts of review writing but it has to be done in a focused and unhurried manner. The reader should find a logical flow from one point to another in the review. It should appear cohesive and not dis-jointed. Typically, the review is covered in following three parts:

1. Introduction
2. Main body
3. Summary

The Introduction describes the background of the study. It contextualises the research question by briefly mentioning about the knowledge gap in existing literature. It brings forth the clinical importance of the study and the possible impact which it can have on current practice. It also mentions how the literature search has been conducted and how the review is going to be organised.

The body of the review comprises of the surveyed literature and its critical analysis and synthesis. The data is classified into themes and subheadings. It describes the background of the study along with the evidence and brings forth the justification of the study which has been undertaken.

The conclusion and summary may be clubbed together or written separately. It covers the key findings of the review in a concise manner. It describes the controversies and inconsistencies in literature and gaps in the knowledge. It also suggests scope for future research.

Pitfalls

There are some common errors while conducting a review of literature. One such mistake is to collect and summarize the collected data and not critically analyse it. This leads to only collection of information without any addition of new information. Another common error is, not to do an extensive literature search. This leads to incomplete review of the topic as there is a chance of missing important relevant information on the topic, this leads to selection bias. Bias also creeps in because the reviewer decides to include only those studies which support his or her view on the topic. Alternative views should also be included in the review to get an unbiased view of both perspectives.

Referencing and Plagiarism

Referencing is a very important part of academic writing. Laws of intellectual property right apply to all academic writing. All quoted or paraphrased material taken from other articles has to be properly referenced. If this is not done it would mean the reviewer is taking credit of an article which is written by another author, this, amounts to plagiarism, which is academic dishonesty. The original author must be given due credit by proper referencing to avoid plagiarism. The journal is also quoted along with the author, this, helps in improving the impact factor of the journal. The reader can access original articles from the references and verify the points being made or try and get a deeper insight into a particular area of study. There are two common methods of referencing. The Harvard style (author-date) which uses the author and date format, quotes bibliography in alphabetical order of author. The Vancouver style (author-number), uses citation number which is quoted in bibliography in the numerical order as it appears in the text [12].

References have two parts. One part is citing of the reference in the text and the other part is a detail reference in the list which is appended at the end of the text.

Plagiarism

Plagiarism is regarded as academic dishonesty or fraud. It amounts to breach of copyright law. Plagiarism can be of many types but most commonly an author's work is quoted without due recognition. Thus, the current author knowingly or unknowingly takes the credit of another author. Inadvertent plagiarism can be avoided by good note-keeping and proper referencing. Passing off your own previous work as new also amounts to self-plagiarisation. You can however, quote yourself with due reference of old work. Likewise, publishing research work in two different journals simultaneously is also plagiarism. The consequences are very serious if one is found guilty of plagiarism. The action could range from retraction of the study to blacklisting from the journal to informing the employer of the author which may result in loss of dignity and in some cases loss of job [13].

One must take all efforts to avoid being accused of plagiarism. The best way to achieve this goal is to cite as one writes, to follow publication guidelines and avoid the cut-paste technique. There are tools available which can help detect similarities between an article and the published literature. A few commonly used softwares are, Turnitin, Safe Assign, WCopyFind and Cross Check [14]. It's a good practice to check the degree of similarities ourselves before submitting the work for assessment.

Case Scenarios

1. You have been allotted a topic of "Pre-operative predictors of a difficult laparoscopic cholecystectomy", by your guide. What is the first step you will take?
   (a) Go and meet the most prolific Laparoscopic surgeon in town.
   (b) Try and contact someone who has done a similar thesis.
   (c) Use appropriate keywords and search the Pubmed.
2. You are doing a literature search. Comment on the appropriateness of the following actions:
   (a) Reading articles and leaving referencing for a later date.

(b) Reading articles which seem to be more interesting than your research question.
(c) Keeping deadlines for literature search.
(d) Using a referencing software.

References

1. Hart C. Doing a Literature Review. London: Sage Publications; 1998.
2. Arksey H, O'Malley L. Scoping studies: towards a methodological framework. Int J Soc Res Methodol. 2005;8(1):19–32.
3. Coughlan M, Cronin P. Doing a literature review in nursing, health and social care. London: Sage Publications; 2017.
4. Booth A, Papaioannou D, Sutton A. Systematic approaches to a successful literature review. Los Angeles, CA: Sage; 2012.
5. Higgins JPT, Green S (editors). Cochrane handbook for systematic reviews of interventions version 5.1.0. [updated March 2011]. The Cochrane collaboration. 2011.
6. Gash S. Effective literature searching for research. 2nd ed. Aldershot: Gower Publishing Ltd.; 1999.
7. Mahid SS, Hornung CA, Minor KS, Turina M, Galandiuk S. Systematic reviews and meta-analysis for the surgeon scientist. Br J Surg. 2006;93(11):1315–24.
8. SearchCIO.com Acronym and term Definitions: Boolean. http://searchcio.techtarget.com/gDefinition/0,294236,sid19_gci211695,00.html. (Last accessed: 27 Aug 2017).
9. Ridley D. The literature review: a step-by-step guide for students. Los Angeles, CA: Sage; 2012.
10. Parkes J, Hyde C, Deeks J, Milne R. Teaching critical appraisal skills in health care settings. Cochrane Database Syst Rev. 2001;3:CD001270.
11. Khalid K, Regina K, Jos K, Gerd A. Systematic reviews to support evidence-based medicine. 2nd ed. New York: CRC Press; 2011.
12. British Medical Association. Reference styles: Harvard and Vancouver. Available from: http://www.bma.org.uk/library_medline/electronic_resources/factsheets/LIBReferenceStyles.jsp [last accessed on 27 Aug 2017].
13. Das N, Panjabi M. Plagiarism: Why is it such a big issue for medical writers? Perspect Clin Res. 2011;2(2):67–71.
14. Kumar PM, Priya NS, Musalaiah S, Nagasree M. Knowing and avoiding plagiarism during scientific writing. Ann Med Health Sci Res. 2014;4(Suppl 3):S193–8. https://doi.org/10.4103/2141-9248.141957.

Drawing Observations from Data and Making Conclusions

Rajesh Panwar and Peush Sahni

It is important to get results from the experiment, but the most important is the process in getting that results.—Nik Ahmad Nizam

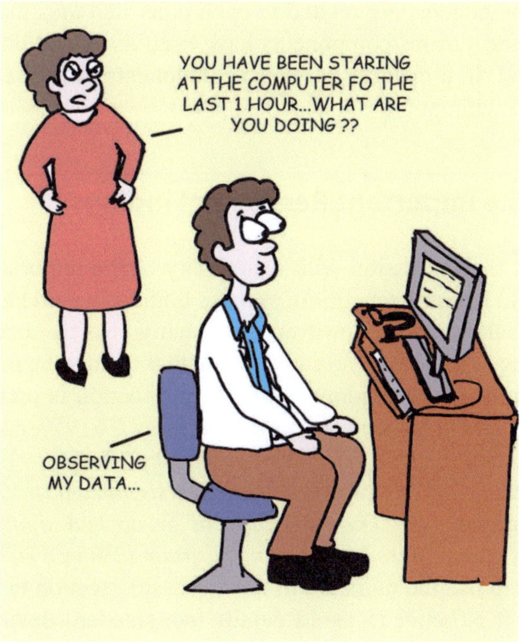

R. Panwar
Assistant Professor, Department of Gastrointestinal Surgery and Liver Transplantation, All India Institute of Medical Sciences, New Delhi, India

P. Sahni (✉)
Professor and Head, Department of Gastrointestinal Surgery and Liver Transplantation, All India Institute of Medical Sciences, New Delhi, India

S. C. Parija, V. Kate (eds.), *Thesis Writing for Master's and Ph.D. Program*,
https://doi.org/10.1007/978-981-13-0890-1_15

Key Points

- Briefly summarize the observations related to the primary and secondary objectives of the study and some other important incidental findings.
- Compare the findings with the observations from other studies in the literature and provide explanations for the differences.
- Discuss the relevance of these findings and their possible clinical impact.
- State the strengths of the study.
- State the limitations of the study and the effect of those limitations on the interpretation of the results.
- In the conclusion section, the main focus should be on the primary objective.

While the results section describes what the study found, the discussion section helps to convert those findings into meaningful observations. There are usually no set rules or order for presenting and discussing observations drawn from data. Authors often use this as a license to express their thoughts. However, there are some essential components that should always appear in this section (Table 1). Many of these components are related to each other and thus may be inseparable. For this chapter, the various components have been discussed under different subheadings. However, in a manuscript, these components may be presented together in a single section without any subheadings [1–3].

Summary of the Important Results or Findings

It is good to start the discussion with a summary of the important findings of the study. There would be some repetition, as these findings would have been presented in detail in the results section. However, it is usually possible to avoid repetition of the text by framing sentences differently and including only the most relevant information. For example, if the finding in the results section is presented as "*the in-hospital mortality rate in the experimental group was 2% (95% confidence interval: 1.3 to 2.7%) as compared to 5% (95% confidence interval: 3.9 to 6.2%) in the control group and this difference was statistically significant (p=0.001)*". This finding can be summarized as "*The experimental group had significantly lower in-hospital mortality as compared to the control group (2% vs 5%)*" in the discussion section. Whether to use the numbers in the discussion section or not is a matter of personal choice. It is better to avoid details like standard deviations, confidence

Table 1 Essential components of the discussion section

1.	Summary of the important results or findings
2.	Comparison of the obtained results with relevant literature and their explanation
3.	Importance and relevance of the findings
4.	Strengths of the study
5.	Limitations of the study

intervals and p values. However, avoiding the numbers altogether can make the discussion very bland. Providing some details such as percentages (as in the example above) adds another dimension to the findings and makes them more interesting to the reader.

The number of observations that can be included for discussion in a journal article is usually limited by the imposed word limit. Such a limitation is not there in a thesis and it is up to the authors to choose the length of the discussion section. Thus, one may choose to discuss all the findings one by one in the order in which they appear in the results section. However, doing so may actually be detrimental as the most important and relevant observations may get lost in the sea of the other 'not so' important findings. Thus, it is always better to select the most important observations and discuss them in detail.

How to Determine Which Observations Are Important?

The usual mistake that authors make is that they consider only the observations with a significant p-value as important. Most of the observations that are statistically significant would usually find a place in the discussion, however, the most important finding is the one for which the study was actually done. Thus, the observations related to the primary objective of the study should be considered most important and should be discussed first whether statistically significant or not. The secondary objectives are also important but the authors may choose to omit a few of these from the discussion especially if the index study does not add much to what is already known about them. If there are some significant incidental findings, these may also be included in the discussion, e.g. significant findings from a subgroup analysis that was not initially planned.

Comparison of the Obtained Results with Relevant Literature and Their Explanation

All the selected important findings are then discussed one at a time in the light of the available literature. A thorough review of literature done before the commencement of the study should have already discussed, in detail, most of the studies relevant to the discussion section. The authors may also choose to add some new studies that have been published after the commencement of the index study.

In the discussion section, one should try to compare the findings of the index study with other similar studies from the literature. It is not necessary to quote the results of all the studies, especially if, a large number of studies are available on the same topic. In such a situation, the authors should select some of the most relevant studies for discussion. The authors may choose studies that have included a larger number of patients or those that used inclusion criteria similar to the index study. If available, it may be more convenient to include a systematic review or a meta-analysis in the discussion as compared to individual trials.

It should, however, be understood that just quoting the results of other studies is not enough. For example, "*the success rate of the experimental treatment in our study was 70%. The study by X et al., Y et al. and Z et al. had success rates of 68%, 73% and 71% respectively which were similar to our study while the study by A et al. and B et al. had success rates of 80% & 85 % which were higher than our study*". There is more to the discussion than just stating such facts. The authors should also try to provide explanations for the similarities or differences in the observations. The explanation should ideally be based on other findings from the index study or known facts from the literature. A possible explanation for the contrasting results in the above example would be "*the higher success rates in the studies by A et al. and B et al. may be due to the fact that they had only included treatment naïve patients while we and other studies with lower success rate also included a significant number of patients who had failed the initial treatment*". Speculative explanations may also be used but only if no other reasonable explanation could be derived from the study or the available literature. These speculations should have some biological basis and should generate a hypothesis, which could be tested in further studies. For example, "*all studies with higher success rates were from southern India while those with lower success rates (including our study) were from northern India. So, the difference in the success rates may be due to the prevalence of different strains of the causative organism in the two regions*".

Sometimes, it may not be possible to provide any logical explanation for an observation. The best approach, in such cases, is to acknowledge this and move on.

Importance and Relevance of the Findings

After comparing the results with the literature, the authors should try to explain what impact the knowledge gained from the present study would have on the future management of the problem that was studied and whether the study provides a novel finding or reconfirms the previously known results. The authors should state what new insights the study has brought and whether the current practice should change on the basis of the results of the study. For example, "*In this randomized controlled trial, we found that drug A has a significantly higher success rate as compared to drug B in the management of gastroesophageal reflux disease (GERD). So, drug A should replace drug B as the drug of choice for GERD.*"

A strong study has a much higher potential for bringing about a change in clinical practice as compared to a weak study. A large randomized controlled trial or a meta-analysis of randomized controlled trials is much more likely to change clinical practice as compared to a non-randomized or a retrospective study. However, the clinical impact of a study also depends on the quality of evidence that is already available. A study that provides a higher level of evidence than the available literature is more likely to change practice. If there were only case reports and short case series on a topic, even a retrospective study would bring a higher level of evidence and thus may have an impact on management. On the other hand, even a randomized trial may not change practice if there are larger randomized trials or meta-analysis available on the same topic. Thus, the importance and relevance of the findings of a study are intricately related to the strengths and weaknesses of the study in relation to the available literature.

Strengths of the Study

Every research involves investment of a lot of time, effort and money and may also entail potential risk to the study subjects. So, there should be a strong reason to do the study. The gaps in the knowledge that are identified through a thorough review of the existing literature form the basis for doing a study. How well the study actually addresses those issues determines the strength of the study. Thus, all the areas where the index study scores over the existing studies or the flaws in the previous studies that are corrected by the index study should be discussed under the strengths of the study. These may be related to 'a novel finding', 'a better study design', 'a larger sample size', 'longer follow-up', 'more generalizability' and so on. A few examples are, "*To the best of our knowledge this is the first study or first prospective study or first randomized study …*", "*All previous studies had included only a small number of patients….*", "*We have also described the long-term outcome which was lacking in the previous trials…*" etc.

Limitations of the Study

Every study has some limitations. The authors should honestly acknowledge the limitations or shortcomings of their study. Limitations may be related to the study design, sample size, bias, missing data, high rate of dropouts, lack of follow-up, low compliance and so on. The authors should try to explain the reasons behind the limitations and also state the efforts that they made to minimize the impact of those limitations. They should also state what impact the limitations would have on the validity of the findings of their study and suggest what measures can be taken to avoid such limitations in future studies. For example, "*The limitation of our study is its retrospective design. We extracted data from a prospectively maintained database thereby minimizing the issues of recall bias and missing data. The chances of selection bias are also minimal, as we have included all consecutive patients who were treated for this disease in our department. It would be difficult to do a prospective study on this subject at a single centre because of the rarity of the disease. A prospective multicentre study would therefore be required to confirm the findings of our study*".

How to Identify Limitations of the Study

The authors may find it difficult to identify the limitations of the study. They may ask a friend or colleague who is not involved in the study, to review the study and suggest limitations. Another way to identify limitations is to prepare a best possible hypothetical study design to test the research hypothesis of the study in question. All the points (study design, number of subjects, duration of follow-up etc.) where the index study falls short of the hypothetical study would be the limitations of the study. One should, however, ensure that the hypothetical study can be completed in the real world and is ethically acceptable. For example,

What would be the best study design for determining whether smoking increases the risk of lung cancer or not?

- Is a randomized controlled trial feasible for this research question?
  The answer is "No". It would be unethical to ask people to smoke just for the sake of a study.
- Is a prospective cohort study possible?
  Technically and ethically "Yes". But it does not seem practical. As only a small fraction of subjects in each group would develop lung cancer and that too after many years, such a study would require thousands of subjects to be followed for many years.

Thus, the best feasible design for this research question is retrospective and thus a retrospective study design in this scenario cannot be considered a limitation.

The flow of discussion is shown in Fig. 1.

Writing the Conclusions

This section is intended to briefly state the purpose of the study, the most important findings and the implications of these findings. The conclusion should be brief and crisp and should allow the reader to quickly find out whether the study accepts or rejects the hypothesis that was being tested. An easy way to know what to write in the conclusions is to go back to the aims and objectives section and look at the primary and secondary objectives of the study. The primary objective should always be part of the conclusions irrespective of its statistical significance. The authors may choose to include some of the secondary outcomes which are either statistically significant or are incongruent with the literature. Some authors use significant incidental findings or the results of post-hoc analysis in the conclusions section, especially in studies with non-significant primary and secondary outcomes. Since the study was not intended for these results, these should not find a place in the conclusions. In case these have to be included, the authors should mention them in such a manner so that the reader can easily understand that the study has only generated a hypothesis that needs to be tested further. For example, "*We conducted this study to determine the impact of extended lymphadenectomy on overall survival and its safety as compared to conventional lymphadenectomy. We did not find any significant improvement in the overall survival after extended lymphadenectomy as compared to conventional lymphadenectomy. The procedure was, however, safe, as the morbidity and mortality rates were similar in both the groups. Extended lymphadenectomy was associated with improved survival in a subset of patients with locally*

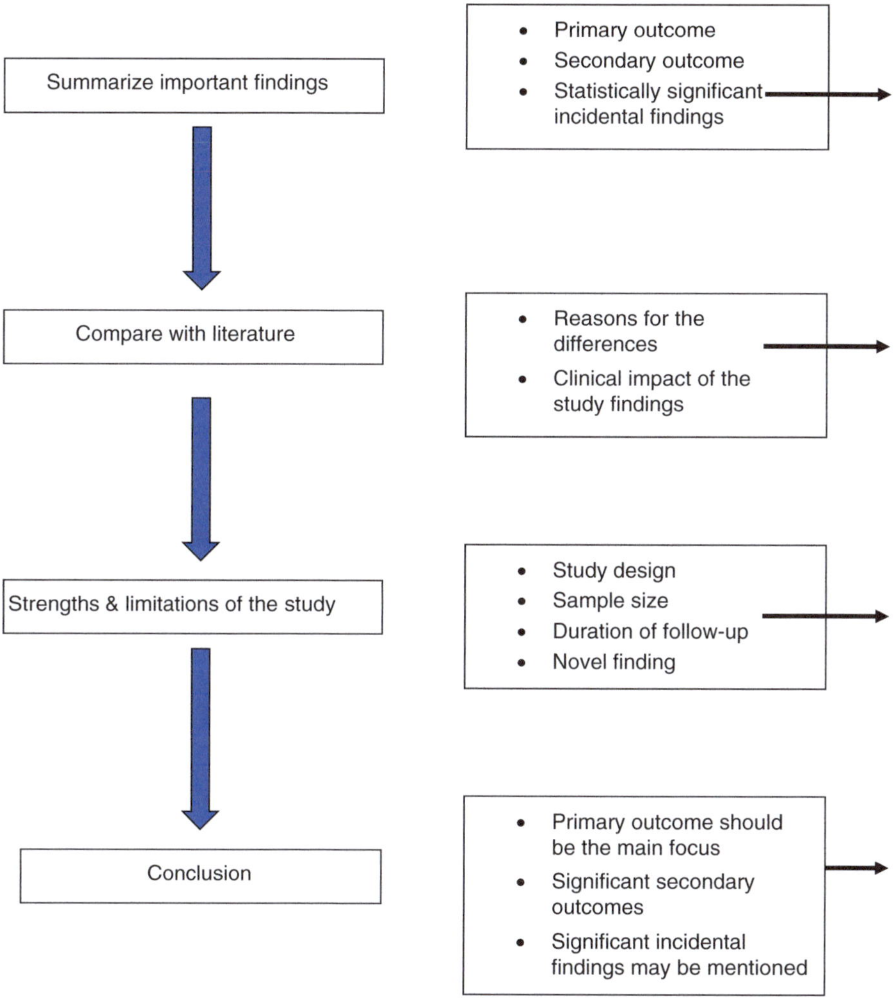

Fig. 1 Flow of discussion

advanced disease. To conclude, extended lymphadenectomy is safe but does not lead to improvement in overall survival. A subgroup of patients with locally advanced disease might benefit from this approach; however, further studies are required to confirm this finding.

Case Scenarios

1. Which of the following observations should be discussed first in the discussion section?
   (a) Observations related to the primary objective.
   (b) Observations related to the secondary objectives.

   (c) Observations with the lowest p-values.
   (d) All statistically significant observations.
2. Which of the following should always find a place in the conclusion section of a manuscript?
   (a) Statistically significant observations from an unplanned subgroup analysis.
   (b) Statistically non-significant observations related to the primary outcome.
   (c) Statistically non-significant observations related to the secondary outcome.
   (d) Statistically significant incidental findings.

References

1. International Committee of Medical Journal Editors. Uniform Requirements for Manuscripts Submitted to Biomedical Journals. Available at http://www.icmje.org/recommendations/browse/manuscript-preparation/preparing-for-submission.html#f. Accessed on 26 Jan 2018.
2. Fletcher RH, Fletcher SW. The discussion section. In: Sahni P, Aggarwal R, editors. Reporting and publishing research in the biomedical sciences. New Delhi: National Medical Journal of India; 2015. p. 43–57.
3. Lange P. How to write a scientific paper for peer-reviewed journals. Available at http://www.ease.org.uk/publications/ease-toolkit-authors/how-to-write-a-scientific-paper-for-peer-reviewed-journals/. Accessed on 26 Jan 2018.

Preparing Figures and Tables

Sudhir Kumar Jain and Rohit Kaushik

The drawing shows me at one glance what might be spread over ten pages in a book.—Ivan Turgenev

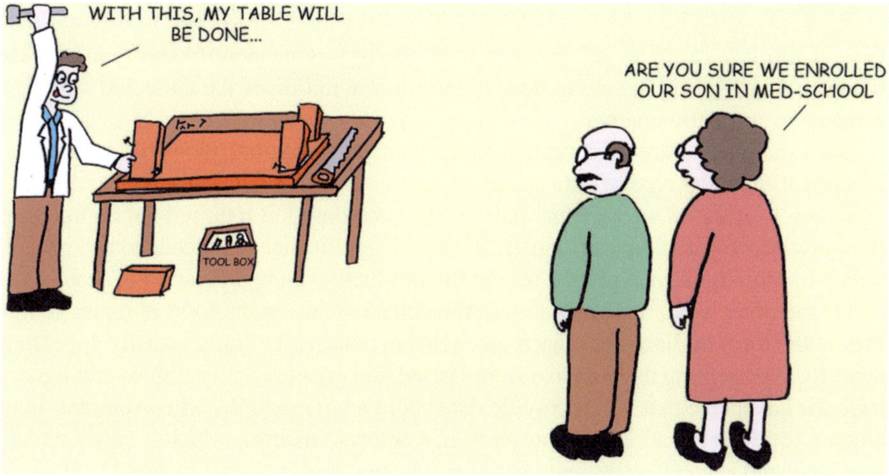

S. K. Jain (✉)
Director Professor, Department of Surgery, Maulana Azad Medical College and Lok Nayak Hospital, New Delhi, India

R. Kaushik
Junior Resident, Department of Surgery, Maulana Azad Medical College and Lok Nayak Hospital, New Delhi, India

S. C. Parija, V. Kate (eds.), *Thesis Writing for Master's and Ph.D. Program*,
https://doi.org/10.1007/978-981-13-0890-1_16

Key Points

- The basic fundamental of research methodology is to identify the type of data and its representation in a systematic way.
- Data may be represented using figures, tables.
- It helps in making the data visually appealing and provides information about a large sample in a concise and understandable way.
- Variables may be qualitative or quantitative. Qualitative variables may be continuous, ordinal or nominal. Quantitative variables are continuous or discrete.
- Information conveyed by tables and figures may be theoretical or data itself.
- Ideal table: (1) Self-explanatory (2) standardised (3) Contains a title (4) Numbered.
- Ideal figure: (1) Title (2) Self-explanatory (3) Scale (4) Legends and axes must be labelled.
- Understanding the use of table and figures helps collaborate results and prevents their misuse or overuse in scientific papers.

Overview

One of the key elements of research methodology is to identify the type of data being collected using the study design and representation of the collected data in a clear and systematic manner.

Both these steps are of paramount importance as each has its own significance. Identification of the type of data collected is important as it has an impact on the final outcome. It provides a rough estimate of the time duration required for completing the study process, the type of statistical tests of significance that needs to be applied, which eventually plays a pivotal role in the production and publication of results.

On the other hand, representation of the collected data in the form of tables or figures in the form of diagrams, charts etc. helps in making the study visually appealing apart from presenting the data in a summarised and organised way. Tables and figures have the advantage that it can provide data about a large sample, whose number may amount to several hundred or thousands, in a compact manner, which is easily understandable and is an effective and attractive way of conveying information [1, 2].

Therefore, it is important that students understand and master the basic concepts involved in designing tables and figures, and at the same time also learn the art to identify which type of figure or table is most suitable for the representation of the data based on the type of data collected and nature of information to be conveyed in the research papers, articles.

Basics of Data Collection

Before we proceed and discuss the fundamental principles involved in designing tables and figures, let us just revise the basic concepts of data collection.

Data

Data is the information gathered by a researcher working on a particular topic of interest. The mode of collecting data is variable. For instance, a laboratory worker may collect data based on the observations made by him during his experiments. Similarly, a field worker or researcher collecting demographic information collect data by filling out forms or pre-designed questionnaires. A doctor may collect data based on patients' lab results or imaging.

All the collected information in this way forms the Data. A proper and complete data forms the framework for the next step in research methodology i.e. data processing and analysis.

Observations

Observations are the measurements carried out on an individual participating in the study. For example, a researcher studying the average height among males takes note of the height of an individual, and each reading accounts for an observation.

Variables

Variables are the traits or the characteristic under study, which can be measured. In the above-cited example, height is a variable.

Variables are further divided into two categories: (a) Qualitative (b) Quantitative.

Qualitative variables are further divided into different types:

(a) Dichotomous
(b) Nominal
(c) Ordinal

Dichotomous

Dichotomous variables as the name suggests may have two values. Also termed as binary variables, these are usually the result of closed-ended or "Yes/No" questions.

Ordinal

Ordinal variables have more than two values and in addition to that, these variables follow a particular order. They can be arranged in an ascending or descending manner. For example: The response to a particular query which may be graded as disagree, agree and strongly agree.

Nominal

They can also have more than two values but they do not follow any set order. For example: eye colour in different individuals, which may be brown, black, blue.

Quantitative variables are also classified as: (a) Discrete (b) Continuous.

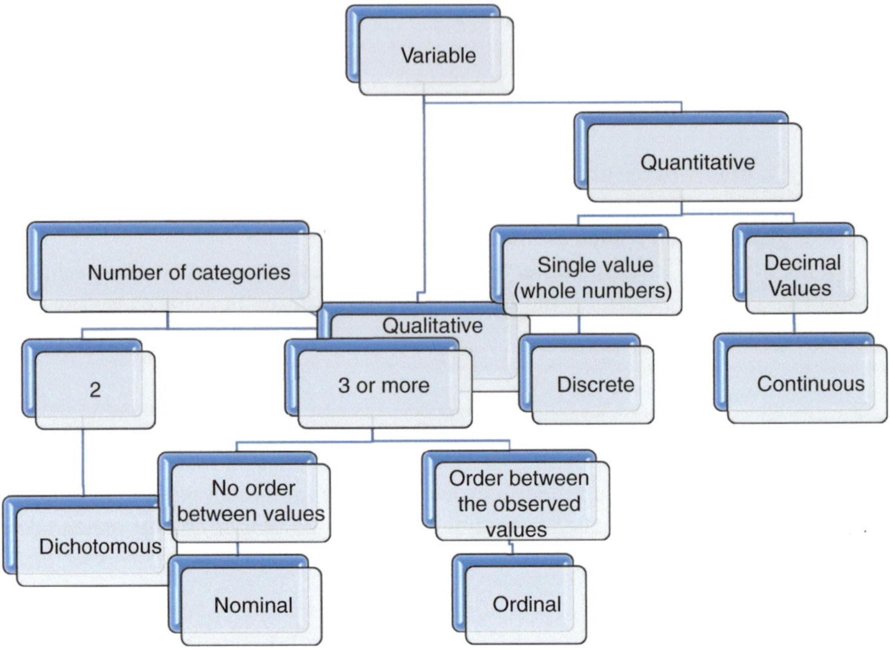

Fig. 1 Types of variables and their classification

Discrete

These variables have a single numerical value. An example would be the age of a person or in common terms the number of siblings or the number of vehicles an individual has.

Continuous

These variables have a numerical value on a continuous grade, which means any value is possible for the variable and the variable can have an infinite number of values. For example: The Blood Pressure of an individual or weight of an individual. Figure 1 shows types of variables [3–5].

Basic Guidelines for the Preparation of Figures and Tables

After having a general understanding of the basics of data collection, the next important step is the representation of the collected data in a schematic way. Figures and tables aid in representing the data, clarify interpretations and to explain concepts.

This part covers when and how tables and figures should be used so that they may convey the desired information to the reader.

Tables

As mentioned multiple times, tables help to represent the data in a more organised way which makes the data visually appealing and more understandable. The information conveyed by a table may be theoretical or data from the observations of a study. It provides a summary of the data.

An ideal table should highlight the following points:

- It should be numbered, using Arabic numerals.
- It should have a title in the beginning, which should be brief, but clearly explaining the table.
- It should be self-explanatory.
- Sufficient space should be present between rows and columns, the layout should be clear and the font used is legible.
- It should have a standardisation, which means, all the values of the different variables depicted in the table should have the same number of decimal places. In general, whole numbers should not have decimal points, p-values and correlations should be rounded off to three decimal places, and all other values (means, standard deviations, t-values) should carry two decimal places.
- It should be included in the article only after being mentioned in the preceding text.
- It should not have vertical lines at its lateral borders.
- Additional information may be given in the table footer if needed.
- The columns should have a title informing what is being described, the sample size for each variable, and relevant information like mean, median, standard deviation whenever available.
- If it is not an original table of the author, the source of the table must be cited in the footnote of the table.
- All acronyms and abbreviations used in the table must be explained in the table footnotes.

An example of a well-formatted table is shown in Table 1.

Note that the title for the table appears **above** the table. The table is well labelled. The first column denotes the parameter under study, with data for DJ stent group and Non-DJ stent group presented separately. The table provides information on means (M), and sample size (N) for two measurements. As the table is well-formatted, it is easy to (a) obtain the required information quickly, and (b) compare different groups and measurements [1]

Table 1 Showing patient demographic and stone details

Parameter	DJ Stent (N-28)	Non-DJ stent (N-28)
Mean age (years)	34.5	36.79
Sex distribution		
Males	16 (57.1%)	17 (60.7%)
Females	12 (42.9%)	11 (39.3%)
Stone size (in mm)	11.00	12.07
Stone location		
Renal pelvis	9	11
Upper calyx	4	5
Middle calyx	9	6
Upper ureter	6	6

Figures

The purpose of figures and diagrams in a research article is not just to make the article more attractive, but it should emphasise on the key elements of the data. Figures, in general, are not a replacement for tables in the research article. However, they may be used to convey additional information in the form of bar diagrams, pie-charts, line diagrams.

Figures come in two types: graphs and images/diagrams. Graphs are included in the research article in order to represent the data which becomes easy for the reader to understand while images and diagrams serve the purpose to explain theories.

Similar to tables, figures should include:

- A title, below the figure, conveying the necessary information as to what the figure is depicting. This is in contrast to a table where the heading comes on the top of the table.
- It should be self-explanatory, making the graph or diagram easy to understand.
- Figures should be mentioned in the text.
- If it is not an original figure of the author, the source of the figure must be cited in the footnote of the figure.
- The scale used in the figure must be explained clearly.
- Figures and graphs should be numbered.
- With context to a graph, the axis must be labelled appropriately and should start from zero. It should be kept in mind not to include too much information in a single figure. Rather, multiple figures can be included.

An example of a well-formatted figure is shown in Fig. 2. The vertical axis starts from zero. The figure is aptly labelled. The vertical and horizontal axis are duly labelled.

Figure 3 shows the basics of data collection and representation [1, 6].

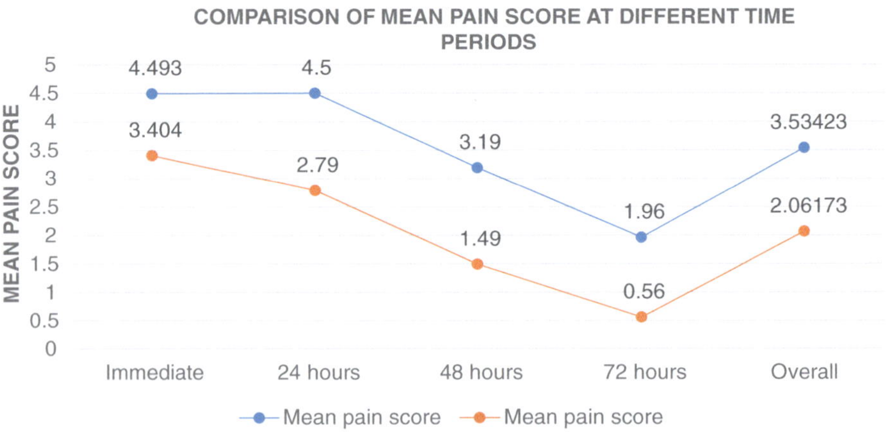

Fig. 2 Comparing mean pain scores at different time intervals post lithotripsy

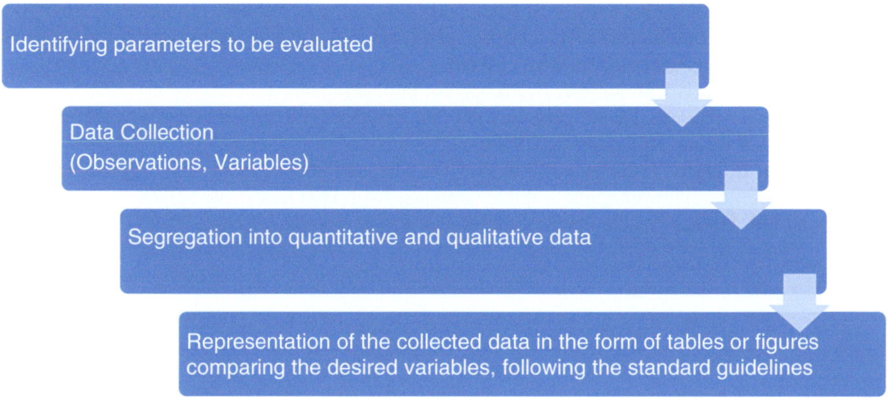

Fig. 3 Basics of data collection and representation

Conclusion

Understanding the fundamentals of data collection, and how to represent them in the form of tables and charts are important elements of reporting the findings of your research.

Mastering this topic collaborates to synthesize research results and prevents the misuse or overuse of tables and figures in scientific papers.

Case Scenarios

1. Characteristics of an ideal table are all except:
   (a) Numbered
   (b) Self-explanatory
   (c) Concise
   (d) Should have a preceding text
2. Which of the following diagram would best represent the monthly variations in prices of diesel, in the city of Delhi over a period of 1 year?
   (a) Pie chart
   (b) Histogram
   (c) Line diagram
   (d) Scatter chart

References

1. Duquia RP, Bastos JL, Bonamigo RR, González-Chica DA, Martínez-Mesa J. Presenting data in tables and charts. An Bras Dermatol. 2014;89(2):280–5.
2. Browne JE. Getting started with research "Writing-up the results of your research". Ultrasound. 2014;22(1):70–2.

3. Boushey C, Harris J, Bruemmer B, Archer SL, Van Horn L. Publishing nutrition research: a review of study design, statistical analyses, and other key elements of manuscript preparation, Part 1. J Am Diet Assoc. 2006;106(1):89–96.
4. Boushey CJ, Harris J, Bruemmer B, Archer SL. Publishing nutrition research: a review of sampling, sample size, statistical analysis, and other key elements of manuscript preparation, Part 2. J Am Diet Assoc. 2008;108(4):679–88.
5. Bruemmer B, Harris J, Gleason P, Boushey CJ, Sheean PM, Archer S, et al. Publishing nutrition research: a review of epidemiologic methods. J Am Diet Assoc. 2009;109(10):1728–37.
6. Ahmad HR. How to write a doctoral thesis. Pak J Med Sci. 2016;32(2):270–3.

Citations and References with Citation and H-Index

Nisha V. Parmar and Divya Gupta

When you have a wit of your own, it's a pleasure to credit other people for theirs.—Criss Jami

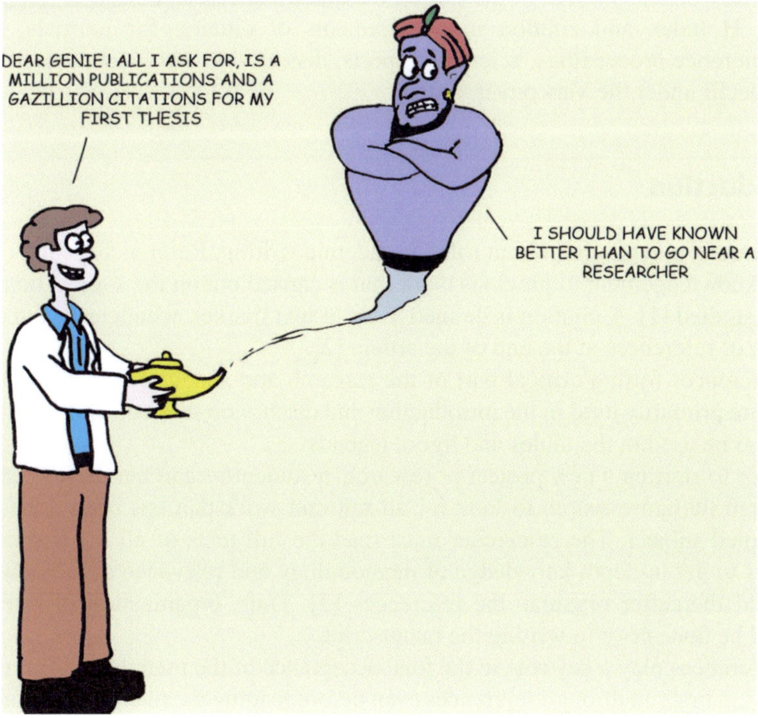

N. V. Parmar
Specialist Dermatologist, Rashid Hospital, Dubai Health Authority, Dubai, UAE

D. Gupta (✉)
Consultant Dermatologist, Oliva Skin and Hair Clinic, Bengaluru, India

S. C. Parija, V. Kate (eds.), *Thesis Writing for Master's and Ph.D. Program*,
https://doi.org/10.1007/978-981-13-0890-1_17

Key Points

- Referencing forms a critical part of the research and reflects the thoroughness of literature search.
- Important referencing systems include note system (e.g. Vancouver system) and parenthetical system (e.g. Harvard system).
- Many reference management software like EndNote, Zotero, Reference manager and Mendeley have been developed to help authors organize and change the order of references.
- Indexing agencies are online database systems that compile information on journal titles and authors. Common indexing agencies are Medline/PubMed, SCOPUS, EMBASE, DOAJ, Hinari and Index Copernicus.
- Quality of scientific output is measured by various scientific indices like impact factor, H index and citation index. These influence both the author impact and journal ranking.
- This chapter discusses the principles of referencing, referencing systems, indexing and various indices of measuring the quality of research such as impact factor, H index and citation index. Elements of citation for journals, books, conference proceedings, scientific reports, dissertation and patent are discussed in detail under the Vancouver system.

Introduction

Referencing plays an important role in academic writing. Referencing refers to giving acknowledgement to previous work that is carried out on the subject being currently studied [1]. A citation is defined as an in-text marker, which leads a reader to the list of references at the end of the article [2].

References form a critical part of the research and should not be taken lightly. They are primarily used in the introduction and discussion sections of an article, and can also be used in the tables and figure legends.

Prior to starting a new project or research, a student/researcher has to perform a thorough literature search to look for all relevant work that has been done on the concerned subject. The researcher must read the full texts of all the accumulated articles to get in-depth knowledge of methodology and relevance of previous studies, and thereafter organize the references [3]. Thus, organization of references should be done prior to writing the manuscript.

References play a key role in the final acceptance of the manuscript. Editors and reviewers first run through references even before reading the manuscript or abstract to see the thoroughness of the literature included and the authors' intentions. Hence utmost precision and time should be dedicated to reference writing. This chapter discusses in depth the art and science of reference writing, impact factor, various indices of measuring the quality of research such as H index and citation index and reference management systems.

Referencing

Referencing includes two elements:

1. An in-text marker, either in parentheses or as a sequential superscripted number, which informs the reader that the information is borrowed from previously, carried out work.
2. A list at the end of the article, which compiles all the citations used in the manuscript.

Referencing Systems

Referencing systems are of two types [4]:

- Note systems
- Parenthetical systems

Note Systems

Note systems include in-text citations in the form of sequential numbers, which then guide the reader to notes either at the end of the page (footnotes) or paper (endnotes).

Examples of note systems include the Vancouver system and the Chicago 16th A system.

Parenthetical Systems

In this form of referencing, the in-text marker is provided in parentheses and includes the author's name and year of publication. The complete reference list is then provided at the end of the text.

Examples of parenthetical systems include the Harvard system, American Psychologists' Association style (APA) system, and the Modern Language Association (MLA) systems.

In medical writing, the Vancouver and Harvard systems are the most commonly used referencing systems.

Vancouver System

In 1978, a group of general medicine journal editors held an unofficial meeting in Vancouver, Canada to devise strict guidelines for manuscripts submitted to their journals, hence giving birth to the Vancouver style of reference writing [5]. This is the most commonly used referencing style used in medical publications and is also referred to as the author-number system.

The Vancouver system utilizes a superscripted in-text consecutive Arabic numeral as the citation, which then directs the reader to the complete numerical list of references at the end of the paper.

Presenting References Using the Vancouver System [5]

1. ***Standard journal article***

   For up to six authors:

   Sarkar TJ, Feldman M, Law E, Pitts YH. Hepatitis B reactivation associated with immune suppressive and biologic modifier therapies: current concepts, management strategies and future directions. World J Gastroenterol 2015; 115(1): 1000–1013.

   For more than six authors:

   Anistell MH, Taylor D, Pfeifer A, Kim R, Rostini T, Mcmayor M et al. Impact of preoperative serum creatinine on short-and long-term mortality after renal surgery: a case-control study. Br J Anaesth 2017; 100(3): 75–83.

Note

The use of issue number in parentheses is optional depending on the journal.

2. ***Organization or group as an author***

   Association of Anaesthetists of Great Britain and Ireland. Peri-operative management of the surgical patient with diabetes. Anaesthesia 2017;77:1630–1650.
3. **Volume with supplement**

   Jackson T, Pollock C. The role of gut and skin microbiota in the development of atopic eczema. Australas J Dermatol 2015; 175;Suppl 3:19–24.
4. ***Issue with supplement***

   Depp J, Weng HG. Response patterns of recurrent glioblastomas treated with tumor-treating fields. Semin Oncol 2012; 95 (6 Suppl 4): S25–S35.
5. ***Volume or issue with part***

   Older versions of some journals had parts in place of issues; the parts were placed in parentheses e.g. Vol (Pt 6). Most journals have now replaced the parts with issues. In case of issue with parts, it is written as Vol (Issue Pt 6).
6. ***Issue with no volume***

   Deb DM, Kassir H, Nouri GS. Intraoperative frozen section analysis in revision total joint arthroplasty. Clin Orthop Relat Res 2010;(301): 440–448.
7. ***Article with no volume, issue or authors***

   Methamphetamine and HIV. HRSA Careaction 2005 July: 7–15.
8. ***Type of article as required***

   Ritchie G, Kashyap A. International approaches to the prescription of long-term oxygen therapy [letter]. Eur Respir J. 2009; 25(1): 541.

9. ***Retracted article***
Sinna H, Rafael I, Rana A, Abdul-Aziz T. Intralesional immunotherapy of plantar warts: report of a new antigen combination. Cutis. 2012; 28 (1): 95–7. Retraction in Cutis. 2012; 29(5): 600.
10. ***Article published in erratum***
Suzuki Y, Motoya S, Hanai S, Hibi T, Nakamura S, Lazar A et al. Four-year maintenance treatment with adalimumab in Japanese patients with moderately to severely active ulcerative colitis. J Gastroenterol 2017.
11. ***Article published electronically ahead of print***
Abassi J. Can a diet that mimics fasting turn back the clock? JAMA 2017 Jun 28 doi: https://doi.org/10.1001/jama.2017.6648. [Epub ahead of print].
12. ***Article in a language other than English***
For articles, which are not in English, NLM translates the title to English and encloses it in square parentheses. The original language of the publication is mentioned at the end of the reference.

Books and Other Monographs [5, 6]

The standard format for the citation of an entire book includes:

1. ***Personal author(s)***
This refers to one or more individuals who are responsible for writing the book. The format of referencing is as follows.
Author(s) of book. Title of book. Edition. Place of publication: Publisher; Year of Publication
2. ***Organization(s) as author***
Name of the organization. Title of the book. Place of publication: Publisher; Year of Publication.

3. ***Chapter in a book***
When the author of the book writes the chapter:
Author(s) of book. Title of book. Edition. Place of publication: Publisher; Year of publication, chapter number, chapter title; page numbers.
When an author in an edited book writes the chapter:
Author(s) of chapter. Title of chapter. In: Name(s) of the editor(s). Ed(s). Title of book. Edition. Place of publication: Publisher; Year of publication, Page numbers.
4. ***Chapter in an online book***
When a chapter is contributed by the original author of the e-book:
Author(s) of the book. Title of the book. [book on the internet]. Edition. Place of publication: Publisher; year of publication. Chapter number, chapter title [date of update/revision; date of citation];page numbers. Available from: URL or database name.
When a chapter is written by a contributing author in an edited online book:
Contributing author(s). Title of the contribution. In: Name of Author(s)/Editor(s) of the book. Title of the book [book on the internet]. Edition. Place of publica-

tion: Publisher; year of publication [date of update/revision; date of citation]; pages. Available from: URL or database name.

5. ***Conference papers and proceedings6***

   A conference paper is an individual paper presented at a conference whereas a conference proceeding refers to a collection of conference papers published in journal issues usually as abstracts in supplements.

   (a) **Conference papers**

      The format for referencing is as follows:

      Author of paper. Title of paper. In: Name of Editors of proceedings, Title of proceedings book, Conference title, Conference date, place of conference, place of publication, publisher, date of publication. Pagination

   (b) **Conference proceedings**

      The format is as follows:

      Editor(s). Title of the proceedings book. Title of the conference; Year Month Date Of the conference; Location of the conference. Place of publication: Publisher, Year of publication. Pages

6. ***Dissertation***

   The standard format for citing a dissertation is:

   Author of the dissertation. Dissertation title [indicator]. [Place of publication]: Name of the University; year of publication. Total number of pages.

   Lara B. Characterisation of alpha-thrombin-induced rapid phase of PI 3-kinase [dissertation]. St. Louis (MO): Saint Louis University; 2004. 141p.

7. ***Scientific or technical report***

   A scientific report is a document elaborating the details of scientific research. The format of referencing a scientific report is as follows:

   Authors. Title of report. Place of publication: publisher; date of publication in the year month format. Total number of pages. Report number.

   Cannes A, Finn S. Health hazard evaluation report. Cincinnati (OH): National Institute of Occupational Safety and Health (US); 2001 Feb.24p.Report NO.: HETA2000–0139-2824.

8. ***Patent***

   A patent is identified with two types of authors, the inventor(s) per se and the assignee, which refers to the organization or individual with the legal right to the patent. The referencing format is as follows:

   Inventor(s); Assignee. Title of patent. Country document type Country code patent number Date issued.

   Myers K, Nguyen C, Inventors; 3F Therapeutics, Inc., assignee. Prosthetic heart valve. United States patent US 6,911,043.2005 Jun 28.

The Harvard System of Referencing

The title of the system is a misnomer, as there is no official connection with the Harvard University. Some Harvard faculty were amongst the first users of this system in the late nineteenth century and hence the name prevailed [7].

In this system, author and date are cited within parentheses in the manuscript e.g. (Cheung J, 2001) [8]. A list of citations is then provided in alphabetical order at the end under the section designated as "References." If the work has up to three authors, all are included in the citation. If the work has four or more authors, the abbreviation 'et al.' is used after the first author's name. If any author has two publications in a given year and both are being cited, a lower case letter after the date is used to differentiate between the works, e.g. (Thappa, 2008a; Thappa, 2008b) [7, 8].

Advantages of Harvard system:

- A reader familiar with a field is likely to recognize a citation without having to check in the references section.
- It helps the reader easily identify sources that are outdated.
- If the same source is cited more than once, it quickly becomes obvious if the publication is relying heavily on a single publication.
- There is no renumbering hassle when the order of in-text citations is changed.

Disadvantages of Harvard system:

- Parenthetical references take up space in the main body of the text and are distracting to a reader, especially when many works are cited in a single place.
- Rules can be complicated for non-academic references, particularly those where the personal author is unknown, such as government-issued documents and organization guidelines.
- The use of the author–date methods can be confusing when the cited authors are very prolific in their publications in any field.

Principles of Referencing [3, 5]

- References should be accurately written ensuring correct spelling and order of authors as well as correct citation in the manuscript.
- Adhere to the referencing style accepted by the journal that the article is being submitted to.
- Citing abstracts as references and personal communications should be avoided.
- When citing papers accepted but not yet published, the authors should designate the article as 'in press' and verify that the article has been accepted.
- Secondary referencing should be avoided.

Figure 1 depicts the various steps in referencing.

Reference Management Systems

Reference management refers to the organization of the list of references in a systematic manner in the order of appearance in the manuscript [9]. Several software have been developed to aid in the management of references, both web-based and

Fig. 1 Algorithm showing the steps in referencing

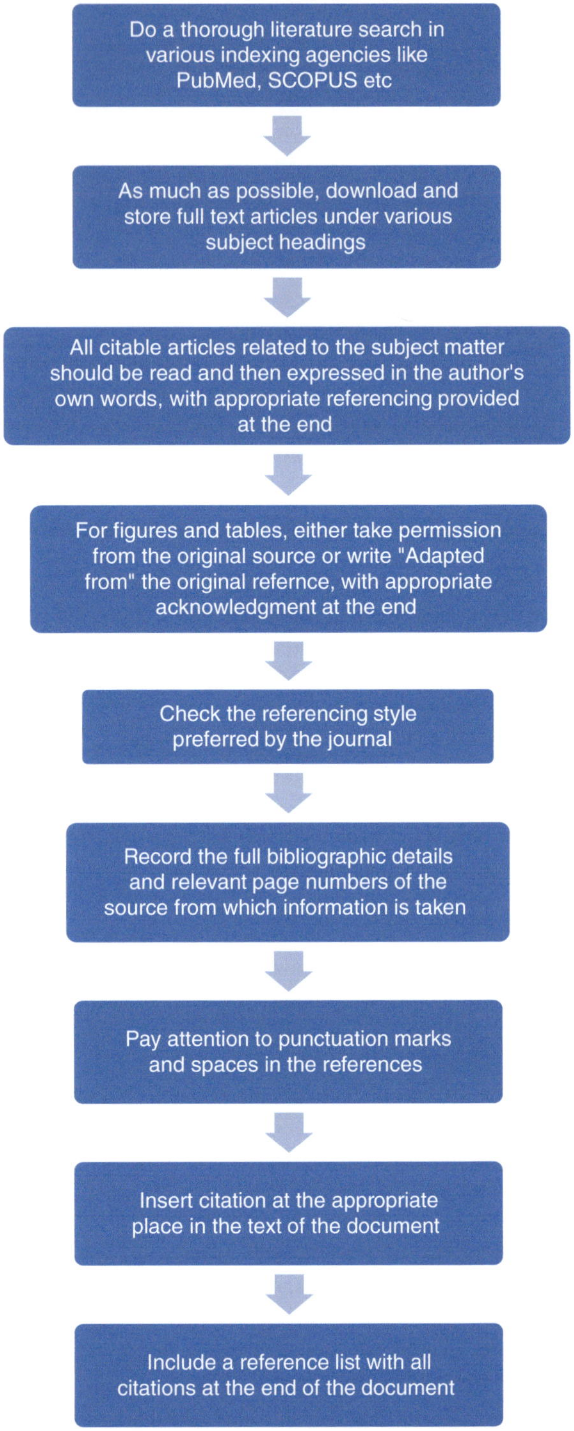

Table 1 Details of various referencing software

	Zotero	EndNote	Mendeley	Reference manager
Developer	Roy Rosenzweig Center for History and New Media	Thomson Reuters	Elsevier	Thomson Reuters
Availability	Free	Commercial	Free	Commercial
Supported operating systems	Windows, Mac, Linux	Windows, Mac, IOS	Windows, IOS, Mac, Linux	Windows
Organization	Installable PC software	Installable PC software	Installable PC software	Installable PC software
Connectivity to PubMed	Yes	Yes	Yes	Yes
Word processor integration	Yes	Yes	Yes	Yes
File attachment, tags/keywords, notes	Yes	Yes	Yes	Yes
Online storage	Yes	None	Yes	None

non-web-based. Students and researchers utilize these and to avoid mistakes while referencing and simplify the painstaking process of organizing references.

The commonly used reference management systems include EndNote, Zotero, Reference manager and Mendeley. Table 1 below summarizes the various reference management systems and their features.

Indexing

When any researcher wants to find information about a topic from a published journal, they usually check for that information on a website on the internet that compiles data about authors, titles, journals, and subjects. This specific online bibliographic database system is known as an index.

Indexing of a journal within a database is very important as it often reflects the quality of a journal, with indexed journals considered to be of higher scientific value as compared to non-indexed journals. With the progressively increasing emphasis on publications by academic institutions, authors prefer to publish in indexed journals [10, 11]. All indexing agencies adopt stringent criteria for journal indexing [12].

Indexing Agencies

Some commonly known and used bibliographic databases or indexing agencies are:

1. MEDLINE/PubMed (see below).
2. SCOPUS (Elsevier).

3. EBSCO Publishing Databases.
4. EMBASE database (Elsevier).
5. DOAJ (Directory of Open Access Journals).
6. Hinari-set up by the World Health Organization and major publishers to enable developing countries to access biomedical and health literature free or at low cost.
7. Index Copernicus.

Performing simultaneous searches through more than one database overcome the inherent limitations of each one and add to the quality of writing, reviewing and editing [11, 13].

MEDLINE/PubMed

One of the most popular, rapidly updated, free and easy-to-use databases is MEDLINE® (Medical Literature Analysis and Retrieval System Online). PubMed content is broader and in addition to MEDLINE citations, includes: citations from old MEDLINE files (from 1950 to 1965), articles of journals that are not included in MEDLINE etc [10, 14].

The process of applying for indexing in MEDLINE is often handled through the journal publishing company. One of the main advantages of MEDLINE is its reliance on the Medical Subject Headings (MeSH) thesaurus, which facilitates retrieval of articles through keywords.

Thomson Reuters Scientific

Thomson Reuters Scientific is a division of Thomson Reuters, and used to be called Thomson ISI (Institute of Scientific Information). One of Thomson's products is the ISI Web of Knowledge, a database that covers over 9000 publications in every area of the sciences, arts and humanities. Once a journal is indexed in ISI Web of Knowledge, it can be assigned an "impact factor" by Thomson [14].

Impact Factor

The Impact Factor (IF) is a tool to identify the journals most cited by researchers and was created by Eugene Garfield, the founder of the Institute for Scientific Information. It is a ratio of the number of citations received in a given year by all articles published in the two previous years (in the numerator) and the number of articles published in the same years (in the denominator). Impact factor of most of the journals can be checked at the journal webpage itself. It is published annually in *Journal Citation Reports* (JCR), by Thomson/ISI publication [10].

Only research articles, technical notes and reviews are "citable" items. Editorials, letters, news items, and meeting abstracts are "non-citable items" for the purpose of calculating the denominator, but can be counted in the numerator [15]. In addition, IF cannot be computed for journals that are less than 2 years old [16]. It is currently used as an indicator for quality of the scientific output. It plays a role in hiring, academic promotions and research grant policy. Hence, authors are forced to publish their research in journals of high IF at the cost of a specialist or national journal that might actually be more appropriate. Increasingly, journals are being designed in such a way so as to make them citable than readable, putting forth the needs of researchers before the needs of ordinary doctors who far outnumber researchers as readers, which might result in a rise in IF but with a decline in the readership [17].

Hence, the usage of IF as a solitary method to assess the quality of the journal is not recommended. Limitations of using the IF are:

1. The predominant type of article published in a given journal, e.g. reviews and original articles (cited more) vs. case reports (less cited);
2. Many journals limit the number of citations and, therefore, it is not possible to cite all that has been read;
3. Authors from developed countries tend to cite articles published in their countries but in developing countries, authors mostly cite journals published in developed countries;
4. Journal with high IFs may not be more useful in daily practice of doctors;
5. Citation behaviours can be influenced by online availability, publication lag, and self-citation by journals [11].
6. A two-year period can inflate a journal's overall impact if only a small number of articles in rapidly changing areas of research account for the vast majority of citations. (e.g. stem cell biology, genomics etc. [18]) Also, a longer period provides a better picture of journal stature than a short period of 2 years.
7. Generally, the basic sciences and broader speciality journals have a higher IF than the clinical sciences or narrower speciality journals.

H-Index

The *h*-index is an index to quantify a body of scientific research output and was suggested by Jorge E. Hirsch, a physicist at University of California. The *h*-index is also called the Hirsch index or Hirsch number. It is an index that attempts to measure the apparent scientific impact of a scientist. An author with an index of "h" indicates that the author has h publications, which has been cited h times. It takes into account factors like the number of co-authors in an article; the average number of citations received by a scientist, and is based on the set of the most cited papers. The *h*-index can be calculated for any group of scientific papers. Most frequently the *h*-index is used to measure the scientific output of an author, but the *h*-index can also be calculated for an institution, country or journal. It has been recommended that the h-index should be used to complement or correct the traditional impact factor [19].

Citation Index

A citation index is a bibliographic database, an index of citations between publications, allowing the user to easily establish which later documents cite which earlier documents. The first citation index was introduced in 1960 by the ISI - the Science Citation Index (SCI). Later, it was expanded to produce the Social Sciences Citation Index (SSCI) and the Arts and Humanities Citation Index (AHCI). The other citation databases include Elsevier (Scopus), CiteSeer, Google Scholar, Ebscohost and Compendex. Citation indexes help understand the author impact in a subject and also journal ranking by giving information about what articles and topics are being published, cited, or ignored [20].

Case Scenario

1. You are required to rate two authors by calculating the H index of their publications.

   Author A has 25 publications to his credit; three of his publications have each been cited once and one of his publication has been cited twice. Other publications are not cited.

   Author B has 15 publications to her credit; two of her publications have each been cited twice and two of her other publications have each been cited once. Other publications are not cited.

   (a) What is the H index of author A?
   (b) Which of the two authors above has a higher H index and why?

References

1. Giving credit: citations and references. Annesley TM. Clin Chem 2011; 57(1): 14–17.
2. Bryson D. Using research papers: citations, referencing and plagiarism. J Vis Comm Med. 2012;35(2):82–4.
3. Peh WCG, Ng KH. Preparing the references. Singap Med J. 2009;50(7):659–61.
4. EndNote: Citation guides. [Internet].Sydney: The University of Sydney Library. Last updated: July 7, 2017 Cited on 15 July 2017. Available from http://libguides.library.usyd.edu.au/endnote.
5. Uniform requirements for manuscripts submitted to biomedical journals. International Committee of Medical. Journal Editors N Engl J Med. 1997;336(4):309–15.
6. Patrias K. Citing medicine: the NLM style guide for authors, editors, and publishers [Internet]. 2nd ed. Wendling DL, technical editor. Bethesda (MD): National Library of Medicine (US); 2007 - [updated 2015 Oct 2; cited 2017 July 15]. Available from: http://www.nlm.nih.gov/citingmedicine.
7. Chernin E. The 'Harvard system': a mystery dispelled. BMJ. 1988;297:1062–3.
8. Citing and referencing: Harvard style Imperial College London 2016 August. p. 1–21.
9. Kali A. Reference writing: a critical element of scientific writing. J Adv Pharm Technol Res. 2016;7:27–9.
10. Castro RC. Journals in surgery and gastroenterology: indexing in databases and bibliometric indicators. Acta Cir Bras. 2006;21(3):122–32.
11. Balhara YP. Indexed journal: what does it mean? Lung India. 2012;29(2):193.

12. Kim H. How to index journal in Scopus and WoS. The 2nd Asian science editors' conference & workshop Hanoi University of Science and Technology Hanoi, Vietnam. August 20–22, 2015.p. 1–42.
13. Akhigbe RE. Scientific journals: indexation and impact factor. Lung India. 2012;29(3):300–1.
14. Getting your journal indexed and using resources for editors. In: Freda MC and LH Nicoll. The editors' handbook: an online resource and CE course [book on the internet]. 2nd ed. Lippincott, Williams and Wilkins. 2010.Chapter 10, P 1–11; Available from: http://www.nursingcenter.com.
15. Robert RS, Gnanavel S. Impact factor: the holy grail of research. Indian J Psychol Med. 2015;37(2):248–9.
16. Shrivastava SR, Shrivastava PS, Ramasamy J. Assessment of the quality of a journal: scientific approach. Int J Adv Med Health Res. 2015;2(1):61–2.
17. Malathi M, Thappa DM. The intricacies of impact factor and mid-term review of editorship. Indian J Dermatol Venereol Leprol. 2012;78(1):1–4.
18. Verma IM. Impact, not impact factor. Proc Natl Acad Sci U S A. 2015;112(26):7875–6.
19. Scopus Journal FAQs: Helping to improve the submission & success process for editors & publishers. P1–17. Available from: https://www.elsevier.com.
20. Nigam A, Nigam PK. Citation index and impact factor. Indian J Dermatol Venereol Leprol. 2012;78(4):511–6.

Part IV

Editing the Thesis

Editing for Language and Avoiding Ambiguity in Data Presentation

Savio George Barreto

You might not write well everyday, but you can edit a bad page.
You can't edit a blank page.—Jodi Picoult

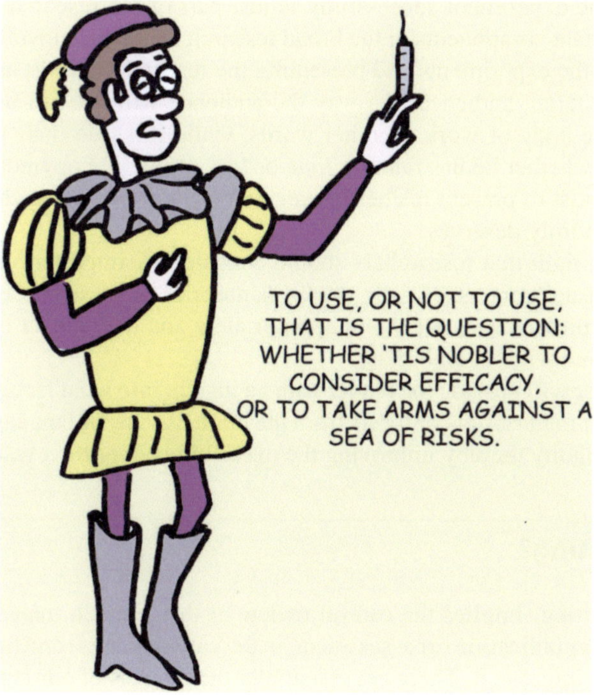

S. G. Barreto
Clinical Fellow, Hepatobiliary and Esophagogastric Unit, Division of Surgery and Perioperative Medicine, Flinders Medical Centre Bedford Park, Adelaide, South Australia

S. C. Parija, V. Kate (eds.), *Thesis Writing for Master's and Ph.D. Program*,
https://doi.org/10.1007/978-981-13-0890-1_18

Key Points

- Performing experiments is only part of the job, accurately interpreting the findings and then presenting them appropriately is just as important, if not, more so.
- The first step to editing is to plan the structure of the text, tables and figures in terms of the flow of the document.
- If the researcher lacks formal writing skills in the language in which the document is prepared, then seeking help from professional editing services is suggested.
- The keys to avoiding ambiguity when dealing with quantitative and qualitative data are to keep an open mind when performing research and interpreting the results, and to subject one's findings to informal peer review before writing them up.
- Courses on how to edit documents are available. Attending these course is recommended.

Introduction

Performing the experiment successfully is just part of the research exercise. Two equally important components of the broad research experience involve interpreting the data from the experiments and presenting the research findings and their implications to the target audience in a way the audience will not just understand, but appreciate, the body of work. In other words, while it is true that 'It takes a wise man to know whether he has *found a rope* or *lost a mule*' (anonymous), it takes an eloquent scientist to present his/her research work in a way in which it will attract the attention it truly deserves.

It is in this light that researchers should consider the importance of editing the textual and visual content of their work (manuscript or thesis) to ensure that the message is expressed accurately and appropriately and the manner of presentation is consistent and without ambiguity.

This chapter will provide the reader with an insight into what is required in terms of editing their manuscripts or thesis from the point of view of language content and avoiding ambiguity thereby improving the overall impact of their research.

What is Editing?

The word 'editing' implies the careful review of the research material prior to its submission for publication (or assessment, in the case of theses) and making changes to correct and improve it. There are essentially three levels of editing, namely, substantiative editing, copyediting and proof reading [1].

How Must One Approach Editing of a Document?

To enhance the message of the document and to avoid redundancy in presenting data, the first step involves '*Substantiative or structural editing*'. The aim of this initial step in the preparation of the document is to clarify meaning, improve flow and smooth language [1]. Essentially this involves an assessment of the textual data as well as the tables and figures to determine the sequence of their representation and then organising them in a manner that best 'tells the story' to the reader. A widespread practice in presenting research documents is that the tables and figures are placed at the end of the manuscript/thesis during the preparation of the initial drafts. It is thus not uncommon for the person drafting the manuscript to duplicate information in the text and tables. While this may not be appreciated even after the final revision or at the time of submission, once the proofs of the document are available, the redundancy can get rather annoying to the trained reader. Thus, carrying out a structural edit at the outset (placing tables and figures in between the textual data in the order in which the researcher would like them placed in the final published/ printed document) will ensure that none of the data from the tables and figures are duplicated in the text and vice versa. Moreover, for those researchers using reference manager software like Endnote ®, this step will ensure that the references are cited in the appropriate order, too. Just prior to submission, the tables and figures can then be copied and pasted wherever they require to be as per the submission guidelines.

The next step involves ensuring consistency, accuracy and completeness of the document, or what is better known as '*Copyediting*' [1]. Copyediting focusses on aspects such as the appropriate use of language in terms of grammar and style (including syntax, spelling, punctuation and clarity of expression), consistency of language (including Structural parallelism, terms used, spelling, capitalisation, hyphenation, abbreviations, numbers and quantitative data and references), consistency of visual content (including typography, heading hierarchy, page layout, figures, tables, and captions), referencing (including accuracy of cross references within text, between text and figures, between list of contents and body of document as well as conformity and completeness of textual references, bibliography and quotations), and acknowledgement of sources [2].

If the researcher is presenting the document in a language that is not his /her native tongue or a language in which the researcher does not possess formal written skills, then it is advisable to seek advice and assistance early in the process of document preparation. Researchers who are not native language speakers can certainly consider enlisting the services of commercial copyediting firms. Most commercial copyediting firms charge a fee for their service. On the other hand, researchers who are not native speakers of the language but are competent with the spoken and written language as a result of their school education, may consider using language editing softwares that are available on the worldwide web. Some of these sites require the document to be uploaded and the output containing the edited document is then made available to the researcher as a downloadable file. Others possess a more formal approach with an interactive service provided. Some examples of copyediting services/software available include Elsevier's English Language editing service ®, Wendy Monaghan Editing Services ®, Whitesmoke ®, ProWritingAid ®. (*The author of this chapter has neither used the services of the aforementioned sites, nor does he endorse them, but has only stated these as examples.*)

Work submitted to a commercial copyediting service generally does not undergo scrutiny for the accuracy of the data. Thus, the onus of presenting accurate and complete information in manuscripts submitted for publication and for theses, as well, rests with the researcher and not the copyediting firms.

It is the responsibility of the researcher to ensure the accuracy and completeness of the data being presented. While some journals and Universities will publish work based on data that is readily accessible for scrutiny, most others rely on the honesty and integrity of the presented data. It is thus paramount that researchers honour and respect the faith entrusted to them and present only data that is true to the best of their capabilities. Raw data must always be stored in a secure place/server in the event that the data is requested for scrutiny at a later date.

The last step in language and content editing is *'Proof reading'* which involves examining the now near final document after completing the layout to correct errors in textual and visual elements [1]. This step essentially draws from the initial structural plan (developed at the time of substantiative editing) and involves going through the entire document in great detail to ensure that the content (textual and figures and tables) and the layout conforms to what the researcher set out to do in terms of telling the reader 'a story'.

How to Avoid Ambiguity When Presenting Qualitative and Quantitative Data

Before presenting any data, it is of utmost importance that the researcher appropriately interprets the findings. It is very easy to go overboard when drawing inferences from one's findings often leaning towards a polarised viewpoint. This is often the result of the researcher having set out with a predetermined notion or a theory, instead of a 'hypothesis' and then carrying out the experiments to 'prove' his/her theory rather than keeping an open mind when performing the experiments. It is paramount to let 'science' rather than the 'scientist' do the talking! At the other extreme when drawing inferences is the 'diffident' researcher who either does not understand the meaning of the findings, is unable to interpret them, or simply lacks the confidence to take a stand in the face of the results obtained. Such researchers often land up presenting their results in an ambiguous manner, or adopt the 'middle' path in academic writing referred to as 'hedging'.

When interpreting findings, one should neither be tentative, ambiguous, nor exaggerated nor make unwarranted claims. While errors in interpretation may occur with both, qualitative and quantitative data, the risk of overstating or exaggerating findings is more likely when dealing with qualitative data if one lacks the balance of mind when questioning the basis for the assumptions. The risk of hedging or ambiguity is more likely when dealing with quantitative data, which seek the use of statistics to answer questions.

The solution to avoid ambiguity when presenting data is to firstly 'keep an open mind'. In terms of qualitative analysis this would mean doing a thorough search of literature and evidence and not dismissing evidence that may be contrary to personal 'beliefs'. When dealing with quantitative analysis, this would mean selecting the appropriate statistical tests to answer the question being asked and NOT to support the theory in the researcher's mind. The next step is to ensure the completeness, accuracy and certainty of the analysis. This is followed by a critical analysis of the data with an aim to drawing inferences. These data and inferences should then be subjected to an informal peer review process. In the case of researchers pursuing a masters or Ph.D. degree, presenting these findings in an open forum to members of the laboratory or department, as well as researchers from other departments would be the way to go. Often, a researcher will be so embroiled in their work that it inadvertently spawns the lack of a balanced approach that can be obtained from seeking the advice of another researcher or even researchers. The feedback at such meetings is priceless so long as the researcher presenting the information is open to criticism and suggestion. Taking on board comments, advice, and suggestions from peers and senior colleagues is one of the best ways to avoid ambiguity. The other useful technique employed by the author is to put the results away for a week and do something altogether different and return to the data in a week to 10 days. Approaching the data with a 'fresh' mind can infuse a sense of open mindedness that is truly refreshing!

A practical algorithm of the steps for editing language and content and for avoiding ambiguity is shown in Fig. 1.

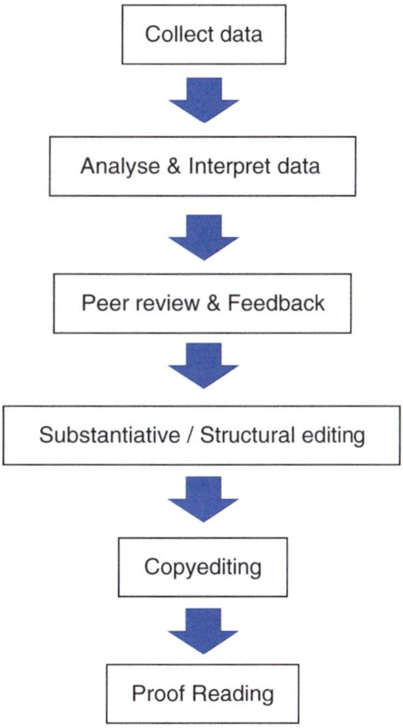

Fig. 1 Algorithm for the steps in language and content editing to avoid ambiguity

Discussion

Sand-Jensen decided to address the problem of poorly written manuscripts by discussing the top 10 things that should necessarily 'doom' a scientific paper [3]. These include lack of focus, originality and personality, writing long contributions, removing implications and speculations, leaving out illustrations, omitting necessary steps of reasoning, using many abbreviations and terms, suppressing humour and flowery language, degrading biology to statistics, quoting irrelevant or trivial references. While I would largely support Kaj's viewpoint, I have a different viewpoint in terms of the use of language. Humour and 'flowery' language would certainly not win favour with readers of science as much as they possibly would in English literature. Rather, the use of grammatically correct English following the 'KISS' principle (Keep it Simple Stupid) suggested by the United States Navy in 1960 would be the way to go!

It is advisable to attend courses, workshops or tutorials that enhance one's skills in editing large documents as these training sessions could empower the researcher with the understanding and necessary skills required to present their research in the best possible manner.

Conclusion

Performing experiments is only part of the job, interpreting the findings accurately and then presenting them appropriately is just as important. The first step to editing is to plan the structure of the text, tables and figures in terms of the flow of the document. The keys to avoiding ambiguity when dealing with quantitative and qualitative data are to keep an open mind when performing research and interpreting the results, and to subject one's findings to informal peer review before writing them up.

Case Scenario

Mohit has completed the experiments for his Master's degree and he is now ready to write up his thesis. The University guidelines stipulate that the thesis is written in English. It provides 'in house' editing support to students who are not native speakers of the language. Mohit has completed most of his education in Hindi but speaks English with his friends and even watches English movies. What should Mohit do?

1. Write the Master's thesis himself since he believes he is very fluent in English.
2. Seek help from the 'in house' editing team at the University for his thesis preparation.
3. Enlist the help of a professional copyediting service he has come across online and provide the receipt for the cost to his supervisor.

References

1. Australian standards for editing practice: Institute of Professional Editors Limited; 2013. Available from: http://www.iped-editors.org/site/DefaultSite/filesystem/documents/ASEP%20 flat%20onscreen%20version.pdf.
2. Wendy Monaghan Editing Services. Available from: http://www.wendymonaghan.com.au/ copyediting.html.
3. Sand-Jensen K. How to write consistently boring scientific literature. Oikos. 2007;116:723–7.

Plagiarism and Copyright, Acknowledgements, Disclosure and Conflicts of Interest

M. K. Ravindran, Balaji Zacharia, and Antony Roy

He who receives an idea from me, receives instruction himself without lessening mine; as he who lights his taper at mine, receives light without darkening me.—Thomas Jefferson

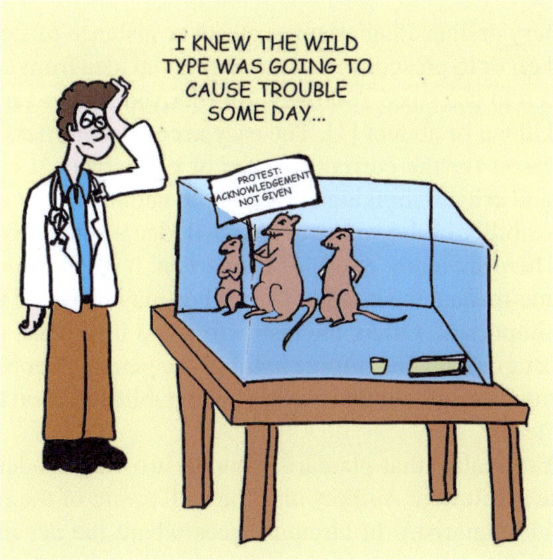

M. K. Ravindran (✉)
Professor and Head, Department of Emergency Medicine, Government Medical College, Kozhikode, Kerala, India

B. Zacharia
Additional Professor, Department of Orthopedics, Government Medical College, Kozhikode, Kerala, India

A. Roy
Former Senior Resident, Department of Orthopedics, Government Medical College, Kozhikode, Kerala, India

S. C. Parija, V. Kate (eds.), *Thesis Writing for Master's and Ph.D. Program*,
https://doi.org/10.1007/978-981-13-0890-1_19

Key Points

- It is the responsibility of the writer to acknowledge a source, context and genres of their writing.
- Plagiarism can destroy the self and academic reputation of an author.
- Copyright violation is not the same as plagiarism, though both are closely related.
- Copyright protects and rewards the creativity of the original author. Legal action can be taken by the owner against anyone who engages in infringement of the copyright of his/her own work.
- Conflict of interest is important in any research work because it can interfere with trustworthiness of a researcher's judgement
- Consent can be either implied consent or expressed consent. It is necessary for photographing, revealing the identity of the patient while publishing and enrolling patients for clinical trial and research project

Introduction

Webster's dictionary defines Plagiarism as an act or instance of stealing or using, to commit literary theft or to present as a new and original idea from an existing source. This word has been in use since 1600 AD. It is derived from a Latin word *plagiare* which means to kidnap or abduct [1]. The easy access to limitless material through internet is one reason for the current menace of plagiarism. It can also affect the writing, reading and critical thinking ability of the author.

It is the responsibility of the writer to acknowledge a source, context and genres of their writing. There are many causes of plagiarism. It may be due to fear of failure or due to poor time management skill. The author may consider the consequences of cheating as unimportant. Often, the instructors and institution may fail to report it when it does occur or may not enforce appropriate penalty. People often think that copying a little from vast amount of resources and publications on the web will most likely go undetected.

It is important to realise that plagiarism can destroy the academic reputation of the author and the institution. Authors must be well aware of the copyright law and measures to avoid plagiarism. In circumstances where the act involves monetary gains to the plagiariser or a loss to the original author, a fine or a compensatory restitution may be warranted respectively. The Committee on Publication Ethics (COPE) has issued guidelines to deal with suspected acts of plagiarism [2]. Once under scrutiny for plagiarism, the peer review process is suspended and in cases of published work a retraction will ensue. The penalty may also include a ban from further publication of research work.

Types of Plagiarism

- Direct plagiarism-A word for word reproduction of prior research.
- Self-plagiarism-Repeating portions from one's own prior work to pass off as new.

- Mosaic plagiarism- It simply refers to presenting plagiarised data or text in a new fashion, using synonyms, changing syntax etc.
- Accidental plagiarism-Occurs when the inexperienced author forgets, misquotes or fails to provide due citation.

Legal Implications of Plagiarism

Plagiarism does not amount to a criminal or civil offence but it is deemed illegal and considered as act of intellectual dishonesty [3]. It intrudes into the author's intellectual property right. It is very difficult to prove plagiarism. Search engines on the internet can detect plagiarism. Anti-Plagiarism softwares like Wcopy find and EduTie.com as well as online prevention services like iThenticate, Turnitin, Amazon 8–9 can be used [4]. Plagiarism is not limited to academic and literary material, it also can involve ideas, art forms such as storylines, music, videos etc. [5]. Paraphrasing is a subtle form of plagiarism. Just by changing or replacing few words, doesn't change the original text in verbatim, so the author remains guilty of plagiarism. Direct quotes are not considered plagiarism if they are properly written in quotation marks and cited.

Although plagiarism and copyright infringement have the same sentiment to put forward, they are in essence different. A blatant use of another's work without providing due attribution is plagiarism whereas copyright infringement involves a narrower perspective of simply reproducing data on a "cut copy paste" basis. Reproduction of information that is available for public access freely does not constitute copyright infringement.

How to Avoid Plagiarism?

An author can avoid plagiarism by citing the source within the text of a manuscript. Effective management of time can also reduce plagiarism. If the author has to meet a deadline to complete an article, he is likely to plagiarise knowingly or unknowingly. Good scientific writing comes with experience. A team approach and involvement of experienced authors helps to educate the young researcher the nuances of prudent scientific writing and the importance of thorough homework and collection of sources of information cannot be overemphasized. It is good practise to set aside separate time for a review of prior literature and for penning down original work as this reduces plagiarism. A good piece of research work is in many ways like rare aged whiskey, takes time to mature, recognised by few and leaves a lasting impression. A flow-chart depicting steps to overcome plagiarism is shown in Fig. 1.

Copyright in Clinical Research-What the Author Needs to Know?

Copyright is a right entrusted by the law for works in literature, theatre and art to the person/persons involved in its making. This right protects and rewards the creativity

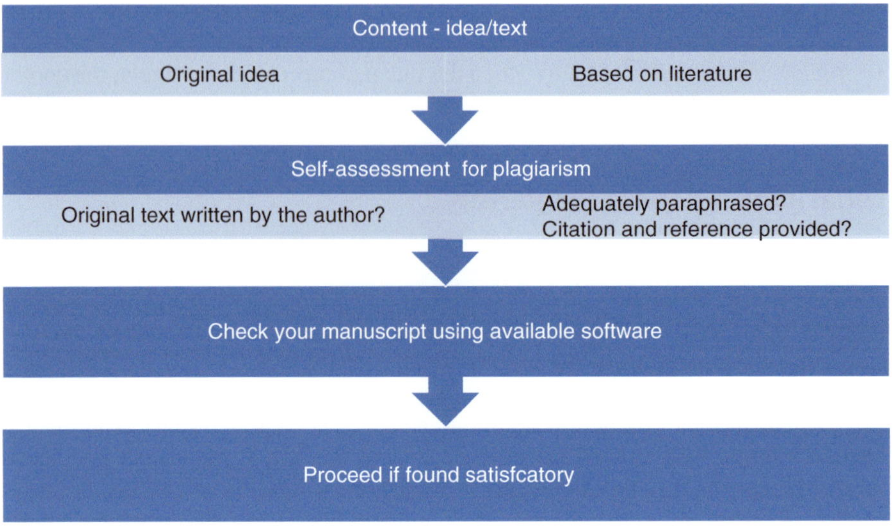

Fig. 1 How to ensure your thesis manuscript is not plagiarised?

of the original creator. If applied rigidly copyright protection can hamper the progress of society. But copyright laws are enacted in such a way to ensure that a balance is maintained between the interest of the creator and the community. Copyright protects the rights of authors. Sometimes an author can relinquish all or any of the rights comprising the copyright in the work by giving notice to the registrar of copyright. In the case of a literary work, the author has the right to reproduce, issue copies of the work to the public, to perform, communicate the work in public, to translate the work and to make any adaptation of his/her work. Computer software are protected and treated as literary work. The author also enjoys the right to sell or give on hire, or offer for sale the software. Copyright acquisition doesn't require any formality as it is automatic. But to serve as prima facie evidence in a court of law the author has to get a certificate of registration of copyright. The copyright of an author usually lasts for sixty years following the death of the author. The commonly known acts of copyright infringement include making infringing copies for sale or hire, permitting any place for performance of work in public, public exhibition of the copyrighted material, importation of infringing copies etc. Legal action can be taken by the owner against anyone who engages in infringement of the copyright of his/her own work. The copyright infringement is under jurisdiction of the district court. Under section 63 of copyright act it is considered to be a criminal offence [6, 7].

Some medical journals may ask the authors to transfer of copyright for all types of contents like audio, video, protocols etc. while some other journals require transfer of publication license. It is the publishers' or journals responsibility to make clear the type of copyright under which it will publish the manuscript. Some contents cannot be copyrighted. The copyright of certain journals sometimes will prohibit the authors the right to own, reproduce, publish, republish, prepare, foreign language translation, distribute, prepare derivative works and publically display the copies. A transfer of copyright is usually included along with the process of submission of the article for review. This is usually done via copyright transfer forms which are usually provided in an online link from the publishers website. All authors are required to sign the form. The transfer agreement usually includes clauses pertaining to the originality of the article and a declaration that the work has not been published or accepted elsewhere.

Reproduction of published data (Figures, flow-charts, schematics, etc.) may be facilitated via a letter of permission. Most publishers have online forms for permission which can be downloaded and mailed to the editor. The letter should convey the article from which information is being sought and the article in which it is to be reused. The letter would also include an affidavit as to the purpose and scope of permission. Open access content and material available from unrestricted public domains may be used without a permission letter. Most publishers will have defined guidelines for the same. Irrespective of the manner in which the material is obtained it needs to be recognised in the article either via a citation along with the references or a footnote.

Conflicts of Interest in Research

Conflicts of interest are defined as a situation where a person's professional judgments or actions concerning a primary cause are affected by his/her involvement in multiple interests, which include economical or non-economic benefits [8]. Conflict of interest is important in any research work because it can interfere with trustworthiness of a researcher's judgement. The term 'competing interest' is occasionally used instead of conflict of interest. For the development of medications and medical devices, it is essential to have a cordial partnership among industry, academicians and government. But there are evidences that this type of a relationship has a risk of decreasing transparency in sharing data and withholding negative results. A well-known example of conflicting interests was the case of the MMR (Mumps, Measles, Rubella) vaccines which were alleged to be linked with autism, investigations later proved that the author of the article had received financial gain from it and had not disclosed a conflict of interest [9, 10]. Such stigma towards the MMR vaccine remains even today. Another example is the case of the anti-diabetic drug rosiglitazone wherein a probable cardiovascular risk was overseen by investigators with undisclosed benefits from pharmaceutical companies [11].

We cannot label the judgement of person with some conflict of interest as unethical. There are many ways in which conflict of interest can affect a researcher like direct employment, grants/research funding, consultancy, travel grants, stock ownership etc. In most situations, the conflict of interest is financial in nature. Sometimes a researcher will have multiple roles such as the role of an administrator and a researcher, these types of obligations can confound results although they are not tangible. The institutional research committee and the ethical committee have authority in investigating any conflict of interest. The best way to avoid concern regarding any conflict of interest is to disclose them prior to starting the project. The manuscript based on the project should also include the statement for conflict of interest to avoid concern for the reviewers and readers when published. Disclosures relating to any potential conflicts of interest such as financial or logistic support for the study should be submitted at the time of review. This is of utmost importance for maintaining the ethics of publishing and for bringing out valid and accurate data. Disclosures in a scientific work should include both relevant financial and non-financial benefits and relationships.

In the Indian scenario, the Good clinical practise guidelines issued by Central drug standards and control organisation deal with conflict of interest [12]. Conflicts of interest are a reality in quality medical research. Prudent disclosure and management of conflicting interests will ensure transparent and ethical research. International committee of medical journal editors provide templates accessible online for disclosure of conflict of interest in matters related to clinical research.

De-Identification of Data

De-identification of data refers to the process used to prevent personal identity from being connected with information. The researcher should ensure to avoid disclosure of personally identifiable information from their records. Whenever the institution/university wants to share data for a research project to another research, certain strategies to prevent disclosure of personally identifiable information need to be adopted. Anonymisation, blurring and de-identification are common strategies used for this purpose. Manually erasing/whitening out medical records, usage of software to delink electronic data are methods of de-identification. There are various methods used in de-identification strategy/disclosure limitation [13].

1. Perturbation-Is used to mask original values in data to avoid disclosure.
2. Masking-Used to mask original values in a data set to achieve data privacy protection.
3. Record code-Unique descriptor which can be used to trace individual level records across de-identified data files.
4. Redaction-Expunging sensitive data from the records prior to disclosure.

Personal identifiers such as name, biometric data, government and personal identification numbers, photographs, address etc. need to be removed from data being shared. Data re-identification becomes essential is some special situations and can be achieved by reversing the process although the entire data may not be retrieved.

Informed Consent in Research

Consent can be defined as "an instrument of mutual communication between the physician and patient with an expression of authorisation/permission/choice by the latter for the doctor to act in a particular way" [14]. The ethical principle of patient autonomy and basic human right gave birth to the idea of consent [15, 16]. No one has the right to touch/let alone treat another person without due permission and this is considered as physical assault and is punishable [14]. Consent can be either implied consent or expressed consent. It is necessary for photographing, revealing the identity of the patient while publishing and enrolling patients for clinical trial and research project [17, 18]. Patients participating in research should be competent to give consent, an adult with sound mind and a parent in case of minors can give consent. Every effort must be made to provide information to vulnerable segments to assist informed decision making. Children and elderly can be assisted in being part of decision making. Nothing shall be done to hinder independent decision making. Illiteracy of the patient shall not be held as a defence in not providing adequate information to the patient or the participant. The balance of risk and benefit must be fully explained to the subject. No facts are to be suppressed. The subjects must be given full freedom to withdraw from the study at any time they choose.

The institutional research committee and the ethical board is responsible for and ensures that a legally valid consent encompassing the principles of voluntarism and intelligent decision in the light of completely transparent patient information is obtained. Common practice of obtaining informed consent involves distribution of patient information sheets, interviews to clarify doubts and procurement of a duly signed informed consent form [19].

Case Scenarios

1. You want to use a quote within the text you are writing. How do you avoid plagiarism for that?
   (a) Paraphrase the quote.
   (b) Use the quote but within inverted quotes and cite reference.
   (c) Use the quote but avoid citation so that it is not identified.
   (d) Use the quote only after taking the permission from the copyright holder.
2. You want to re-use a previously published table/figure from an article where you are the primary author. How do you avoid copyright violation?
   (a) Get documented permission from the copyright holder of the previous article for using the content.
   (b) Use the table/figure as required and add citation.
   (c) Re-frame the table/figure with modifications.
   (d) Use the table/figure without taking permission of the journal.

Acknowledgments Acknowledgement is a gesture that allows us to thank all the individuals who helped to make the project a successful one. A standard pattern for writing an acknowledgement letter has not been described. In thesis, a single page usually following the contents page is allotted for acknowledgement. The investigator mentions gratitude to the individuals who helped in the research in order of their importance. The usual format includes acknowledging the guide and co-guides, followed by other faculty in the department in order of seniority. This is then followed by acknowledging the administrators of the institute for facilitating the research. The colleagues, family members and the involved patients are then acknowledged. The rendering must be concise and without emotion. However, when the thesis is converted to a manuscript for publication, acknowledgemnt as two to three concise statements is included at the end of manuscript, before the references. This will include acknowledgements for the funding sources if any and to other contributors to the study who, however, doesn't satisfy the authorship criteria. All the contributors to the project need not be co-authors and in such circumstances the statement of acknowledgement becomes a polite gesture of recognising their assistance. It is common practise in many institutions to provide a copy of the completed research project to the contributors. Acknowledgements boost researcher morale and promote further cooperation especially when one or more of the contributors do not receive authorship.

References

1. Das N, Panjabi M. Plagiarism: why is it such a big issue for medical writers? Perspect Clin Res. 2011;2(2):67–71. https://doi.org/10.4103/2229-3485.80370.
2. Flowcharts. Committee on Publication Ethics. Available from http://publicationethics.org/resources/flowcharts.
3. Lands R. Plagiarism is no crime published by the association of illustrators (AOI). Quotation: Plagiarism may be a taboo in academia, but in art is almost essential; 1999.
4. Badke W. Training plagiarism detectives: the law and order approach. Online. 2007;31(6):50–2.
5. Brehm AS. Defendants in idea submission claims are increasingly winning summary judgment by demonstrating independent creation. Los Angeles Lawyer. 2010;33:28.
6. The Copyright Act 1957. Accessed from http://copyright.gov.in/documents/copyrightrules1957.pdf.
7. The Information Technology Act, 2000. Accessed from-http://www.dot.gov.in/sites/default/files/itbill2000_0.pdf.
8. Lo B, Field MJ, editors. Conflict of Interest in Medical Research, Education, and Practice. Washington (DC): National Academies Press US; 2009. Available from: http://www.ncbi.nlm.nih.gov/books/NBK22942/
9. Wakefield A, Murch S, Anthony A, Linnell J, Casson DM, Malik M, et al. Ileal-lymphoid-nodular hyperplasia, non-specific colitis, and pervasive developmental disorder in children. Lancet. 1998;351(9103):637–41. *Retracted 05–09-2007*
10. Flaherty DK. The vaccine-autism connection: a public health crisis caused by unethical medical practices and fraudulent science. Ann Pharmacother. 2011;45(10):1302–4.
11. Wang AT, Mc Coy CP, Murad MH, Montori VM. Association between industry affiliation and position on cardiovascular risk with rosiglitazone: cross sectional systematic review. BMJ. 2010;340:c1344.
12. Ghooi RB. Conflict of interest in clinical research. Perspect Clin Res. 2015;6(1):10–4. https://doi.org/10.4103/2229-3485.148794.
13. Privacy technical assistance center.US department of education. Available from: http://ptac.ed.gov/.
14. Satyanarayana Rao KH. Informed consent: an ethical obligation or legal compulsion? J Cutan Aesthet Surg. 2008;1(1):33–5. https://doi.org/10.4103/0974-2077.41159.
15. Beauchamp TL, Childress JF. Principles of biomedical ethics. 5th ed. Oxford: Oxford University Press; 2001.
16. Madhava Menon NR. Medical ethics and health care - issues and perspectives. Karnataka Med J. 2000;71:2–9.
17. Joga Rao SV. Medical Ethics, A Ready Referencer. 1st ed. Bangalore: Legalaxy Publications; 2004. p. 84.
18. Medical Ethics Manual. World Medical Association, Inc. 2005. p. 105. Available from: http://www.wma.net/.
19. Gupta UC. Informed consent in clinical research: revisiting few concepts and areas. Perspect Clin Res. 2013;4(1):26–32. https://doi.org/10.4103/2229-3485.106373.

Part V

Publishing and Presenting the Research Work

Preparing Manuscript from Thesis Material and Selecting Journals for Submission

Vikram Kate, Sathasivam Sureshkumar, and Akhila Kavirayani

You don't write something because you want to say something, you write because you have got something to say.—F. Scott Fitzgerald

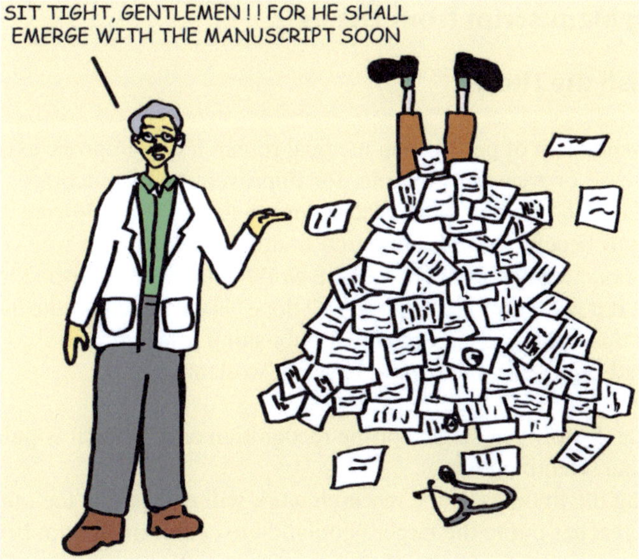

V. Kate (✉)
Professor and Head, Department of Surgery and Senior Consultant General and Gastrointestinal Surgeon, Jawaharlal Institute of Postgraduate Medical Education and Research, Pondicherry, India

S. Sureshkumar
Associate Professor, Department of Surgery, Jawaharlal Institute of Postgraduate Medical Education and Research, Pondicherry, India

A. Kavirayani
Consultant Paediatric Rheumatologist, Nuffield Orthopaedic Centre, Oxford University Hospitals NHS Foundation Trust, Oxford, UK

S. C. Parija, V. Kate (eds.), *Thesis Writing for Master's and Ph.D. Program*,
https://doi.org/10.1007/978-981-13-0890-1_20

Key Points

- The best way of getting the thesis work and the research outcome known to the rest of the world is to get it published in a scientific journal.
- The skill of preparing an article out of a dissertation can be acquired and mastered by familiarizing oneself with original articles published in various journals.
- The International Committee of Medical Journal Editors (ICMJE) provides assistance in preparing the manuscript and the submission process.
- Indexing often serves as the officially recognized database where researchers and scholars can reliably find high quality scientific journals for publication.
- Predatory, scholarly open-access journals generally have weak peer-review system and often charge the authors a heavy processing fee. Submission to these *questionable* open-access standalone publishers to be avoided.
- Familiarizing oneself with manuscript submission and tracking system helps in publishing the thesis work in a shorter time frame.

Preparing Manuscript from Thesis

Why Publish the Thesis?

The fundamental aim of performing medical research is to improve existing knowledge on disease or treatment options for improvement of outcomes. This is best achieved when the research work reaches out to the wider healthcare provider network who will benefit from the research findings [1]. The best way of getting the research outcome known to the rest of the world is to get it published in a scientific journal. [2] "If it wasn't published, it wasn't done" is the famous quote by E.H. Miller 1993 which underpins the importance of publishing research work.

Specific advantages in publishing research work are:

1. The research work per se gets prime recognition only when it is published in an appropriate scientific journal.
2. Publishing the findings of the research work will ensure that the outcome of the research reaches out to the target population to confer maximum benefit.
3. Facilitates career progression of the researcher in the specific research field.
4. Lucrative to funding agencies who might be interested in the particular area of research.
5. Influences the professional recruitment of the researcher in teaching medical institutions and also aids promotional avenues [3].
6. Enhances reputation amongst peers in addition to a sense of personal academic achievement.
7. Last but not the least, it is the moral responsibility of the researcher to disclose the findings of the research as it might benefit the medical fraternity and society as a whole, by positively or negatively influencing current knowledge of the disease or treatment strategies. The most effective means of achieving this would be via publication in a reputed scientific journal.

Manuscript Preparation from Thesis

The thesis is an outcome of carefully planned and executed research work, which details all the aspects of the project ranging from the protocol to the conclusion. The detailed thesis project is often voluminous and can range from a hundred pages to a thousand pages depending on the 'base' project i.e. a master's degree thesis or a PhD thesis. It is not practical to publish the thesis work in its entirety in any scientific journal, as an individual issue of a journal generally publishes around 15–20 manuscripts. Hence to publish the thesis in a specific journal, the content needs to be edited as per the journal's requirements. Every journal has different requirements in terms of manuscript style, type of font, size of the font, spacing and word/character count [4]. These details can be found in the section on "Instructions to authors" in the journal's web page. Most journals limit the word count to 2500–3500 for original research work, which generally extends over four to five pages. It is no less than a herculean task to edit the contents of the thesis, which often runs into hundreds of pages, to a manuscript of 4000 words, whilst preserving the core essence. However, the skill of preparing an article out of a dissertation can be acquired and mastered by familiarizing oneself with original articles published in various journals, which will make the student familiar with the manuscript style and the expectations of the reader, the reviewer and the editor [5, 6].

The typical article in medical journals is said to follow the IMRAD pattern, which stands for Introduction, Methods, Results and Discussion. However, most current scientific journals have adapted the guidelines laid out by the International Committee of Medical Journal Editors (ICMJE). The first recommendation of the ICMJE on Uniform requirements for manuscripts submitted to biomedical journals was framed in 1997 and the guidelines are updated at regular intervals [7]. The latest version of "Recommendations for the Conduct, Reporting, Editing and Publication of Scholarly Work in Medical Journals" guideline was updated in December 2016 and the Portable Document File (PDF) is available free to access for the researcher [8]. The document sets out clear guidelines to be followed when reporting the research and the specific statements to be made during the manuscript submission to ensure proper conduct of the research and adherence with ethical standards. The ICMJE also provides assistance in preparing the manuscript and the submission process, which can be accessed free-of-charge via the home page link of ICMJE [9]. It is prudent to read and understand the guidelines before preparing the manuscript to avoid multiple revisions or rejection of the article.

As part of standard reporting of research, a specific format is recommended to be followed depending on the study design. The mandatory reporting and checklist includes Strengthening the Reporting of Observational studies in Epidemiology for observational studies (STROBE), Standards for Reporting of Diagnostic Accuracy (STARD) and Consolidated Standards of Reporting Trials (CONSORT) for clinical trials [10–13]. Table 1 describes the mandates for the manuscript and compares the style of thesis and the typical manuscript submitted and published in the journal.

Table 1 Mandates for the manuscript and compares the style of thesis and the typical manuscript submitted and published in the journal

Contents	Thesis	Manuscript
Certificate of thesis completion	In the front page	Not required
Acknowledgement	Usually in second to fourth page	At the end of the manuscript, in two to five lines
Abstract	Not mandatory	Mandatory, 150–250 words in most journals
Introduction	500–1500 words	150–200 words
Review of literature	Ranges from 100 to 150 pages	Not required
Aim and objective	Should be spelt out separately i.e. Aim, primary and secondary objective(s)	Objectives are usually incorporated at the end of the introduction or in the beginning of methodology
Methodology	Detailed methodology including the year and duration of the study, department and institution where it was carried out, patient details, procedure/ intervention details, primary/ secondary outcomes and the scale used to measure the outcomes, ethical/ legal aspect etc., ranges between five to ten pages	Brief methodology focusing on 1. Study design 2. Inclusion/ exclusion criteria 3. Randomization, blinding, allocation concealment etc. depending on the study design 4. Brief description of intervention, duration of follow up/ data collection 5. Outcome variables and methods/scale for the assessment of outcomes 6. Declaration of Helsinki for human studies and clinical trial registration if applicable 7. Brief mention about ethics committee approval and informed patient consent The methods section is usually written in 500 to 750 words
Statistical analysis	Detailed statistical aspect of the thesis including details of sample size calculation and rationale for selection, all the variables, statistical tests used for outcome variables etc., ranges from four to five pages	Brief statistical analysis written in a paragraph ranges between 50–100 words focusing on 1. Sample size calculation 2. Primary and important secondary outcome variables and the statistical tests used for the same 3. Defining cut off for statistical significance

Table 1 (continued)

Observations and Results	Details of all possible analysis of the research variables and write up for all the tables and figures. Usually written between ten to twenty pages	Results written as paragraphs between 150 to 200 words, citing the table number where necessary. There should not be an overlap of contents between the text and illustrations. The brief results need to focus on 1. Number of patients included and eventually analyzed 2. Tables which need to be explicit and self-explanatory 3. Brief write up of results which have not been included in the tables or figures
Discussion	Detailed discussion which compares methods, all the parameters/variables studied and the outcomes. Written between 10 and 20 pages	Focused discussion on the important outcomes, written in 750–1500 words
Summary	Briefing the thesis including the objective(s) of the study, methods, results and discussion	Not required
Conclusion	Written in detail stating the rationale and justification of arriving at the conclusion	Written in 50–100 words stating the final outcome of the study. May include recommendations based on the outcome
Limitations	Detailing the hardship faced and the weakness of the conducted research, with possible suggestions to overcome such issues in future studies	Included at the end of the discussion, stating the important limitation(s) which could possibly affect the study outcome
Tables and figures	Between 20 and 40 tables and figures	Restricted to 4–6 tables/figures in most journals. Few journals allow extra content (tables, figures etc.) to be published as "supplementary material" available online along with the article
References	Ranges from 50 for a master's degree thesis to 250 references for a PhD project. Vancouver style is commonly followed	Restricted to 30–50 references depending on the individual journal requirements. Referencing style may vary among the journals, however, most journals follow the Vancouver style of referencing

(continued)

Table 1 (continued)

Contents	Thesis	Manuscript
Annexure	Includes the following 1. Protocol submitted 2. Institutional review board/ ethics committee certificates 3. Patient information sheet and consent form 4. Description of scale, classification/ definitions of items used in the thesis detailing the source 5. Data collection Proforma 6. Master data chart	None of the mentioned items required. A small number of journals request a statement from the corresponding author stating that the original data collected can be produced when solicited
Details of contribution of authors/ investigators	Not required	Generally required in brief stating the contribution toward, conceptualization, literature search, designing the study, data collection, analysis, write up of the manuscript and agreement among the included authors
Statement of conflict of interest, copyright- transfer agreement, financial disclosure	Not mandatory	Required as a mandatory part of submission. Some journals also require confirmation from the corresponding author that the article is not already published or under review in any other journal at the time of submission and that all the authors have viewed and approved the manuscript before submission. Most journals require declaration of the conflict of interest and disclosures from all the authors individually
Various statements on adherence to standard research reporting	Various statements on adherence to standard research reporting like Helsinki Statement for human studies, Data sharing statement for clinical trials, STROBE reporting and checklist, CONSORT reporting and checklist are desirable but not mandatory	Required as a part of Uniform requirements for manuscripts submitted to biomedical journals

Selecting the Journal for Submission

Searching for the Journal to Publish the Thesis Work-Where to Begin?

The selection of the journal for publication of the thesis work is a crucial step in eventual successful publication. It begins with searching for similar or related published research work [14–17]. Medical research search engines like PubMed are freely available and serve to find journals which have published related research work [17, 18]. PubMed searches the database from PubMed Central and Medline, where a majority of the published medical researches are indexed. Similarly, Google Scholar and Elsevier supported tools such as Mendeley also provide a good number of accessible publications from many journals. The journals that have published similar allied research work are more likely to consider the work for potential publication. Identifying journals in this manner is most likely to be beneficial for young research scholars with limited experience in publication.

Scope of the Journal and the Thesis Content

After shortlisting potential journals, it is important to visit the home page of each of the selected journals to check out the aim and scope of the journal. It is important to be aware that some journals such as the *Journal of Gene Medicine, Molecular Oncology* etc. publish only basic research, whereas other journals like the *International Journal of Surgery, World Journal of Gastroenterology, New England Journal of Medicine etc.* publish both basic and clinical research work. If the submitted manuscript does not fall within the scope of the journal, it will be rejected at the editorial screening itself, prior to being sent for peer review [16–18]. Hence, selecting the most suitable journal will avoid multiple rejections and thereby the unnecessary time delay [19].

Another easy method to search for journals with a similar scope of publication is to simply check the journals, which were quoted in the literature review of the thesis. If a journal is cited multiple times in the review text of the thesis, it is likely to have a similar aim and scope as the research work in question.

Multidisciplinary or Speciality Journal

Multidisciplinary journals like the *New England Journal of Medicine, International Journal of Advanced Medical and Health Research* etc. tend to publish research work from all fields of medicine. Specialty journals like the *International Journal of Surgery, Annals of Surgery, JAMA Surgery* etc. predominantly publish surgical research work. Journals such as the *Journal of Gastroenterology and Hepatology; Canadian Journal of Kidney Diseases* etc. publish mainly organ-oriented research.

Multidisciplinary journals have the advantage of wider readership and a high impact factor, however, publications in these journals are often multicentric research studies of high academic calibre [14–18]. The speciality and organ oriented journals often have a select target audience who will derive maximum benefit from the published research. Selection of the journal should be done after considering the above criteria and the field in which the thesis work was done. Search engines such as https://www.biomedcentral.com/journals may also be used to fetch the existing journals in a particular speciality [20].

Indexed Journals and Indexing Agencies

Much is spoken and discussed regarding indexed journals amongst the academic fraternity. Young researchers often have no clue as to what is considered an indexed publication. A majority might be under the impression that journals available on PubMed are indexed and the rest are not. The indexing process will help the author in avoiding the predatory journals. In these journals, there is generally a weak peer-review system and often the quality of accepted articles may not be up to the standards. These journals often charge the authors a heavy processing fee as well. The list of predatory journals can be found at https://web.archive.org/web/20170112125427/https://scholarlyoa.com/publishers/" [21]. Since the originality and legitimacy of the published research work in any journal entirely depends on the stringent peer review system, indexing agencies follow strict guidelines for the peer review system and conduct regular checks to ensure adherence.

Indexing often serves as the officially recognized database where researchers and scholars can reliably find high-quality scientific articles. Indexed journals adhere to the austere manuscript publication criteria which includes a transparent blinded peer review system which prevents research work of lesser standard from being published [21, 22].

Recognized indexing databases include the following

1. Embase/ExcerptaMedica
2. IndMed
3. Medline (Index Medicus)
4. PubMed Central
5. Scopus
6. Science Citation Index

The recognized indexing agencies make the article easily and widely available to researchers and provide a surrogate guarantee of the quality and reliability. This will also help in improving the citations of the article. Hence while choosing the journal for manuscript submission it is vital to check the home page of the journal with regards to the status of indexing and the agency with which it is indexed.

Open Access Publication

Open access gives researchers the opportunity to make their research work universally available by paying an open access fee. This usually ranges from 200 USD to 2500 USD in line with the reputation of the journal. The readers, however, will have access to the article without paying a subscription fee to the journal. If the publication is freely accessible online, it will have a wide readership and the researcher thereby gets the highest recognition for the work done as it reaches out to the maximum possible audience [23–25]. Many journals do not charge for manuscript processing and publication, for authors not opting for open access. A few journals charge for colour illustrations. It is to be noted that the open access fee is charged over and above the publication charges and the charges for publishing colour images if any. Some funding agencies make it mandatory for the researcher to opt for open access publication and include these charges as part of the funding. In non-funded thesis work, the author has the option to opt or decline the open access publication depending on the charges and/or the agreement amongst the other investigators.

International/Regional Journals and Language of Publication

Publishing the thesis work in an international journal like the New England journal of medicine, Nature medicine etc. gets wider recognition for the researcher as it reaches out to all parts of the world [23, 24]. Publication in English assures a higher readership as it serves as the common language for exchanging modern scientific knowledge. However, the work, which is concerned with or benefits a highly specific finite geographical area is less likely to get accepted in an international journal. Non-native English speaking authors might need to make use of language editing services provided by recognized agencies for preparing the manuscript, which increases the chance of acceptance [26].

Behavior of a disease/drug or distribution/pattern of health issues related to a particular race or geographical population can better serve its purpose if it gets published in regional/national journals (e.g. *European journal of medicine, Tropical Gastroenterology* and *Indian Journal of Surgery*). The researcher needs to assess the crux and the core message of the thesis to decide in appropriately selecting a regional, national or an international journal.

Journal Impact Factor

Journal Impact Factor (JIF) serves as a comprehensive tool to assess the quality, reliability and reputation of the journal [27, 28]. It is calculated from the average number of citations per paper published in the particular journal in the preceding two years. A higher impact factor indicates that the articles published in the journal are of adequate quality to be read and cited by many researchers [29, 30]. Publishing in a high impact journal increases the chances of getting more citations for the article and wider recognition for the research work [31, 32]. However, the rejection rate in most high impact factor journals is significantly high, to the extent of 70–80% of submissions being rejected, as these journals strive to publish the highest quality research work. Most journals provide information on the current impact factor in the home page. This can be confirmed by the journal citation report (JCR) before submitting the manuscript, as falsified impact factors have been found to be reported by a few fraudulent journals.

Author Guidelines and Checklist

Before submitting the manuscript, it is mandatory to read and understand the author guidelines of a particular journal as every journal has different submission requirements with respect to word count, manuscript style and content, structure of the abstract, number of tables and figures, authorship criteria, copyright and legal processing etc. Reading and preparing the manuscript as per the journal guidelines reduces the duration of submission to eventual publication by avoiding multiple revisions at editorial screening [33]. Most journals provide a check list to be verified before final submission which includes number of files such as the title file, blinded manuscript file, tables and figures file, conflict of interests statement, authorship statement, statement on originality and non-submission to other journals and other supportive/specific documents. Preparing and arranging all the required files before submission will reduce the time spent in uploading the manuscript. Figure 1 illustrates the preparation of manuscript and submission process for a journal.

Manuscript Submission Process and Tracking System

Most journals follow an online manuscript submission system, which is an easier and faster method of publishing research work. The submission is then diverted to a common manuscript processing system such as Manuscript Central (Scholar One) and Editorial Manager in which the manuscript can be submitted and tracked using the assigned manuscript number during further course [34].

In summary, publishing one's thesis work is a task made easier by being systematic and organised. Also, 'being fore-warned is being fore-armed'. Familiarising oneself with the process and being aware of potential problems will save precious time and effort and go a long way towards ensuring successful publication of the thesis work.

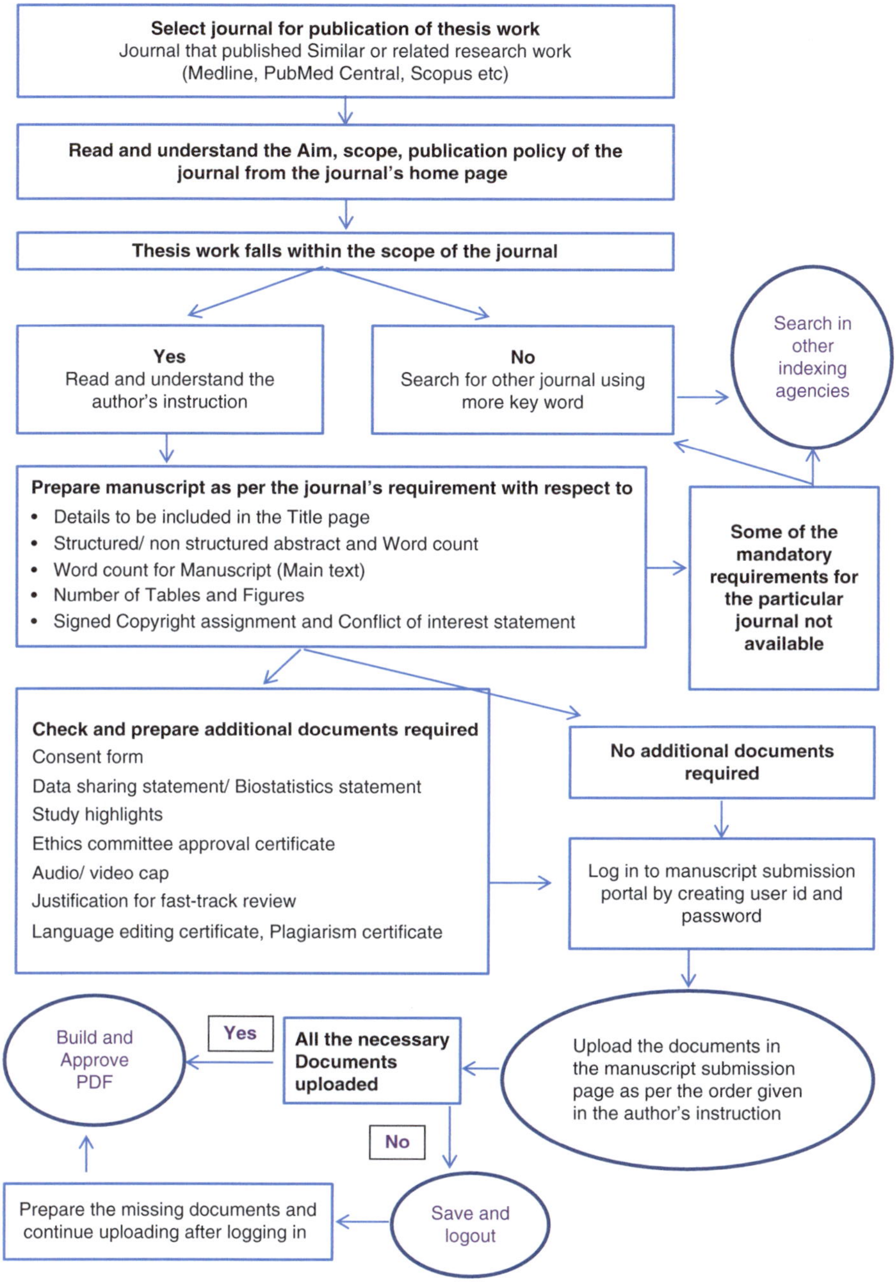

Fig. 1 Preparation of manuscript form thesis and submission process for a journal

Case Scenarios

1. After submission of manuscript to an indexed journal, the editor returns back the manuscript stating that it is not as per the journals requirements. Which of the following is the appropriate step?
   (a) Consider a different journal for publication.
   (b) Check the instruction to author of that journal and prepare the manuscript accordingly.
   (c) Attach study highlights and data sharing statement.
   (d) Reduce the word count and number of figures and tables.
2. You receive a mail from editor of a journal stating that they are interested in publishing your original article, and will provide concessional publication fee if you submit the manuscript in next one week. What would you do?
   (a) Immediately accept the invitation and submit the manuscript.
   (b) Check the article processing fee/publication fee and submit the manuscript if affordable.
   (c) Check the indexing status of the said journal by visiting the home page and read the details of editorial board, instruction etc.
   (d) Check the possibility of potential/probable Predatory, scholarly open-access journal before considering it for submission.

References

1. Lancaster FW, Smith LC. Science, scholarship and the communication of knowledge. Lib Trends, Winter. 1978;27:367–88.
2. Russell JM. Scientific communication at the beginning of the twenty-first century. Int Soc Sci J. 2001;53(168):271–82.
3. Aggarwal R, Gogtay N, Kumar R, Sahni P. The revised guidelines of the Medical Council of India for academic promotions: need for a rethink. Natl Med J India. 2016;29(1):1–5.
4. Welch HG. Preparing manuscripts for submission to medical journals: the paper trail. Eff Clin Pract. 1999;2(3):131–7.
5. Peh WC, Ng KH. Preparing a manuscript for submission. Singap Med J. 2009;50(8):759–61.
6. Ghahramani Z, Mehrabani G. The criteria considered in preparing manuscripts for submission to biomedical journals. Bull Emerg Trauma. 2013;1(2):56–9.
7. Uniform requirements for manuscripts submitted to biomedical journals. Writing and editing for biomedical publication. J Pharmacol Pharmacother. 2010;1(1):42–58.
8. Recommendations for the Conduct, Reporting, Editing, and Publication of Scholarly Work in Medical Journals- Updated December 2016. Available from: http://www.icmje.org/icmje-recommendations.pdf. Accessed 29 Aug 2017.
9. International Committee of Medical Journal Editors- Manuscript preparation Available from: http://www.icmje.org/recommendations/browse/manuscript-preparation/. Accessed 29 Aug 2017.
10. PLOS Medicine Editors. From checklists to tools: Lowering the barrier to better research reporting. PLoS Med. 2015;12:e1001910.
11. Hopewell S, Clarke M, Moher D, Wager E, Middleton P, Altman DG, et al. CONSORT for reporting randomized controlled trials in journal and conference abstracts: explanation and elaboration. PloS Med. 2008;5(1):e20. https://doi.org/10.1371/journal.pmed.0050020.

12. Von Elm E, Altman DG, Egger M, Pocock SJ, Gøtzsche PC, Vandenbroucke JP, et al. The strengthening the reporting of observational studies in epidemiology (STROBE) statement: guidelines for reporting observational studies. PLoS Med. 2007;4(10):e296.
13. Bossuyt PM, Reitsma JB, Bruns DE, Gatsonis CA, Glasziou PP, Irwig LM, et al. Towards complete and accurate reporting of studies of diagnostic accuracy: the STARD initiative. BMJ. 2003;326:41.
14. Shokraneh F, Ilghami R, Masoomi R, Amanollahi A. How to select a journal to submit and publish your biomedical paper? Bio Impacts. 2012;2(1):61–8.
15. Fahy K. How to get published in an international journal. Women Birth. 2010;23:43–4.
16. Frank E. Authors' criteria for selecting journals. JAMA. 1994;272:163–4.
17. Thompson PJ. How to choose the right journal for your manuscript. Chest. 2007;132:1073–6.
18. Thyer BA. Targeting one or more potential journals. In: Preparing research articles. New York: Oxford University Press; 2008. p. 13–32.
19. Ali J. Manuscript rejection: causes and remedies. J Young Pharm. 2010;2(1):3–6. https://doi.org/10.4103/0975-1483.62205.
20. Errami M, Wren JD, Hicks JM, Garner HR. eT-BLAST: a web server to identify expert reviewers, appropriate journals and similar publications. Nucleic Acids Res. 2007;35(Web Server issue):W12–5.
21. Scholarly Open Access. List of Publishers: Beall's List. Available from: http://scholarlyoa.com/publishers/. Accessed 25 Aug 2017.
22. Index Copernicus International. Available from: http://en.indexcopernicus.com/. Accessed 25 Aug 2017.
23. Garfield E. Which medical journals have the greatest impact? Ann Intern Med. 1986;105:313–20.
24. Garfield E. Citation indexes to science: a new dimension in documentation through association of ideas. Science. 1955;122:108–11.
25. Llewellyn RD, Pellack LJ, Shonrock DD. The use of electronic-only journals in scientific research. Issues Sci Tech Librarian. 2002; https://doi.org/10.5062/F41V5BZM.
26. Lozano GA. Ethics of using language-editing services in an era of digital communication and heavily multi-authored papers. Sci Eng Ethics. 2014;20(2):363–77.
27. Hirsch JE. An index to quantify an individual's scientific research output. PNAS. 2005;102(46):16569–72.
28. Makeham JM, Pilowsky PM. Journal Impact Factors and Research Submission Pressures. ANZ J Surg. 2003;73:93–4.
29. Garfield E. When to cite. Libr Q. 1996;66(4):449–58.
30. Maffuli N. More on citation analysis. Nature. 1995;378:760.
31. Bellini C. Cited or read? Lancet. 2012;379(28):314.
32. Reedijk J. Citations and ethics. Angew Chem Int. Ed. 2011;50:2–3.
33. Wager E. Do medical journals provide clear and consistent guidelines on authorship? Med Gen Med. 2007;9(3):16.
34. Bishop MJ. Manuscript central interactive online system and issue summary. Brief Bioinform. 2007;8(6):381.

Presenting Thesis in Conferences: Oral and Poster Presentation

Santhosh John Abraham

If you don't know what you want to achieve in your presentation, your audience never will.—Harvey Diamond

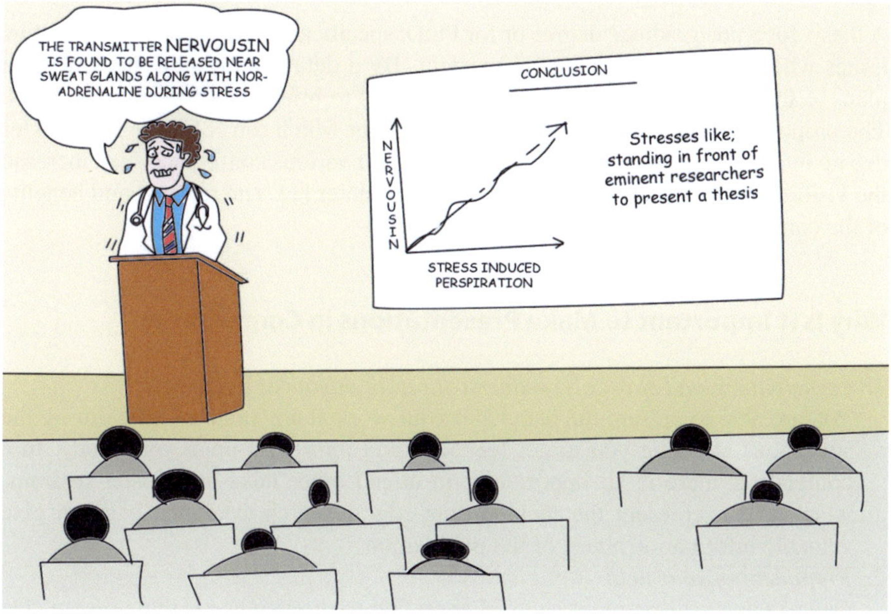

S. J. Abraham
Head, Department of Surgery, Lourdes Hospital, Kochi, Kerala, India

S. C. Parija, V. Kate (eds.), *Thesis Writing for Master's and Ph.D. Program*,
https://doi.org/10.1007/978-981-13-0890-1_21

Key Points

- The task to convert the voluminous thesis data, its analysis and the conclusions drawn over few years to a ten minute oral or a poster presentation is too demanding.
- The process starts with in depth discussion of the doctrine under proposal with colleagues and seniors, refining the proposal and submission for presentation in an appropriate conference.
- The initial presentation may better be a poster which gives the presenter ample informal time to defend his concept with the viewers in different ways thus improving the presentation skills, confidence levels and finally lead to a chance for making an oral presentation.
- The increasing visibility the candidate makes by continued presentation will make the profile of the presenter better.

Introduction

A thesis for a postgraduate degree or for Ph.D. specifically addresses an issue or few issues where differing theories are existent. By a detailed research the candidate plans to find a better solution to the issue or tries to bridge the differing doctrines. The proposal will be a new explanation or thought which can solve the issue under debate in a better way. Presentation of the work at various conferences can increase the visibility of both the work as well as the presenter [1]. The rewards and benefits of the conference presentations are innumerable.

Why Is It Important to Make Presentations in Conferences?

1. *Contribute to and learn about the most recent advances in the field*
   You are able to present the data from your work at any point of time during the study thus allowing you to get feedback and improvise upon your study. In a conference, there is an opportunity to attend other talks and poster-sessions, which often represent the most cutting-edge research available, and can give valuable information ahead of the publication.
2. *Proponent of your field*
   One of the most important gains of attending the conference is that you are able to act as an advocate of your science. Presentation can bring the doctrines and your thoughts into the notices of other researchers, policy makers and even public to improve your visibility.
3. *Learn how to talk about your data*
   Your presentation skills will substantially improve with each presentation. More importantly when you are confronted with extempore questions, you get prepared to handle the question in a much more organized fashion. As each presentation gets over, your skills improve which will aid in the final defense of your research.

4. *Contribute to your own profile*
   In a competitive job market, your presentation and publications will make a sizable contribution. "Travel Bursary and Fellowships" help to improvise the resume in addition to providing the financial support. There is hardly anything to choose between oral or poster in terms of visibility and hence avail every opportunity to improve your curriculum vitae.
5. *Opportunity to meet your colleagues & seniors*
   Conferences will provide ample opportunities to meet peers and leaders in the same field, to have discussions, to clear certain issues and to get some new inputs. Fostering the relationship will pave the way for future collaborations; joint works and even job opportunities.

How to Convert Thesis Work into a Presentation?

Conversion of a thesis where the issues under consideration are proved or disproved on the basis of a huge data into a 10-min oral presentation or to a poster of limited space is a demanding task [1, 2]. The following steps will enable an author to convert his thesis into presentation in conference.

1. The author should first understand the problem he is trying to analyse in depth—its relevance (clinical/theoretical), the different hypothesis and explanations with their merits and shortcomings, how the proposed solution or theory will help in solving some of the concerns. He should be well versed with the methodology used, interpretation of the data with significance, conclusions with rationale and enough references which can support the outcome. It is also important to make sure that others who are working in the same field are able to use his proposal partly or entirely to take up similar work to find solutions to related issues [3].
2. The author needs to discuss with his mentor/s and colleagues about the proposal to make a presentation of his work and take their opinion on the project to consolidate or refine or even change. Often the frank opinion of the colleagues will give a better insight and the entire plan may be changed [4].
3. Most of studies have primary and secondary aims at the proposal stage. But as the research proceeds it may also yield some valuable observations which may not be relevant to the thesis under consideration but certainly will be worth bringing out for the understanding of the people or may be of use to another study either already on or worth considering to begin. May be these corollary findings of the thesis will also find a suitable place in some conference and any discussion with the colleagues can be of great help.

The steps in converting a thesis into a presentation are shown in Fig. 1.

How to Choose the Conference for Making the Presentation?

The conferences available today are either general in nature or a specific theme-based one or many times disease and organ based. The level of these conferences

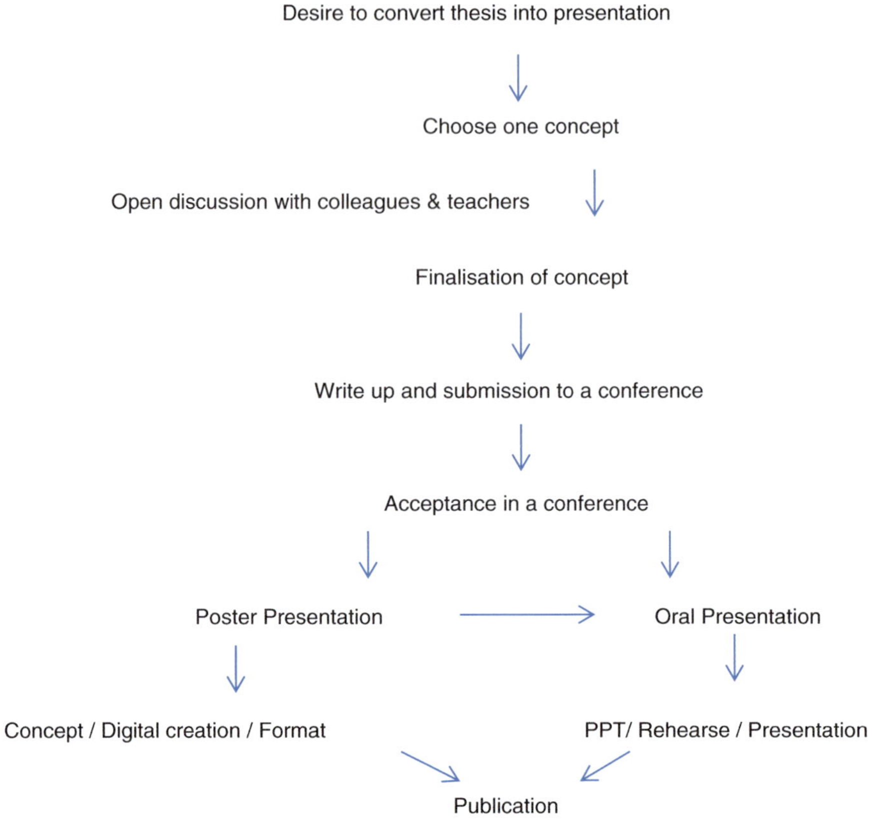

Fig. 1 Steps in converting thesis work into a conference presentation

varies from local to state to national and international levels. It is easier to choose the conference based on the topic of the study. For instance, "A thesis on Gastric Ulcer" can find acceptance in any general or gastrointestinal tract related conferences. The most difficult issue will be the level or nature of conference in which the candidate can send the presentation and can get an acceptance. A conference where fundamental research is the primary area of discussion, a clinical observational study may not find its place. But if the research findings are valid and highly relevant, be it clinical or theoretical, the presentation may be accepted. The presenter hence needs to choose the conference based on his own realistic assessment about the strength or credibility of his thesis. A look into the kind of papers in previous conferences may help the presenter to make a better assessment on the level of acceptance [2, 5]. It is also important to look at the theme of the conference as anything in the same lines might get accepted fast.

While the candidate is keen on a particular conference, it is important to realize that acceptance of the paper also becomes a challenge. An appealing title with a well-drafted abstract, which is submitted in time, will be contributory. The credibility of the institution and the support group involved in the paper will be yet another deciding factor in many situations despite the strength of the paper itself.

What Is the Appropriate Format of Presentation and Preparation for Each?

The presentations in any conference can either be in the form of oral podium presentation or in the form of a poster, which from physical format is moving to its e-version. In some or even in most of the conferences among the e-versions of poster, the selected few or sometimes all are given a short time to explain or defend themselves to the assessors [5, 6]. Even if these are not for competition, the author is often given time for defending himself to the questions asked by the viewers. Posters have the space limitation while oral presentation has an added time limitation too. Both have different types of impacts- Oral presentation is limited to a specific audience in the specific time while posters do get prolonged time of exposure and a larger viewership. Both get augmented in terms of time and viewership, if there is an e-version on the proceedings where the papers and posters are included. Sometimes the choice has to be made on the basis of availability and on any statutory requirement. At times the policies in selection of papers by the organisers also will make an influence as to which category the paper gets accepted- oral vs. poster. Double-blind controlled studies, prospective studies and thesis with basic research are better conceived than clinical observational studies or studies like clinico-pathological co-relation where the professional expertise of a group of specialists comes into assessment. Papers where the demographic pattern is purely an institution based is less likely to be accepted against a population based data.

A poster presentation may be the best way to start a research being brought into notice. If you keep an open mind, inputs can be received and collated to give a direction to the work. It often gives you an opportunity for an informal talk with all levels of participants, more time to receive questions and answer them in a more relaxed way without much pressure of time. It also will help you to defend the thoughts in different ways and help you to choose the best way. As you proceed with the collection of data, analysis can be periodically done to make some preliminary observations. These can be presented better on oral presentation and get further inputs into the work. The final result can go to publication.

How to Make an Impact on Presenting the Thesis?

The impact a presentation can make in the conference depends on multitude of factors.

1. Choosing an appropriate title for the presentation is an important issue. The title needs to be framed in such a way that with a single glance, it will attract the reader, will give a rough idea on the topic and possibly will give a glimpse how

the conclusions can impact the future. Lot many of the participant delegates choose the lectures based on its title alone. It is recommended to frame the title after many times of writing or most practically even after writing the whole paper.

2. Making the presentation in any conference is an art. The "nervous" presenters need to be differentiated from "liars". The anxiety of making a presentation can be overcome by the following points.
   (a) Understanding the audience is an important factor—their level of knowledge on the subject, their possible interest in the topic and the possible influence of the conclusion in their thought process and in their daily clinical practice.
   (b) Preparing the lecture with the available audiovisual aid in the conference. An alternate plan B also need to be kept as backup, in case there is a last minute change at the venue in terms of timing, format etc. One should also look at the guidelines already given by the organisers and complying with it will help the whole presentation. Technical challenges posed by the presenters such as making the presentation in incompatible software, often works against them in terms of valuable time allotted, loss of tempo of presentation and above all the interest of the audience [7]. It is advisable to check the compatibility of slides, videos etc. prior to the presentation to avoid interruptions in the presentation. It is important to make the presentation using the commonest method and technique in contemporary practice.
   (c) Proven or specified formats are to be used. The contents in the slide need not contain the entire narration of presentation which in fact only drags the listener. It is better to have highlighted points by bullets and the narration can be better drawn out of that. Repeated spell checks need to be done before making the final presentation. A busy slide will be difficult to be read [6]. All animations and multiple colours are better avoided and are only modes to distract the concentration of the readers.
   (d) Rehearsing the talk is to be done early so that the flow and delivery of lecture can be smooth and attractive. It is important to always adhere to the time allotted. It is usually seen that the last few slides are hurried through for want of time, which generally contains the most valuable points in the presentation. In such circumstances of pace at the end of the talk will turn out to be counterproductive.
   (e) The presenter must conduct himself at the podium and must be presentable. Greeting the Chair, facing the audience with a smile and with an attempt to make an eye contact will help draw the audience to the presenter.
   (f) The language, the diction and the tone of delivery of the talk matters a lot in keeping the audience with the presenter. Though scientific presentations are not tests on one's linguistic skills, but still the language counts a lot in keeping the tempo and flow of presentation. Emphasis is to be done when it is needed. In an unexpected break in the flow during presentation, it is a wise pattern to narrate the matter in the slides verbatim rather than panicking on the stage so as to get the presentation back in track.

(g) Answering questions after the lecture is an art, especially in an award paper session as it is expected that the presenter independently defends the study. Genuine questions raised need specific answers. It is important to identify experts on the topic, who raise questions, with whom you need to have discussion later on for redefining your thoughts and taking your thesis further. Inputs from them may also throw light on some hidden aspects of your research. Developing contacts with seniors and important people among the audience and maintaining the rapport in days to come is a skill as well a talent. This will pave for the entrance to other similar conferences and for many presentations. However, sometimes, comments are from those who want to make their presence noticed. Such comments should be answered tactfully without any direct offence against the person.

3. Providing relevant references from the literature related to the study is important. However, too many references may also be confusing and will just finish the valuable time you have been given for presentation.
4. Some conferences will bring out a proceedings book with abstracts of the conference presentations. However, the authors have the liberty to publish the article independent of the conference supplement.
5. The continued presence, repeated presentations and contributory discussions in the topic of your area of research will make you better known in the concerned area [8].

Conclusion

Although the task of converting a thesis work into a short presentation is demanding, it's equally rewarding. The conference presentation not only aid in improvising the study, but also sharpen one's presentation skills and confidence level as well as help in expanding the contact circle which may prove beneficial in future.

Case Scenarios

1. When one plans to convert his thesis to a presentation, the author needs to discuss the attempt with his colleagues to refine the presentation. True/False.
2. Graduation from poster presentation to oral presentation to publication is a natural process. True/False.

References

1. Star L. Written Papers into Oral Presentations, HDR & ECR research seminars. 2015.
2. Boza T.-G. How to give a fabulous academic presentation: five tips to follow. Get a life, Ph.D. 2011.
3. Cohen BP, Kruse RJ, Anbar M. The social structure of scientific research teams. Pacific Sociological Review. 1989;25(2):205–32.
4. Jarvinen PH. Research questions guiding selection of an appropriate research method. Proceedings of the 8th European Conference on Information Systems; 2000. p. 124–131.

5. Sanida O, Milutinovic M, Saso T, Milutinovic V. The best method for presentation of research result. IEEE TCCA Newsletter 1996; p. 1–6.
6. Milutinovic V. A good method to prepare and use transparencies for research presentations. IEEE TCCA Newsletter. 1997; p. 72–79.
7. Falkovych K, Lynda H, van Rossum G, Bultermanet DCA. Context aware guidance for multimedia authoring: harmonizing domain and discourse knowledge. Multimedia Systems. 2006;11(3):226–35.
8. Fowler F. J. Survey Research Methods. Thousand Oaks: Sage Publications 2002; 14 (4): 329–336.

Part VI

Thesis for Master's Degree/Specialty And Sub-Specialty Courses in Medicine/Doctor of Philosophy Course

Writing Thesis for Speciality Courses in Medicine

Vikram Kate, Nina V. Kate, and Mohsina Subair

This is how you should do it, you sit down at the keyboard and you put one word after another until it's done. It's that easy and that hard.—Neil Gaiman

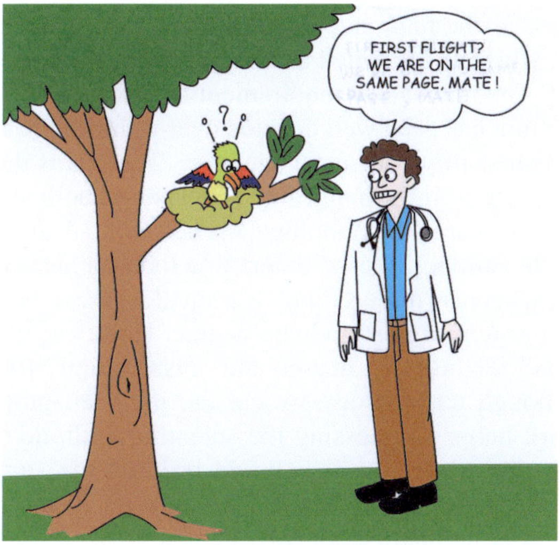

V. Kate (✉)
Professor and Head, Department of Surgery and Senior Consultant General and Gastrointestinal Surgeon, Jawaharlal Institute of Postgraduate Medical Education and Research, Pondicherry, India

N. V. Kate
Senior Consultant Obstetrician and Programme Coordinator, National Board of Examinations, Rajiv Gandhi Government Women and Children Hospital, Pondicherry, India

M. Subair
Senior Resident, Department of Plastic and Reconstructive Surgery, Postgraduate Institute Medical Education and Research, Chandigarh, India

S. C. Parija, V. Kate (eds.), *Thesis Writing for Master's and Ph.D. Program*,
https://doi.org/10.1007/978-981-13-0890-1_22

Key Points

- The thesis is defined as the final outcome of systematic research on a topic, which is presented as a requirement for acquisition of an academic degree.
- Thesis work helps in assessing the scientific aptitude of the candidates rather than their clinical ability.
- Careful planning and execution of the work includes various steps and a systematic approach to these can help in successful completion.
- Thesis work should be presented in a way that captures the reader's imagination and not as an assortment of facts.
- The conventional structure of a thesis comprise title page, certificates, table of contents, acknowledgment, introduction, aims and objectives, review of literature, methods, results, discussion, conclusion, summary and appendices.
- The student should be aware of the various "Don'ts of thesis writing" to avoid last minute hassles and rejection/revision.
- MD/MS thesis is carried out under the affiliation of a university, whereas DNB is affiliated to the National Board of Examinations.

"Thesis" is defined as the final outcome of systematic research and experimentation on a topic, which is presented as a requirement for acquisition of an academic degree [1]. The mandatory requirement for completion of the thesis as a part of the curriculum has been well debated over years and has now become the part and parcel of speciality courses in medicine. The words thesis and dissertation have often been used interchangeably [2]. Though both aims at training the student in the basic research methodology, the academic degrees obtained varies between regions. In Europe, "thesis" refers to a focused piece of work to obtain a doctoral degree whereas "dissertation" is a smaller research on a broader topic for a attaining a masters or postgraduate degree. However, in the US, it's vice versa, i.e., "thesis" for master's degree and "dissertation" for doctoral degree respectively. Although terminology varies, the intended purpose remains the same. Thesis work helps in assessing the scientific aptitude of the candidates rather than their clinical ability. It helps in training the student in the basic research methodology and hence kindles the interest in the candidate. It can contribute to the existing medical knowledge in a great way. The basic requirement for a successful thesis is the enthusiasm for taking up a topic and studying in its depth.

For a postgraduate student, successful completion of their thesis is a matter of pride and satisfaction, as it involves an in-depth study of the topic and years of hard work. Writing thesis is the most daunting task a postgraduate student faces, especially with time constraints due to clinical patient care and other academic activities. Thesis work and writing is, many a times, like a 100 m race for the amateur researcher, the course being quite quick with hardly any time for thinking as required. However, with proper guidance and planning, it can be a 400 m race which is neither too quick nor too long.

Planning a Thesis/Dissertation

The postgraduate students are often overwhelmed right from the beginning of their course with constant worry regarding their thesis/dissertation. Peer pressure and short-cut advises seems tempting and often leads into detrimental situations later on. Careful planning and execution of the work can help tide over the "nightmare" easily as, in thesis work and writing, "well prepared is half done".

The various steps in pre-planning a thesis involve the following:

- Choosing a topic
- Choosing a guide/mentor
- Verifying the guidelines
- Preparing a protocol and approval of the study
- Gathering information
- Well planned execution
- Writing thesis work

How to Choose a Unique Thesis Topic?

This is the most important part of thesis writing. Getting it right will ensure the candidate enjoying the work and will set the pace for the work. A visit to the library and glancing through the theses accepted in the previous years can help in formulating a brain-map for undertaking the daunting task. A thorough discussion with the guide about areas appealing to you can also be productive.

An ideal thesis should be original work and should not be a disjointed work related to previously done vague topics. It should offer scope for creativity and choice for the student. Even though the initial idea is promulgated by the guide, an enthusiastic student should be able to take control in determining its directions. The topic should be able to bring out a few fresh perspectives and should be relevant to the workplace. It is important not to be overambitious while choosing a topic. It should be feasible to be completed over the set time period and should have adequate resources available. These are important criteria to be ensured before setting on the journey. The topic should be appealing both for the student as well as the guide so as not to lose interest half-way through. It is advisable to take up a topic that is gaining popularity over time. Though it sounds obvious, the fresh postgraduates may be unaware and may get excited with topics that were controversial few years back and hence adept guidance plays a role. It is advisable to choose a topic that is central and well connected to the areas the candidate would like to explore in future. This will provide with an opportunity to branch out interests in the course of their career. However, this is not mandatory as it's the basic learning of the process that sets the pace for future research and writing.

Choosing a Guide/Mentor

The adept and professional guidance is the keystone for successful completion of a thesis. A good guide would sculpt out a researcher in his/her resemblance. Right from choosing a topic to helping with troubleshooting during the research work to writing and publishing, the role of the guide is inexplicable. The students are allotted guides based on their course speciality and are often not provided with an opportunity to choose amongst the available faculty. Hence, it's important to establish a good rapport with your guide so as to ensure smooth progress of your work. If, unfortunately, there is a lack of adept guidance, the students can always tactfully approach faculty they prefer for suggestions and advice.

Verifying the University Guidelines

This step is vital before going ahead with the thesis proposal and the work per se as it helps in keeping up with the deadlines for the various steps as well as helps in formulating an outline of the process. The administrative guidelines are usually available on the websites of the university/institute or can be obtained by writing to the registrar. A research monitoring committee is formulated in the university/institute to assess and approve proposals for thesis, to assess the need for funding for the work and for monitoring and supervising so as to enable timely submission of the postgraduate thesis [3].

The students are often required to provide a detailed protocol of the study to the research monitoring committee for assessment within the stipulated time period, which is roughly 3–4 months from the beginning of the course. Few institutes require the students to physically present their protocol for approval. This helps in assessing the feasibility and adequacy of the projects, as well as help in modifying the protocol based on the inputs from the assessors. The protocols approved by the research committee will then have to be submitted to the ethics committee of the institute/university for approval, only after which the study can be commenced. The process of getting approvals and actual commencement of the work may take upto 6 months from the onset of the course. This process may however be more tedious and time-demanding in institutes/colleges which function under a combined university and hence keeping on time with the deadlines becomes all the more important.

It is advisable to understand the guidelines of thesis submission also right from the protocol stage of the study [1, 3]. Most of the universities usually require 3–5 bound copies apart from the soft copy of the thesis. The theses will then be sent to 3–6 assessors by the dean of the institute/university for decision regarding acceptance. The thesis may be accepted, rejected or revisions may be advised which has to be submitted within a stipulated time period. The valuation usually does not include an oral assessment of the candidate as in case of doctoral degrees [4]. For MD/MS thesis, public defense of the thesis is never carried out. However, some universities carry out an assessment of the candidate's depth of knowledge on the topic and involvement in the work as a part of the viva-voce examination. For speciality MD/MS courses, successful submission of the thesis work and its acceptance is mandatory to enable the student to appear in the final examinations.

Preparing a Protocol and Approval of the Study

The forerunner of thesis writing is the preparation of a protocol. A good grasp on the topic planned and a clear understanding of the goals of the study are essential for writing an effective protocol. A good and effective protocol will help in guiding through the conduct of research work. Well defined goals and objectives and a clear methodology are quintessential for an ideal protocol. The protocol should also define the statistics to be used in the study, the study design and rescue methods in case of unfortunate events.

The proposal has to be presented before the research monitoring and ethics committees to assess its appropriateness and approval for the conduct of the same [3]. However, it's important to keep an open mind and to make changes/modifications to the protocol if found necessary during the course of the study. The administrative guidelines of the respective institutes often provide details of such changes which require the approval of the committee prior to the modification.

Execution of Thesis Work and Writing

This is the crux of the thesis/dissertation work where the postgraduate student sets out to find the answers to the questions raised in the topic. This requires a well-planned execution to avoid last minute hassles and falling behind time. Before setting out, it's important to assess the availability of the resources and plan a timetable. The students' zeal and vigor to devote adequate time in a divided fashion is important to ensure the adequate data and information to be collected in time.

As the study progresses, it's advisable to read and learn about the topics in-depth as this can help in making timely and useful modifications to the project. It is wise to start writing the thesis work simultaneously as the study progresses, especially the review of literature. The benefits of such an approach are manifold. Firstly, scientific writing is not based on talent, but on practice. Hence sooner the better so that there is ample time to make revisions and will provide time for improving the quality of writing. Secondly, writing as the thesis work is being carried out is an easy and efficient way of structuring the thesis as it takes much less time when things are afresh in the mind. The progress in writing will provide a psychological boost as well for carrying out the work. More importantly, gathering information to write the review will help develop new ideas to improvise/modify the thesis before it's too late for the same.

Structure of a Thesis

There is no single format for thesis writing and the general guidelines vary between universities [5]. Hence, verifying the guidelines for details such as layout, font type and size, word limits etc. is important. However, the conventional structure of a thesis is as follows:

- Title page
  - This should include the title of the dissertation/thesis, name of the student and the degree which is being applied, the time period of the work and date of submission.
- Certificate
  - These should be prepared in the format described in the thesis guidelines of university/institute. The conventional format certifies that the student carried out the work during the set time period for acquisition of the degree. Often, there is a declaration by the guide stating the originality and the conduct of work under his/her guidance.
  - Table of contents
- Acknowledgements
- Introduction
  - This should include a background and the rationale for conducting the study. It should emphasize on the contribution that the study can add to the medical knowledge and how it addresses any pre-existing lacunae.
- Review of literature
  - This section should discuss in detail the evidence available in the literature about the topic being studied. It should also summarize the findings of the relevant studies in the literature.
- Methods
  - This section should give in detail the methodology adopted during the study including all specific details such as name of instruments, drug used etc. The rule of thumb to be followed is that the methodology should be explicit and should be reproducible by another researcher who wants to carry out the study.
- Results, Tables and Figures
  - This is the most important part of the study as it describes the findings of the study. The conventional method is to describe the result in text as well as in form of tables and graphs. However, a concise writing like the results section of journal articles without repetition of data can also be adopted.
- Discussion
  - This section describes the bigger picture by comparing the results of the study with the available literature. There should be active critiquing of one's own study with an open mind. The students should be able to analyze their own study in depth and draw a conclusion.
- Conclusion
  - This section should provide an answer to the research question that was raised and should be drawn based on the results of the study.
- Summary/abstract
  - This section provides a brief overview of the study and should be written after completion of the entire work. This section may be added either at the beginning of the thesis or at the end based on the pre-set guidelines.
- References
  - A list of references should be provided at the end for a wider reading. It is advisable to follow a consistent pattern of writing references such as

Vancouver style or Harvard style. It is important to understand that the strength of the study is not gauged by the number of references and hence should avoid unnecessary citations.

- Appendices
  - This section should include other information to be presented such as the master chart, data collection proforma, consent forms used etc.

How to Write Thesis Effectively?

Writing and presentation of the thesis work is the key skill to ensure the success of any project. As once told by a psychology professor at Oklahoma University, scientific writing can be compared to advertising [6]. An advertising agent tries to sell his product whereas the researcher tries to sell his results/findings. It should not, however, be misunderstood as good advertising can sell faulty products, but to persuade the public to buy a high-quality product it should be presented in a convincing manner. Similarly, thesis work should be presented in a way that captures the reader's imagination and not as an assortment of facts.

As mentioned earlier in the chapter, it is always a wise plan to start early alongside as the study progresses. It's better to start with sections of the thesis, which the author is confident of first rather than following a chronological order. This will sharpen and improve the writing skill and hence enable to tackle the difficult portions with ease. The first draft should be prepared as early as possible as it's highly unlikely to be perfect. Hence, prepare the first draft and submit to your guide for revision and feedback. Multiple attempts at working and re-working on the draft will be needed to sharpen the thesis and to improve the writing skills. Referring previous theses also will help by giving an idea on the structure, style and the pattern. Attention should be paid to managing references as they are read. Using software such as Zotero, Endnote etc. to create a database of the bibliography will be helpful while writing a structured thesis [7]. Though the task of learning to use these is cumbersome to start with, at the end of the dissertation/thesis it will prove useful. Avoiding plagiarism is another important part of effective writing. It is important that students understand what accounts for plagiarism and methods to avoid it. Plagiarism, though accidental, might even cost the degree. For non-native speakers for English, many universities offer courses or support for academic writing which may be beneficial. Many theses writing tools are now available online such as Boom Essay, Mendeley, Sparrho etc. which can help in easing the overwhelming task of writing the thesis [8]. Sharing the writing with peers for feedback is also an effective method for modifying the writing. This is more important as with time, it becomes difficult to maintain a critical distance from your work and hence typos and inconsistencies in arguments can be easily picked up by others. The various steps in writing a thesis effectively are shown in Fig. 1.

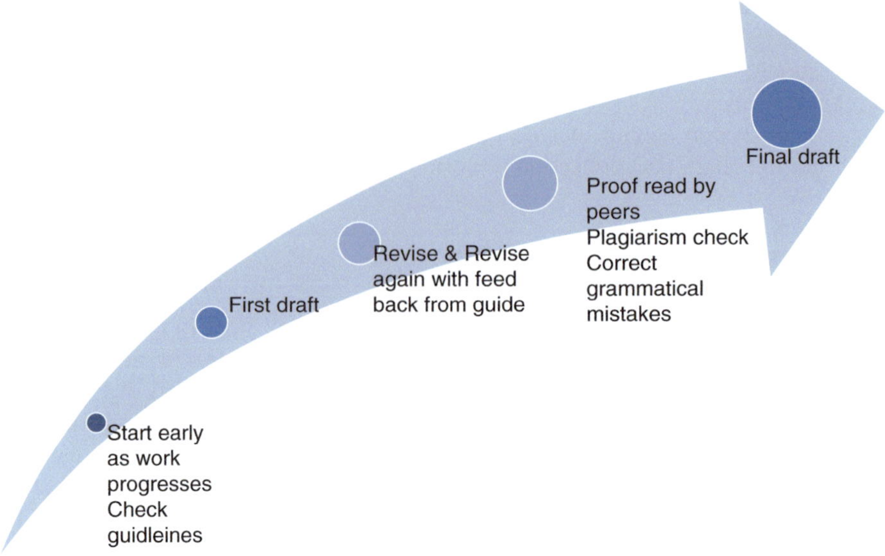

Fig. 1 Steps in writing thesis effectively

Don't's of Thesis Writing

- *Avoid grammatical errors, as they are a sign of carelessness*
- *Don't try to sound too technical, the goal of writing should be clarity*
- *The paragraphs should not be written as disjoint entities.*
- *Writing can be stylish, but care should be taken not to lose the ideas in between the pomposity and verbosity*
- *The thesis-writing task should not be at the cost of time for relaxation as this instills a sense of exhaustion and will hamper progress and can adversely affect the quality of writing.*

Pattern and Schedule of Thesis Writing for the Speciality Courses for the Diplomate of National Board of Examinations (DNB)

The Ministry of Health of Government of India established The National Board of Examinations (NBE) an autonomous body in 1975 at New Delhi so that the post-graduate medical education in India could be standardized. The degree awarded by the board is called as Diplomate of National Board (DNB) [9].

The selection of candidates under this programme is through the Centralized Entrance Test (CET) conducted at the national level twice a year. Graduate in medicine (MBBS-Bachelor of Medicine and Bachelor of Surgery) candidates are eligible to write the DNB-CET entrance examination for an entry into a DNB course which is for a period of 3 years. If a candidate has a Diploma in a speciality, then the person is eligible to write an entrance for the postdiploma CET for an entry into a DNB course which is for a period of 2 years.

Once selected, the candidates start the course at their respective centres carrying out the DNB speciality courses in India. As a mandatory requirement to be awarded the DNB degree, the candidate has to carry out the thesis and complete it in the stipulated time frame which is varying according to the course of 2 and 3 years.

On starting the course candidates have to select the thesis topic and have to prepare the Thesis Protocol as per the guidelines set by The National Board of Examinations. Workshops are arranged by the NBE to sensitize the candidates in protocol and thesis writing at periodic intervals across the country. The format suggested for protocol includes synopsis, background and introduction, review of literature and lacunae, research question and aims and objectives, material and methods, references, data collection forms and clearance certificates from the Institute Scientific and Ethics Committee. Once the protocol is ready it has to be sent to the NBE for approval by the experts appointed by the NBE. Many a times the protocols are sent back to the candidates for revision by the NBE and the necessary changes have to be made and resent. The quality of the protocol can be improved if its critically reviewed by the guide or co-guide as the candidates are new to the field of research.

Following the approval from the NBE the thesis work on the research is started by the candidate under the guidance of the guide/co-guide. An interim analysis is conducted so as to get an idea of the work done so far and to suggest or correct lacunae's if any.

Once the work is completed, candidates have to send their completed thesis to the NBE board for approval, 6 months before their theory exams. The theory examinations by the NBE are usually carried out in the month of June and December. Submission of the thesis is mandatory to become eligible for theory exams, however, as opposed to the University guidelines for speciality examination for MD/MS courses, approval is not needed to appear for the examinations. Theses are sent by the NBE to subject experts at the national level for evaluation and approval, and once approved its conveyed to the candidates. In case the experts find some lacunae in the study its sent back for necessary corrections and has to be sent again for evaluation.

Approved thesis and successfully passing the theory and clinical exams is necessary for the award of the degree by the NBE. The candidate receives the degree at the central convocation of the NBE held at national level for the award of all the degrees.

Causes for Revision/Rejection

A thesis is not commonly rejected because of lack of originality, but it often requires revision/rejection when the ideas are disjointed and is poorly presented [10]. Errors such as spelling or grammatical errors, complicated data and statistics without adequate explanations, incorrect references etc. reveal the carelessness of the student. In such situations, the assessor tends to suspect such callousness might have occurred in the conduct of the work and in the data presented. Hence, it's important to avoid these pitfalls. The importance of the writing skill can be well understood by placing oneself in the shoes of the assessor. Reading a long thesis is by itself taxing, however, reading a long and poorly written one can become painful. Hence, a well-presented thesis might get accepted even if the quality of work is of moderately acceptable nature.

Conclusion

Thesis work and writing hence is one of the most daunting yet rewarding tasks that a postgraduate student undertakes. Studying in-depth about a topic and producing a hard-bound copy of one's own findings and arguments can instill a sense of achievement that can kick-start a research career. The key to dispelling the myths about writing the thesis is thus by careful planning and execution, and constant practice to improve the writing skills.

Case Scenarios

1. An ideal thesis topic should all of the following EXCEPT
   (a) It should be original work and should not be a disjointed work related to previously done vague topics.
   (b) The area of research should be able to bring out a new perspective and should be overall relevant and to the place of work of the candidate.
   (c) It should be feasible to be completed within the time period of the thesis and should have adequate local resources and funds available to carry out the study.
   (d) The topic which were controversial few years back also can be chosen as thesis is to familiarize with research methodology.
2. You are required to submit a thesis for obtaining your degree. Arrange the steps in the order in which you will approach:
   (a) Collect literature on the topic
   (b) Choose your guide and decide on the topic
   (c) Write the manuscript
   (d) Submit protocol for evaluation by the research committee.
   (e) Start your thesis work/experiment
   (f) Check university guidelines and prepare protocol.

References

1. International Standard ISO 7144. Documentation—presentation of theses and similar documents. Geneva: International Organization for Standardization; 1986.
2. Breimer D, Damen J, et al. Hora est! (on dissertations). Leiden: Leiden University Library; 2005.

3. Rules for the evaluation of the dissertation. http://collegeinfo.org.
4. Thesis Defense Tips. Dissertation Writing Service. http://dissertationwritingservices.org.
5. Thesis structure. https://student.unsw.edu.au/thesis-structure.
6. Sternberg RJ. Provost professor of psychology at Oklahoma State University. Thesis Writing_ Advice: https://www.postgrad.com.
7. How to Choose: Zotero, Mendeley, or EndNote. http://libguides.wustl.edu/choose.
8. Top Thesis Writing Tools. Thesis Writing Tools_Blog: https://www.postgrad.com.
9. Sharma A, Zodpey S, Batra B. Engagement of National Board of Examinations in strengthening public health education in India: present landscape, opportunities and future directions. Ind J Public Health. 2014;58:34–9.
10. Pearce L. How to examine a thesis. McGraw-Hill International; 2005. p. 79–85.

Writing Thesis for Sub-speciality Courses in Medicine

Lalgudi N. Dorairajan, Ketan Mehra, and Ramanitharan Manikandan

"There is nothing to writing. All you do is sit down at type writer and bleed."—Ernest Hemingway

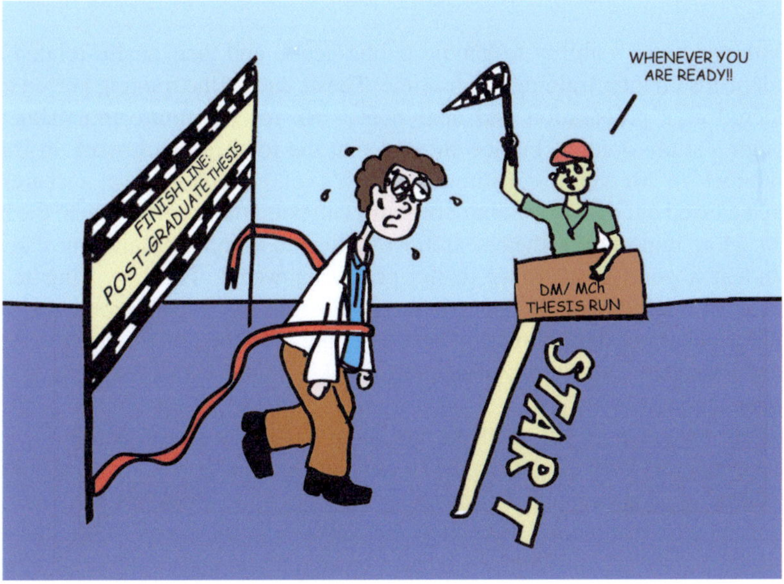

L. N. Dorairajan (✉)
Professor, Department of Urology, Jawaharlal Institute of Postgraduate Medical Education and Research, Pondicherry, India

K. Mehra
Senior Resident, Department of Urology, Jawaharlal Institute of Postgraduate Medical Education and Research, Pondicherry, India

R. Manikandan
Additional Professor and Head, Department of Urology, Jawaharlal Institute of Postgraduate Medical Education and Research, Pondicherry, India

S. C. Parija, V. Kate (eds.), *Thesis Writing for Master's and Ph.D. Program*,
https://doi.org/10.1007/978-981-13-0890-1_23

Key Points

- The need to strengthen research at super speciality level.
- Research work as a part of sub-speciality postgraduate curriculum—The MCI requirements.
- Differences in the requirements of thesis writing in different universities at sub-speciality level courses.
- Variability in the conduct and assessment of dissertation/research project in different universities at sub-speciality level courses.
  - Types of studies permitted as thesis work.
  - Monitoring of research work.
  - Impediments faced by the student in carrying out research work.
  - Timelines for dissertation protocol and final thesis submission.
  - Method of assessment of the research work.

Introduction

A health personnel's ability to handle public health and their health-related questions depends on their training programme. Thesis during the training period can be considered as a preparation and analytical work for the future practising field. Although a study done in France showed that the total research work in training programmes in Medicine constitutes only 5% of overall medical research [1], research carried out during training programs can potentially contribute to the health system. More importantly, the research work done in training programme can make the student a good practitioner in the practising world. Thesis writing requires expertise in various fields. The research done in such conditions are multidisciplinary and not only clinical. These not only help the practitioner sharpen his analytical abilities but the experience also makes him a better team player while rendering care to his patients.

But the objective of any medical education system is to not to solely produce practising doctors with a high degree of clinical skill but also to produce scientists and research workers capable of advancing the field of medicine for the betterment, if not of the whole humanity, at least of the community they serve. Thus, the development of research in different areas must be an integral part of our education system. Unfortunately, this is the weakest in our medical education system. A study done by Nundy et al. looked at the research work published during the period from 2005 to 2014 using Scopus database out of the research work done in 579 Medical Council of India recognised institutions. They found that 25 out of 579 that is 4% of institutions produced around 40% of all research in the 10 years period. Among all the institutions the large institutions like AIIMS, New Delhi produced most of the research output. In India majority of research work is done by publicly funded medical institutes. Even among these, nearly 60% of the institutions had no publication in a full decade. The study found that states like Maharashtra and Karnataka had the largest number of medical colleges but contribute less in the field of research [2].

Another study showed that the top ten medical institutes, most of them being public institutions, produced nearly 41% of the research work in India [3]. The leading 25 private institutions under the National Board of Examinations, New Delhi, contributed a mere 5.6%. Although research in India has improved in the recent past and much has been achieved in the last 20 years, compared to the other developing nations it still is lagging. India ranks below Kenya, China and Brazil in the number of full-time researchers per 10,000 workforce. The reasons include, among others, lack of public support, appreciation and social recognition. Hence the young student is not attracted towards the field of research [3]. It is thus evident that there is a tremendous need to improve research in the medical colleges and educational institutions of this country, both in the private sector and in the public institutions.

There is no dearth of talented students, in India, entering the field of medicine who can produce exceptional research work. There is a lot of competition for entering the medical profession and a lot of respect for health care professionals among the people of the community. In spite of all this, according to an evaluation done by SCImago in 2017 based on the scientific research output, among 500 Asiatic institutions, there are only three Indian medical schools. The All India Institute of Medical Sciences, New Delhi was ranked 276, the Sree Chitra Tirunal Institute for Medical Sciences and Technology, Thiruvananthapuram, ranked 434 and the Postgraduate Institute of Medical Education and Research, Chandigarh ranked 454 [4].

It is, therefore, apparent that there is a need to invest on nurturing the research talent and skills of the postgraduate students in medical colleges and institutions so that interest in medical research can be kindled in at least some the students who can then pursue a career in research. To impart training in research methodology and writing thesis/research articles has been one of the consistent aspects of the postgraduate curriculum in India at the basic postgraduate degree level. In India, a student pursues a sub-speciality clinical course (also known and referred to as super speciality clinical course in the MCI Postgraduate Medical Education Regulations 2000) after obtaining a basic postgraduate degree in a subject such as medicine or surgery. These degrees are called DM (for Doctor of Medicine) in case of medical sub-specialties or MCh (for Magister Chirurgiae) in case of surgical sub-specialities. This chapter explores the status of research work as part of sub-speciality postgraduate curriculum.

Research Work as a Part of Sub-speciality Postgraduate Curriculum

One of the goals of postgraduate medical education as listed by the Medical Council of India (MCI) in its Postgraduate Medical Education Regulations 2000 amended from time to time is to produce competent specialists, medical teachers or both who have acquired a spirit of scientific enquiry and are oriented to the principles of epidemiology and research methods [5]. Towards achieving this goal one of the stated objectives of the postgraduate training program for a student of any discipline is that at the end of the course the candidate is expected to be able to analyse relevant published literature and to be able to demonstrate competence in basic concepts of epidemiology and research methods. Towards further achieving the goals mentioned above and objectives of postgraduate medical education one common major component of all postgraduate curriculum prescribed by the MCI includes writing a thesis or research articles and training in research methodology. Accordingly, the MCI makes it mandatory through clause 13.9 of its regulations that all postgraduate students including those pursuing sub-speciality courses would be required to present one poster, read one paper in a State or National conference and at least submit one research paper for publication during the tenure of his postgraduate studies to be eligible to appear in his final degree examination [5].

While this training in research methodology takes the shape of a mandatory thesis or dissertation writing for students pursuing MD/MS basic postgraduate degree courses, the MCI has not made it mandatory for students of sub-speciality courses but has left it to the discretion of individual universities. Nevertheless, although it appears that writing thesis is not an essential component of sub-speciality training course as prescribed by the MCI, in effect and by the requirements mentioned in clause 13.9 of its regulations, at a minimum the student is expected to conduct the research project/study to enable him to present/publish a paper to be eligible to appear in the examination at the end of his course.

Objective of Research Work as Part of Postgraduate Curriculum

The objective of this research exercise as a part of postgraduate basic or sub-speciality curriculum is not so much as to generate new knowledge, although eminently desirable and every effort is made in that direction, as to familiarise the student in research methodology. It seeks to train the student in the methods of framing the research question and designing the research proposal to answer the question, learn literature search, acquire the discipline required for systematic data search and record keeping, know how to apply simple tests of statistical analysis and when to interact with a statistician for more complex analyses and finally how to prepare a report which may be in the form of a book (thesis) or a manuscript ready for submission for publication. These research skills will help the student later in the career to scientifically analyse problems in her field of practice. The "hands-on" research experience also empowers the student to critically appraise the research articles presented in journals and apply them meaningfully in practice.

The Requirement of Thesis Writing in Different Universities at Sub-speciality Level Courses

Dissertation or thesis writing requirements at DM/MCh degree level is highly variable in different universities in this country. Some universities have a formal thesis writing, while other universities have a less formal "research project" on research activity leading to submission of research manuscript for publication and yet others have no formal requirement spelt out. Some institutions such as AIIMS, New Delhi, have a high degree of variability from department to department in the same institution in this regard [6]. For example, in the DM in Hematopathology, the candidate has to carry out two thesis works, one being an experimental study and the other being a clinical study. In the same institution, the DM in Endocrinology and Metabolism the curriculum requires the candidate to carry out one thesis, and in the MCh Pediatric Surgery course the candidate is expected to conduct research activity that must be submitted "either in dissertation form or a manuscript ready for publication" [6]. Thesis work is a mandatory requirement in the DM/MCh degree courses in JIPMER, Puducherry and in the DNB curriculum for super specialities conducted by the National Board of Examination, New Delhi [7]. Wherever formal thesis writing is recommended the process, standards and timelines prescribed are similar to the MD or MS postgraduate thesis in that University.

Types of Studies Permitted as Thesis Work

The type of study permitted by different universities as part of thesis writing is also variable. Most universities recommend a prospective clinical or laboratory study. However, some institutions such as the National Board of Examinations, New Delhi allow retrospective record reviews and other forms of retrospective studies as acceptable forms of research activity. Certain courses in AIIMS, New Delhi require submission of two dissertation work. In such a case, one should be an experimental laboratory-based study and the other one must be a clinical study. Certain universities such as the Delhi University specify that the topic of study should not have been carried out in that University in the preceding 5 years.

Monitoring of Research Work

There are several concerns that students and guides could have in the process of carrying out dissertation work. The guide is concerned about the integrity of data collection, the regularity with which the study is conducted and the data collected which are crucial to the value of the outcome of the study. To address these concerns a formal system of monitoring the progress of dissertation work should ideally be in place which is sadly lacking in most universities. Although some universities such AIIMS, New Delhi have prescribed a formal system of periodic review of dissertation work in the curriculum, this is variable within the same university. In AIIMS, New Delhi some departments require the candidate's work to be reviewed every month, some departments require this to be done every 6 months, and some other departments have only one mid-term review prescribed formally during the period when the dissertation is carried out. In JIPMER, Puducherry there is an annual review of the dissertation work carried out by the MD/MS postgraduate student but not at the DM/MCh sub-speciality level. In most cases it is treated as a matter between the guide and the candidate and the academic wing does not maintain an oversight. This often results in a last-minute rush for completing the thesis work that sometimes compromises the quality of work. The periodic systematic review would help the student and guide in carrying out the work and permit timely midcourse correction when needed. It would also ensure that the data collected is accurate and add greater reliability of the outcome of the research exercise.

Impediments Faced by the Student in Carrying out Research Work

The student is concerned whether she will get adequate number of study subjects, whether the tests that need to be performed would be feasible, whether the study subjects would stick to the follow-up plan, whether the equipment required for the study would be available over the entire period of about 2 years that the study would span and whether the necessary resources would be provided by the department and the institution. Also required is access to literature specifically full-text articles. Excepting some well-funded universities, most medical colleges in this country do not have a large collection of journals especially back volumes. Electronic access to published articles would make the literature search and consequently research easy, but this is not readily available in most universities and colleges. Furthermore, the MCI continues to prescribe that only subscription to print form of journals are acceptable for recognising the course. This discourages universities from subscribing to electronic forms of journals. To address some of these concerns of the candidates, many universities have cautioned guides not to propose ambitious research projects for their candidates that may result in time overruns. The university also occasionally permits the change of the research project in case of legitimate reasons coming in the way of carrying out the initially approved proposal.

Timelines for Dissertation Protocol and Final Thesis Submission

The protocol typically is expected to be submitted 3–6 months after the candidate enrols in the course. The National Board of Examinations and JIPMER, Puducherry require the dissertation protocols to be submitted within 3 months of the beginning of the course. The protocol is usually approved in the department and then the postgraduate research committee of the university. While some universities require all human studies to be approved by an ethics committee, others don't have a uniform policy. In certain universities, the matter has been left to the discretion of the postgraduate research committee to take a decision in this regard on a case-by-case basis. However, it is prudent to have every project approved by the ethics committee as most standard journals would not publish an original article unless the study has been approved by an ethics committee. This is also the recommendation made by the ICMR guidelines on human research [8]. Animal studies, by law, require the mandatory approval of the animal ethics committee.

Non-submission of the research protocol on time usually incurs a penalty in most universities where formal dissertation is mandatory. An extension of one-month time is often given to the candidate based on the discretion of the academic head. During this period there may also be a financial penalty imposed on the candidate. For example, JIPMER, Puducherry imposes a penalty of Rs. 10,000 for late submission of research protocol by the candidate. The Delhi University imposes a penalty of Rs. 1000. In case of further delay the course may be extended by 6 months or sometimes, in extreme cases, the registration of the candidate for the course is cancelled.

In the case of a formal thesis, on completion of the research work, the entire study is compiled in the form of a book and submitted as thesis work towards the fulfilment of the requirement of the course. Many universities have put a limit on the number of pages that this book can have. Many of them have restricted the number of pages to about 100. In case the research activity has a less formal character of a research project or work that culminates in the submission of a manuscript for publication, it is expected that the manuscript should have been accepted for publication in a peer-reviewed preferably indexed journal. Many universities have relaxed this criterion and have accepted the submission for consideration for publication as adequate.

Be it submission of the thesis work as a book or as a manuscript the deadline for submission as per recommendations of the Medical Council of India in case of MD/MS course or as per recommendation of the university in the case of sub-speciality courses are typically 6 months before the start of the exit theory examination of the course. In case of some universities such as the Delhi University and the Guru Gobind Singh Indraprastha University, Delhi the deadline for submission is one year before the start of the theory examination of the course. In case the candidate fails to submit, she is not permitted to take the examination, and her examination is delayed by 6 months. Some universities allow a grace period of up to one month along with a penalty varying from Rs.1000 to Rs. 10,000 for submission during the grace period.

Method of Assessment of the Research Work

The dissertation so submitted for a DM/MCH course is evaluated by reviewers. While the MCI recommends a standard protocol of review of MD/MS postgraduate thesis consisting of one internal and at least two external reviewers, at the sub-speciality courses, there is no uniform recommendation. The various methods followed include assessment by internal and external examiners who may be the same examiners as for the exit examination, or they may be different. The certification by the head of the concerned department that the work done by the candidate is of sufficiently good quality worthy of publication is adopted by certain institutions. The latter is more common when research activity takes the form of project work. A flow chart for areas needing improvement in the writing of thesis for a sub-speciality program is shown in Fig. 1.

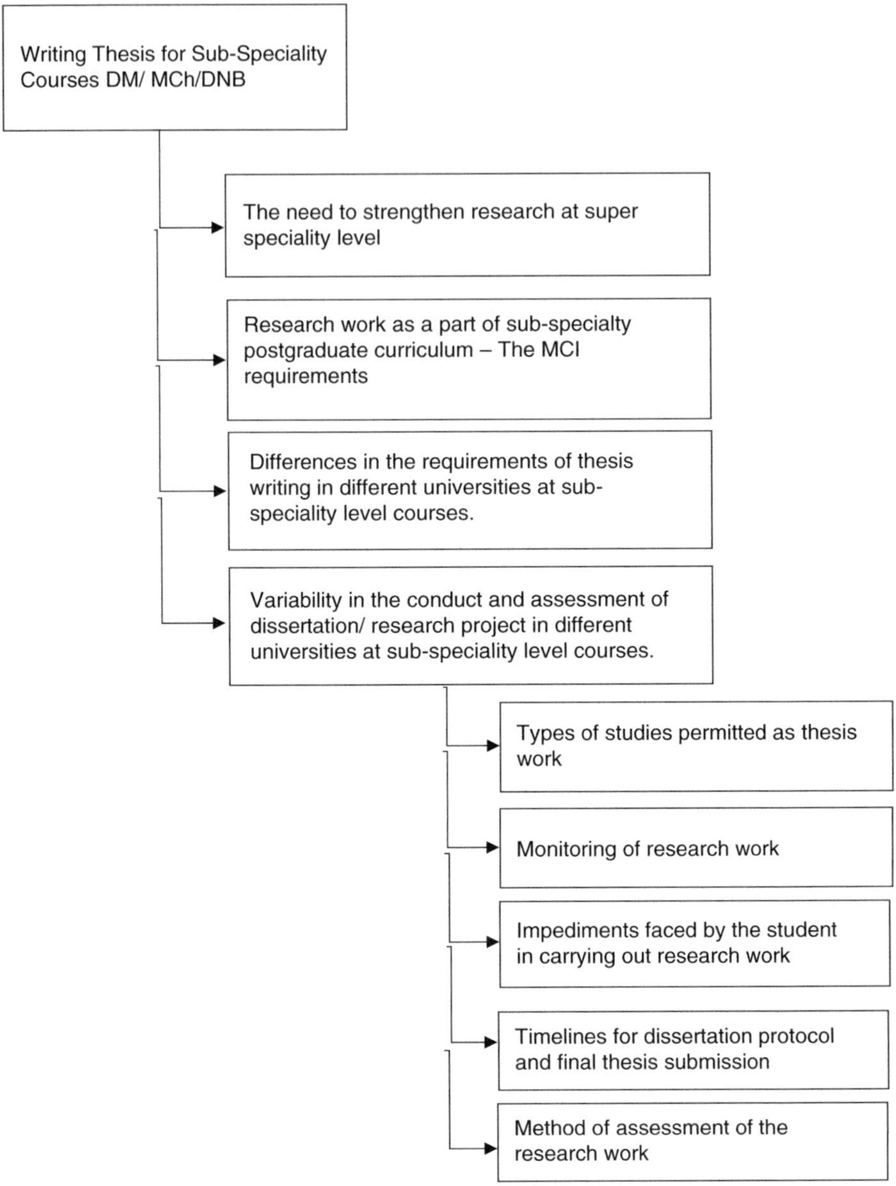

Fig. 1 Flow chart for areas needing improvement in the writing of thesis for a sub-speciality program

In conclusion, dissertation writing at sub-speciality level is highly variable in different institutions in this country. There are differences in the number of research projects to be carried out, nature of work, timelines, and outcome standards in terms of whether the work is submitted as a thesis or as a manuscript for publication and whether the paper should be submitted for publication or should be accepted for publication. There is a need to bring in some uniformity among all universities in this regard. This move can be led either by the MCI or by the institutions of national importance set up for developing modern patterns of medical education such as AIIMS, New Delhi, PGIMER, Chandigarh, JIPMER, Puducherry and NIMHANS, Bengaluru, coming together and developing a common basic curriculum for research in postgraduate medical education at the sub-speciality level.

Case Scenarios

1. You are the Dean of a medical college making the curricula for super speciality programs beginning with DM (Cardiology). The Head of Medicine suggests that the student should submit a thesis as part of the degree requirements, but the Head of Cardiology feels it is not required as per MCI norms. Which one of the following alternatives would you prefer to ensure compliance with MCI requirements?
   (a) Omit research work as a part of the curriculum.
   (b) Include dissertation work as in the case of MD (Medicine) course.
   (c) Include some formal research work in the curriculum leading to publication of a manuscript.
2. The deadline for submission of the thesis as per Medical Council of India is
   (a) Three months before exit theory exams.
   (b) Six months before exit theory exams.
   (c) One year before exit theory exams.
   (d) Can submit along with the exams.

References

1. Levasseur G, Schweyer F-X. Research in general medicine through medical theses. Sante Publique. 2003;15(2):203–12. French
2. Ray S, Shah I, Nundy S. The research output from Indian medical institutions between 2005 and 2014. Curr Med Res Pract. 2016;6(2):49–58.
3. Nagarajani R. Study reveals poor state of medical research—the Times of India [Internet]. [cited 2017 Sep 2]. http://timesofindia.indiatimes.com/india/Study-reveals-poor-state-of-medical-research/articleshow/51920662.cms
4. Scimago Institutions Rankings [Internet]. [cited 2017 Sep 2]. http://www.scimagoir.com/rankings.php.
5. The Medical Council of India. Postgraduate Medical Education Regulations 2000 [cited 2017 Aug 31]. https://www.mciindia.org/documents/rulesAndRegulations/Postgraduate-Medical-Education-Regulations-2000.pdf.
6. The All India Institute of Medical Sciences, New Delhi. AIIMS-Syllabus. [cited 2017 Sep 2]. http://www.aiims.edu/aiims/academic/aiims-syllabus/Syllabus%20-%20DM%20%20M%20Ch.pdf.
7. The National Board of Examinations, Delhi. Surgical oncology curriculum. [cited 2017 Aug 31]. http://www.natboard.edu.in/notice_for_dnb_candidates/Surgical%20Oncology%20currciculum%20final.pdf.
8. Indian Council of Medical Research. Ethical guidelines for biomedical research on human subjects. [cited 2017 Sep 3]. http://www.icmr.nic.in/ethical_guidelines.pdf.

Dissertation Writing for Master of Science Course

Subhash Chandra Parija, Noyal Mariya Joseph, and Madhuri Parija

A good dissertation is a done dissertation
—ancient grad student proverb

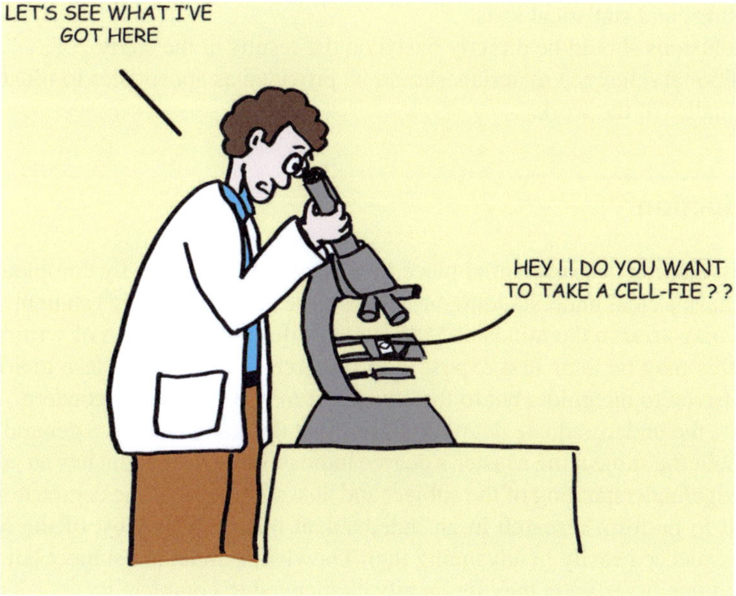

S. C. Parija (✉)
Vice-Chancellor, Sri Balaji Vidyapeeth, (Deemed University), Pondicherry, India

N. M. Joseph
Assistant Professor, Department of Microbiology, Jawaharlal Institute of Postgraduate Medical Education and Research, Pondicherry, India

M. Parija
Senior Resident, Department of Orthopaedics, All India Institute of Medical Sciences (AIIMS), Bhopal, India

S. C. Parija, V. Kate (eds.), *Thesis Writing for Master's and Ph.D. Program*,
https://doi.org/10.1007/978-981-13-0890-1_24

Key Points

- Master's degree signifies that the degree holder has the skill to perform research in an independent manner.
- Time management is crucial for completion of MSc dissertation.
- A strong self-motivation and self-discipline will help the students to stay focussed on their work.
- Working along with a small group of students may kindle a positive competitive spirit.
- Good communication and presentation skills are as important as carrying out a good research work.
- The Guide is meant to facilitate the dissertation process and not to lead.
- The student is primarily responsible for the quality of the dissertation and his/her work will be evaluated prior to awarding the Master's degree.
- Aims of the study refer to what you plan to achieve, while the objectives tell how you plan to achieve them.
- The results should be presented in a logical manner with use of appropriate sub-headings and statistical tests.
- Conclusions should be directly based on the results of the study.
- Additional reference materials should be provided as appendices to illustrate the originality of the work.

Introduction

MSc dissertation is a substantial piece of work, but to successfully complete it, one should have a clear understanding of what is expected of a Master's student. Several queries may arise in the minds of MSc students during the process of writing a thesis, as this may be their first exposure to research [1]. Some of these queries may appear trivial to the guide, but to the student, it may be of serious concern.

While the undergraduate degree signifies that the candidate has a general knowledge about the subject the Master's degree indicates that the person has an advanced knowledge/understanding of the subject and also signifies that the degree holder has the skill to perform research in an independent manner [1]. Most of the Master's students succeed easily in advancing their knowledge about the subject but when it comes to the dissertation they feel really challenged to complete it

Most of the Master's students assume that their guide has the greater responsibility to choose an appropriate topic for research, plan and carry out the study, while their role as a student is mostly passive and they have to blindly write and do what they are being instructed by the guide. Sometimes even the guides have a similar mindset and assign their students certain pre-determined topics for research and utilize the student only to carry out the procedures involved in their dissertation, without guiding them how to plan, carry out and write up a dissertation. But what these students and guides are often forgetting is that the MSc student is expected to master the art of dissertation writing as a part of their curriculum and develop the confidence to carry out independent research in future. The MSc student should be capable of identifying a research topic, framing a research question/hypothesis, performing literature review, carrying out research in par with established standards, analysing the data, drawing conclusions and making recommendations [2]. Successful completion of an MSc dissertation does not depend only on strict adherence to the rules and guidelines of the University, but largely depends on the active involvement of the candidate in the process of planning and performing dissertation work and his/her ability to understand how to write a dissertation. This chapter is intended to provide an overview of the process of dissertation writing and serve as a meaningful guide for the MSc students as well their supervisors/guides.

Steps in MSc Dissertation

MSc dissertation involves several steps as described in Fig. 1 [1, 3]. The initial steps including selection of appropriate topic, study design, methodology and the way the research was performed, primarily influence the quality of the dissertation work. Writing, reviewing and editing the dissertation are the last steps in the dissertation

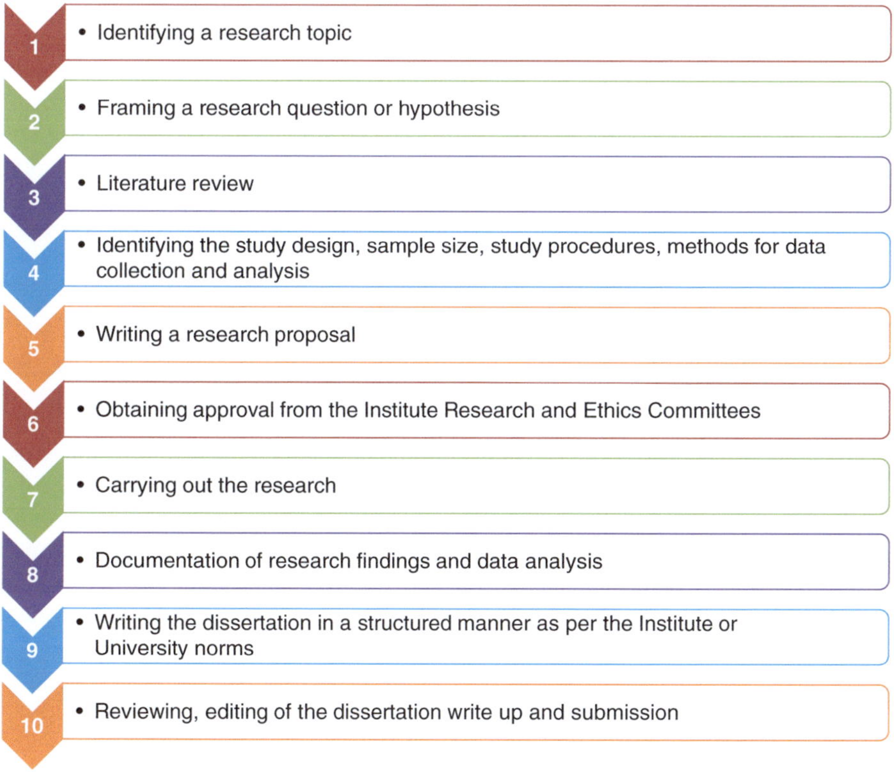

Fig. 1 Steps in MSc dissertation

cycle. But one cannot ignore the importance of the art of writing a dissertation because if the Master's student lacks the ability to write up his/her work in a scientifically sound and lucid manner, the significance of the work can be underrepresented. So, gaining the skill to write a good dissertation is as important as carrying out a good research work.

Skills Required for Writing MSc Dissertation

Time Management

Time management is crucial for completion of MSc dissertation before the submission deadline. The students should be aware of the time when they are expected to submit the dissertation. Accordingly, they should plan their research work and allot sufficient time for writing the dissertation. Adequate time should be allotted for completing each of the individual sections and the student should strive hard to complete all the sections within the stipulated time [1, 3].

Self-motivation

The MSc students during their course may have several distractors such as parties, family functions, holiday trips, and other personal commitments. The supervisor/guide may not mind a student taking some time off for certain important functions or occasional party. But the student should learn to give more importance for completion of the dissertation. A strong self-motivation and self-discipline will help the students to stay focussed on their work and discourage them from getting deviated unnecessarily [1].

Organizing Support

The Master's thesis usually has a short time frame, so the students have to train themselves to work independently in order to concentrate and focus on their research work. However, working independently to complete the dissertation in time can make the students feel lonely. So, it would be beneficial for them to maintain contact with selected students working on related topics or research work [3]. Working this way as a small group may kindle a positive competitive spirit and encourage the students to complete their dissertation in time. Each of the members in the small group can share with each other their experience in tackling practical problems faced by them.

Communication Skills

It is desirable to develop good verbal and written communication skills. The MSc student should be capable of expressing his/her ideas in a simple and effective manner when interacting with the supervisor/guide or their fellow students [1]. Good communication also requires active listening. Whenever the guide/supervisor asks the student to change the way he/she works, the student should understand there is some deficiency on his/her part and heed to the supervisors advise. Paying attention to the supervisors and correcting their ways may help the MSc students in succeeding in their task.

Presentation and Technical Skills

The MSc student should develop good presentation skills in terms of organising their contents and use of appropriate charts/figures/tables while writing the dissertation [1]. A brief discussion with their fellow students who have good presentation skills may be useful. The MSc student is also expected to learn the ways of gathering scientific information required for their dissertation from authentic sources. It is also important to develop the technical skills required for using the word processors, reference citing software and other related tools which may help in effectively writing a dissertation.

Roles and Responsibilities of the Student and the Supervisor

The successful completion of the MSc dissertation depends on both the student and the supervisor. Both of them should understand their roles and responsibilities and work in coordination to produce a significant piece of work known as Master's dissertation.

Role of the Supervisor/Guide

Each MSc student will be assigned a supervisor/guide who has the required expertise in the subject and also a good knowledge about performing research. The supervisor is primarily meant to facilitate the dissertation process and not to lead. The various roles of the supervisor include the following [2, 4]:

1. To advise the student in choosing the most suitable topic for research based on the feasibility, time frame and potential risks.
2. To assist in identification of relevant material to be included in the review of literature.
3. To assist in modifying the thesis protocol in view of the time or resource constraints.
4. To advise on appropriate study procedures/methodology including selection of suitable statistical tests for data analysis.
5. To monitor the progress of the thesis work and alert if there is undue delay or deviation from the proposed work.

6. To facilitate writing of the dissertation as per the Institute/University norms.
7. To review and edit the dissertation before submission mainly to assess if the study results have been appropriately represented and the conclusions and recommendations are based on the study findings.

Responsibilities of the Student

The MSc student should clearly understand that the dissertation is entirely his/her own work. The student should also be aware that he/she is primarily responsible for the quality of the dissertation and his/her work will be evaluated prior to awarding the Master's degree. The following are the responsibilities of the MSc student [2, 4]:

1. To maintain regular contact with the supervisor/guide and inform the progress of the dissertation work.
2. To discuss the challenges faced while carrying out the research work with their supervisor/guide in order to decide a suitable approach to tackle it.
3. To inform the supervisor/guide about any deviations from the proposed work.
4. To seek advice and obtain permission from the supervisor/guide if any extension is required for completing the dissertation due to some unavoidable reasons.
5. To obtain guidance from the supervisor while writing the dissertation.
6. To ensure that the writing style complies with the Institute/University guidelines, there are no grammatical or expression errors and the reference have been mentioned according to standard norms.
7. To incorporate the changes or corrections suggested by the supervisor/guide.

Writing the MSc Dissertation in a Structured Manner

General Instructions

Most Universities/Institute have well-written guidelines for writing MSc dissertation, with a detailed description of the word count, font type and size, line spacing, numbering style, margins, instructions for tables/figures etc [5]. It is mandatory that the students strictly adhere to these guidelines.

There may be certain differences in the structure of MSc dissertation across Universities. In general, the MSc dissertation includes the following sections [2, 5]:

1. Title page
2. Abstract
3. Acknowledgements
4. Abbreviations
5. Contents
6. Introduction
7. Review of literature

8. Aims and objectives
9. Materials and methods
10. Results
11. Discussion
12. Summary and Conclusions
13. References
14. Appendices

Title page

The title page should consist of the title of the dissertation, name of the student, name of the supervisors (guide/co-guides), name of the departments involved, and the month and year of submission. Usually, a standard template for title page will be provided by the University/Institute.

Abstract

A structured abstract is an important component of the MSc dissertation. An abstract is an independent, brief description of the dissertation work. It consists of a short introduction/background, aims of the study, methodology, results and conclusions [5]. It serves as an overview of the dissertation and helps the reader decide whether the dissertation is of interest to him/her.

Acknowledgements

A brief acknowledgement of usually one page should be included in the dissertation. It is intended to duly acknowledge the support or guidance received for carrying out the research work and writing the dissertation [2]. If many have contributed to the study, a general description of their roles would be sufficient [5]. The supervisors should be individually acknowledged for their contributions. It is mandatory to acknowledge the source of funding such as external funding agency and the Institute/University for the financial support received [5]. The acknowledgement page is usually signed by the student.

Abbreviations

It is customary to include a list of all the abbreviations used in the dissertation as an easy guide for the readers to understand the various abbreviations employed [5].

Contents

The contents page should list the title of the different sections of the dissertation. The abstract, acknowledgements, abbreviations should also be listed in the contents page without page numbers. The rest of the sections headers, such as introduction, aims and objectives, review of literature, methodology, results, discussion, conclusions and references should be listed with page numbers. The appendixes can be assigned individual numbers (preferably roman letters) and listed in the contents page [5]. A separate list of tables/figures may be provided along with the contents page [2].

Introduction

The introduction is a short section of the dissertation, which describes in 1 or 2 pages the background of the subject which is being studied. It is written in simple words without the use of unnecessary abbreviations to provide the reader with background information, make him/her understand the lacunae in the existing literature, describe the research problem and rationale for carrying out the study [2, 5]. The introduction usually ends with a short paragraph describing the aim of the study.

Review of Literature

The literature review is intended to critically present the available literature which is relevant to the research topic. The student should review and analyse the existing literature to provide a better understanding of the subject. It serves to showcase the depth of knowledge the student has about the topic and exhibit his/her skills to critically evaluate and present the currently available literature. It also describes the trends in the variables to be studied and the factors that can potentially influence the study parameters [2]. It will provide the background against which the thesis will be assessed to see what problem has been specifically addressed by the study and the information gathered as an outcome. It is desirable to summarize important information in existing literature as tables or figures [5].

The literature review is also important to justify the methods or procedures used in the study [2]. It provides the reader with a better understanding of the available methods, the advantages and limitations of those methods and their utility in specific settings. It helps in rationalising your choice of methods or procedures for the study.

The review of literature should be written in a logical order with appropriate use of subheadings to organize the contents [5].

Aims and Objectives

Although the aim of the study has been already mentioned briefly at the end of the introduction, it is necessary to describe the aims and objectives of the study in this section. The aims are general statements about the overall intended purpose or goals of the study. The objectives are the specific statements about how the aims are to be accomplished. In short, the aims refer to what you plan to achieve by this study, while the objectives tell how you plan to achieve them [2, 5].

Materials and Methods

This section should describe the study setting, study design, sample size calculation methods, study participants, the criteria for inclusion and exclusion, study procedures or methods. It is necessary to describe the way the study was carried out, the phases of the study, the roles of different personnel involved in the study and whether the study involved any blinding procedures if required to obtain unbiased outcomes. It is also mandatory to mention whether the approval from the Institute Research and Ethics committee and other relevant committees have been obtained. If the study involved human participants, the student has to mention whether consent was obtained or waiver of consent was approved by the Ethics committee.

There should be detailed description of the procedures used so that it can be replicated by others while undertaking similar studies. However, if previously well-established procedures were used, a brief description of the procedure would suffice with citation of the standard reference. If there was any deviation from the previously published methods, the modifications adopted in this study should be clearly stated [5]. The statistical methods used for data analysis should also be described.

Results

The results of the study should be presented in a logical manner with the use of appropriate subheadings in line with the objectives of the study. It is always desirable to mention the demographic details of the study participants before presenting the study results. This paves way for comparison of the study findings with the previously published or future studies involving similar study participants.

The data should be preferably represented as tables or figures or charts. Certain data can also be mentioned in a descriptive manner as text, but avoid repeating the information in the figures or tables in the text. The results of the statistical tests employed should be mentioned irrespective of whether the values indicate a significant association or not. Sometimes, the outcome of the study may be opposite of what was expected. Instead of trying to underrepresent such data, the student is expected to mention such contradictory data with the results of the statistical tests, so that the reasons for such findings can be discussed later in the discussion. Reference to the available literature or comparison to published studies should not be done in results [5].

Discussion

The discussion should follow a logical sequence, first beginning with a brief description of the advantages and limitations of the methods used, then discussing the important findings of the study and finally discussing the controversial or new findings [5]. It also makes sense to discuss related findings together.

The student should describe the interpretation of the study results and compare it with the previously published studies. It is necessary to provide a scientific explanation for the outcomes of the study. Although the reasons explaining the study findings are primarily the views of the student (as the primary author), it should be based on the results of the present study and/or aptly supported by the findings of other published studies [5].

The limitations of the study should be written in the last paragraph of the discussion. The limitations such as small sample size, inherent problem of the methods used and other factors that could have potentially influenced or biased the outcome of the study needs to be mentioned.

Summary and Conclusions

This section is intended to summarize the key findings of the study. It should be presented more as a general statement rather than repetition of the results. The student should be able to make appropriate conclusions directly based on the study findings [5]. This section should also describe the importance of the study results and their clinical implications with potential applications. The need for further validation of certain study findings and the scope for further research based on the study outcomes should also be mentioned in this section [2].

References

The references cited throughout the dissertation should be listed here. The student should follow either the Vancouver or Harvard style for listing the references [2, 3, 5]. The in-text citation should be appropriate to the reference style used. Certain modifications in the bibliography style may be suggested by different institutes or universities, it is mandatory for the students to adhere to their institute or university guidelines.

Appendices

This section should be used for providing additional reference material to illustrate the originality of the work [2, 5]. Some of the supporting materials that can be included in this section are the master chart, study questionnaires, consent forms, research and ethics committee approval certificate, etc.

Case Scenarios

1. Your study was approved by the Institute Research and Ethics committee. But after that you come across a new guideline that recommends modification in the standard procedure for performing a test which is part of your study.
   (a) Will you modify the study procedures based on the recent guideline?
   (b) Whom will you inform about this recent change?
2. You observe an unusual finding in your study which is contradictory to the published literature.
   (a) What will you do? Will you mention it in your dissertation or disregard it?
   (b) If you decide to mention the unusual finding in the results, in which section of your dissertation will you explain the probable reasons for getting such conflicting results.

References

1. Biggam J. Succeeding with your master's dissertation: a step-by-step handbook. 2nd ed. Buckingham: Open University Press; 2011.
2. School of Management and Languages. A guide to writing your masters dissertation. School of Management and Languages 2017. https://www.researchgate.net/file.PostFileLoader.html?id=5769c2a840485404cf385288&assetKey=AS%3A375547478724608%401466548904040
3. Kreikemeyer A, Schneider P. How do I successfully write a masters thesis? A practical guide for peace- and conflict- researchers and other social scientists. 4th ed. Hamburg: University of Hamburg; 2007.
4. El-Ansary A. Guidelines for writing a successful MSc thesis proposal. King Saud University 2004. http://www-elec.inaoep.mx/~rogerio/ProposalGuidelines.pdf.
5. University of Eastern Finland. Msc thesis writing instructions. University of Eastern Finland 2017. http://universityoffinland.com/documents/1110526/1539831/101123_MSc_thesis_writing_instructions.pdf/6d8989f6-00bc-45ce-a763-30099b4b7a97.

Writing Thesis for Doctor of Philosophy Course

Jharna Mandal, Subhash Chandra Parija, and Ajay Haldar

"A thesis is a sustained, logical and well evidenced argument."

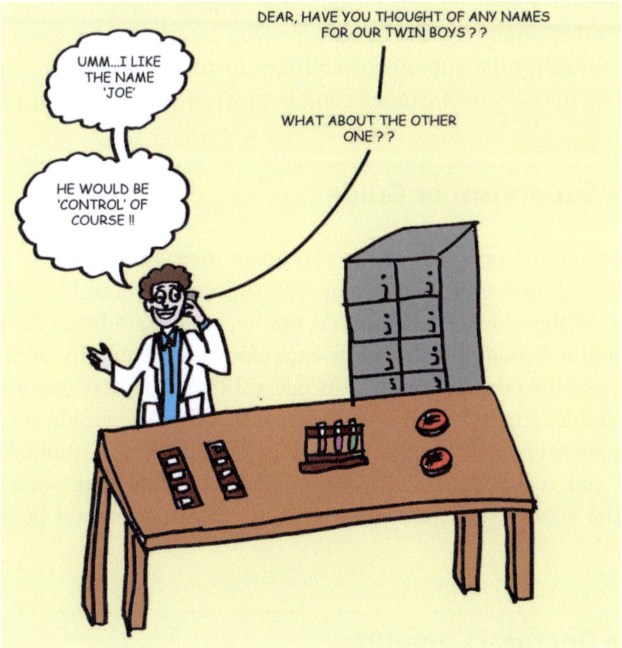

J. Mandal
Additional Professor, Department of Microbiology, Jawaharlal Institute of Postgraduate Medical Education and Research, Pondicherry, India

S. C. Parija (✉)
Vice-Chancellor, Sri Balaji Vidyapeeth, (Deemed University), Pondicherry, India

A. Haldar
Assistant Professor, Department of Obstetrics and Gynaecology, All India Institute of Medical Sciences (AIIMS), Bhopal, India

S. C. Parija, V. Kate (eds.), *Thesis Writing for Master's and Ph.D. Program*,
https://doi.org/10.1007/978-981-13-0890-1_25

Key Points

- This short review describes the roles and responsibilities of the PhD candidate, the guide/supervisor and the doctoral committee.
- Students will be able to get an overview of the process of PhD thesis writing.
- This review will provide the necessary information required for submission of the synopsis.
- This will provide the necessary information regarding the submission of thesis followed by the viva-voce.

Introduction

A PhD dissertation is a documented proof of original research which has been conducted to extensive depths containing a significantly detailed study of the area of research based on sound evidence and with critical analysis. This is actually a monogram written solely by the candidate who has done the research work and formally approved by the supervisor and the doctoral committee. The statements made should be in one's own framed sentences without an ounce of plagiarism.

Role of the Supervisor or Guide

Guiding the academic progress of the candidate throughout the period of study is the chief responsibility of the supervisor. The supervisor should counsel the student in all aspects of the course and provide the necessary guidance on the nature of coursework and research, the standards expected and the quality of work. All matters pertaining to the completion of a successful thesis namely content, originality, research standards, structure and documentation and writing style are the responsibilities of the supervisor. A supervisor has a right to expect substantial effort, initiative, respect and receptiveness towards suggestions and constructive criticisms. Only when the supervisor is satisfied with the thesis, it should be submitted for approval [1–4].

Role of the Doctoral Committee

After the candidate is admitted to the course, a doctoral committee is constituted. The doctoral committee usually consists of three members, namely, a Guide/Supervisor (as Coordinator he/she would initiate the steps for the formation of the Committee), another faculty member from the same department/institute working in the same field as an Internal expert, some faculty working in the related field of work can be assigned as co-guides and one faculty member from outside the institute specialized in a related field as an External expert shall be included in the committee. The number of members for the doctoral committee may vary with the institute depending on their rules and regulations [2, 3].

The members of the doctoral committee in close cooperation with the supervisor should monitor the student's progress from time to time. Doctoral committee meetings are advisable every 6 months to review the student's progress of work. They should also help the supervisor guide the candidate in the selection of the methodologies. They should provide subject matter expertise and serve as a content expert in the student's field of research. The external expert should review the draft version of the protocol or proposal of the work and provide suggestions for revising the content in the areas related to their expertise. All members should actively participate in guiding the student and offer their expertise during the meetings. The external expert should also review the draft version of the thesis and provide suggestions for revising the content related to their area of expertise so that it can be approved for submission and publication [3].

Role of the PhD Candidate

The candidate plays the pivotal role in the PhD thesis. The entire work that has been assigned should be diligently worked upon with full integrity. Commitment on the part of the candidate to devote the time, dedicated efforts to gain the background knowledge and skills needed to pursue the research work successfully and energy to engage in research and to be able to write a thesis. It is always better to develop a plan and timetable for completion of all phases of the thesis work within the appropriate deadlines. Students should do literature review regularly to keep themselves updated about the recent developments in the area of research. All work and protocols should be well-documented and regularly updated. It is always better to have regular discussions with the supervisor regarding the work progress and results. One should pay special attention to the advice and criticisms received from the supervisor as well as the doctoral committee members. Though the supervisor is required to be reasonably available for discussion, it is also the student's responsibility to keep in touch with the supervisor [2, 3].

Selection of a Topic for PhD Research

The very first step in the PhD thesis is a choice of a good topic. This depends on the supervisor most often who with her/his experience suggests a list of the topics/questions that have not been covered/answered or on finding an answer to a lesser studied problem or looking at a particular question from a different viewpoint so as to derive a new answer, etc. It is ideal if both the guide/supervisor and the candidate is able to go through the available literature. In the course of the time, new method or new tool may also be added which can provide a new dimension to the initial concept [2].

Developing a Hypothesis or Framing the Research Question

It originates with the "why" and "so what", and in order to prove or disprove the hypothesis, one has to look for a study design, develop the objectives which can answer the research questions or justify the hypothesis. A hypothesis or a research question, in essence, acts as a guide giving a direction to the research work [2].

Writing a Research Proposal

The hypothesis sets the ball rolling for the proposal writing. A PhD proposal is an outline of the proposed research work that is designed to answer the research question or test the hypothesis. It should define the goals and objectives that are to be fulfilled by the study proposed. It is important to make a note of the existing lacunae in the field and how this study will fill the existing knowledge gaps and highlight the originality and novelty of the work being planned. Thus a background review of existing literature related to the area of work concerned should be made and the experiments are selected accordingly dividing the work into several workable phases. All these should be discussed in the doctoral committee meetings and necessary inputs should be taken after a formal discussion with the subject experts concerned [1–9].

Carrying Out the Work

The proposal should be approved by the Institute scientific and ethics committee before starting the work. A detailed plan of work should be drawn up that is feasible and practical after discussion with the members of the doctoral committee and one should abide by the timelines assigned. Ambitious and too rigid deadlines can be detrimental both to the candidate as well as for the research work. One should remember that a good PhD proposal evolves as the work progresses. Unlike other research proposals, "**A good PhD proposal is not set in stone**" and it is normal for students to refine their original proposal in light of an advancement in the field of work, new literature citing alternative method or research approaches and comments received from the doctoral committee [2].

Data Analysis and Compilation of Results

Analysis of data is a complex task in itself and can give shivers to many. Though this seems quite daunting and unimpressive, it can be managed without much difficulty provided all the findings have been documented meticulously. A good understanding of the various experimental techniques applied is important for a good compilation. It would be worth if on completion of each experiment one tries to analyze how close one is towards fulfilling each objective.

Synopsis

A synopsis is essentially a detailed summary of the work highlighting the important findings. This must be like a good preface to a book and should have all its appealing characters. The synopsis should bring out in abridged form, the aims for conducting research, work done, results, and conclusions drawn. The candidate should present the synopsis in a doctoral meeting in the department before its submission. Usually, within 3–6 months before the submission of the thesis, the synopsis should be submitted so that it can be sent to the thesis reviewers. The candidate shall make a presentation of the synopsis before the doctoral committee. The length of the synopsis can vary with the institute but ideally be six to ten pages. Once the synopsis is accepted by the examiner, the thesis is sent for evaluation. On receipt of the comments, the same is transmitted to the doctoral committee of the candidate. If the thesis examiner/examiners suggest requirement of the revision and re-submission for further examination, then the revised thesis duly certified by the Doctoral Committee is sent to the same examiner for further evaluation [3, 7, 8].

Public Viva-Voce/Thesis Defence

Once the thesis has been approved and on receipt of communication from the Institute, the guide/supervisor shall coordinate the conduct of public viva-voce for the candidate. The Doctoral Committee appoints the examiner (usually the Indian examiner) who will conduct the public viva-voce examination in the presence of interested members of the public. Alternatively, an eminent person, preferably from the panel of examiners submitted by the doctoral committee of the candidate may be appointed for conducting the viva. Once the date of the viva or public defence has been fixed, a notification of the same should be circulated at least ten working days prior to the event on the institute website as well as to all the departments and a copy of the same should be available in the library for public viewing. Ideally, the viva-voce should be conducted within 6 months of consolidation of the reports from the examiners. Once the candidate successfully defends the thesis publicly, he/she is awarded the degree in the subsequent convocation [1–3, 7, 8].

Types of Doctoral Thesis

Once ready, the thesis can be bound as a bound thesis form which is the traditional and classical style, with only one (right) side of the page containing the printed matter while the other (left) side of the page is empty.

The second form is the book form of the doctoral thesis. This has become quite popular as it is practically useful and can be carried anywhere like a book since both sides of the page have printed matter.

Style of Thesis Writing

There are many styles and guidelines of writing a dissertation. Nevertheless, the following divisions/sections are usually applicable universally across the globe. There may be certain additional features like acknowledgements, abbreviations, appendices and publications which should be appended as per the institute/university guidelines.

The **most common style of writing** contains the entire thesis written according to the following sections.

(a) Introduction
(b) Review of literature
(c) Materials and Methods
(d) Results (incl. Figures, images, tables etc.)
(e) Discussion
(f) Summary and Conclusions
(g) References/Bibliography

The **second style of writing** contains the entire thesis written as chapters, each chapter referring to each objective with its methodological details, results and discussion, with a common summary and conclusions in the end. This is easier to write and should be done after fulfilling each objective. This has an advantage over the former as it gives a sense of continuity to the reader without having to refer back to each objective while reading the results and discussion.

Introduction: "Good Beginnings will have Good Endings"

A good introduction is like a window to the research work entailed in the dissertation and its main purpose is to guide the reader towards the specific question being addressed. It lays the background, defines the problem statement, slowly plunging into the genesis of the work and finally telling the reader as to why the work was carried out [1, 6].

Review of Literature: "The Genesis of a Good Study Relies on a Sound Background Knowledge"

This is an important section of the thesis which is directly related to the work as it entails the findings of the available and relevant scientific publications across the globe in the same area of work. It is important to discuss the individual publications that were found appropriate. Every statement made needs to be supported by an appropriate reference. It is pertinent that all the references quoted should be read individually and not merely copied from some already existing literature. In the process, it is important to discuss key papers which have more relevant data than those which offer little information. The depth and extent of review of literature are at one's discretion, but it should neither be too voluminous nor too concise [4, 5].

Materials and Methods: "The Whys and Wherefores of Procedures Followed"

The essentials of this section should answer "What?", "How?" and "Where?" A detailed description of the experimental procedures should be mentioned here so that it can be reproduced by someone else. If the methods have been adapted from another published work, then the same should be cited and a full description of the methods should be made. If any alterations in existing standard procedures are made the same should be mentioned. This will then serve as a ready source of such methods for future students. Very often scholars prefer to place reagent preparation and certain laboratory methods in the appendices. In such a case, one should cite them appropriately so that one is able to follow the same when needed. It is important to note that if references are not cited appropriately, it will automatically reduce the scientific merit [1, 2, 4].

Results: "Compiling Results is like the Art of a Good Storytelling"

The result part should be displayed sequentially which should be meaningful. All tables, figures and images, etc, should be arranged in continuity with the text so that a logical flow is maintained. Many times results are simply compiled without any connectivity. In essence, the building up of the facts based on the analyzed data and stringing them into a single thread one by one needs intellect and concentration. This section should be given utmost importance both by the candidate and the supervisors and along with the doctoral committee members.

All tables should be self-explanatory, have titles indicating the contents and appropriate legends. Figures should be clearly labelled and understandable without having to refer to the text. All data should be explicitly stated which contribute to the study and only the description of the experimental data should be made without any extensive interpretation. It is to be emphasized that the data should be accurately described so as to answer the questions or justify the hypothesis with appropriate caveats where applicable [6–8].

Discussion: "A Compendious Discussion Leads the Reader Maintaining its Pace"

Writing this part is the trickiest of all. This should contain a detailed account of the interpretation and evaluation of the results against the background of the relevant literature. One needs to refer to the results for writing this. This section should only contain the interpretation and should not be a repetition of the data mentioned in the results. If the experimental outcomes are clearly depicted in the results, it is sufficient to refer to them and discuss the significance of these findings. It is important that the written matter be clear, comprehensive and concise using complete sentences [6–12].

Summary and Conclusions: "The Bad, the Good and the Missing"

This is more than just a chapter and is the essence of the entire thesis. The researcher should be able to highlight the achievements of the thesis and relate to the significance of such findings. This should be to the point, without much exaggeration of each finding. The conclusions need to be clearly spelt out with appropriate limitations. This should also mention the possible next steps for further developments in knowledge in the area identified and mention what remains to be done. This is where the opinions of the researcher get a place finally [2, 6, 7].

Bibliography/References: "The Style Speaks for Itself"

The style of writing bibliography can be as per the institute/university guidelines. Mostly it is a question of taste and tradition. There are a number of styles to choose among. Every style has its essential characteristics, but the purpose of all is to aid the reader in follow up. Therefore this list should contain details only of those works cited in the text of the document. These details must include sufficient information so that readers may easily locate and consult these references [2, 7, 8]. The flowchart for writing a PhD thesis is shown in Fig. 1.

"Begin at the beginning," the King said gravely, "and go on till you come to the end: then stop." -Alice's Adventures in Wonderland by Lewis Carrol.

Case Scenarios

1. You have completed two-thirds of your major part of the work and have come across some literature which contradicts your hypothesis. You decide to ignore this finding and stick to your plan only.
   (a) Was this approach correct?
   (b) What should ideally be done?
   (c) How will you incorporate any change in your thesis plan? Whom should you inform before making any changes in the existing proposal?
2. You are in the habit of documenting only the final results of each experiment. But when you start analyzing your results you find that some of the data linking the various experiments are missing.
   (a) What should you do to avoid such problems?
   (b) What are the ways that one can document and store data for future analysis?
   (c) Is it ideal to just document data and analyze it later?

Declaration There are no conflicts of interest.

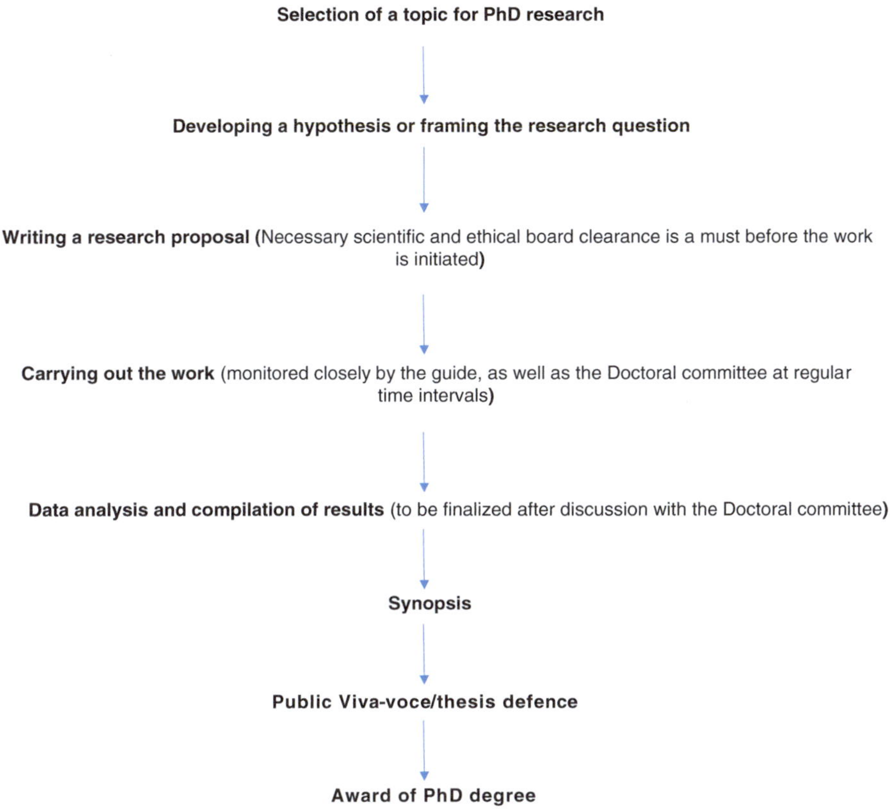

Fig. 1 Flowchart for writing a PhD thesis

References

1. Sternberg D. How to complete and survive a doctoral dissertation. New York: St. Martin's Press; 1981.
2. Ruger S. How to write a good PhD thesis and survive the viva. Knowledge media institute. Kents Hill: The Open University; 2016.
3. Guidelines for degree of doctor of philosophy 2016–19. Puducherry: JIPMER; http://jipmer.puducherry.gov.in.
4. Khan KS, Kunz R, Kleijnen J, Antes G. Systematic reviews to support evidence-based medicine. How to review and apply findings of health care research. London: RSM Press; 2003.
5. Pautasso M. Ten simple rules for writing a literature review. PLoS Comput Biol. 2013;9(7):e1003149.
6. Holtom D, Fisher E. Enjoy writing your science thesis or dissertation!: a step by step guide to planning and writing dissertations and theses for undergraduate and graduate science students. London: Imperial College Press; 1999.
7. Phillips EM, Pugh DS. How to get a Ph.D.: a handbook for students and their supervisors. 2nd ed. Buckingham: Open University Press; 1994.
8. Chandrasekhar R. How to write a thesis: a working guide. The University of Western Australia. http://www.student.uwa.edu.au/__data/assets/pdf_file/0007/1919239/How-to-write-a-thesis-A-working-guide.pdf

9. Giesler M, Boeker M, Fabry G, Biller S. Importance and benefits of the doctoral thesis for medical graduates. GMS J Med Educ. 2016;33(1):8.
10. Browne JE. Getting started with research "writing-up the results of your research". Ultrasound. 2014;22(1):70–2.
11. Fahy K. Writing for publication: argument and evidence. Women Birth. 2008;21(3):113–7.
12. Hardy S, Ramjeet J. Reflections on how to write and organize a research thesis. Nurse Res. 2005;13(2):27–39.

Part VII

Statistical/English Language/ Plagiarism Software

Statistical Packages for Data Analysis

N. Sreekumaran Nair, K. T. Harichandrakumar,
and N. Ravishankar

A statistical analysis, properly conducted, is a delicate dissection of uncertainties, a surgery of suppositions.
—MJ Moroney

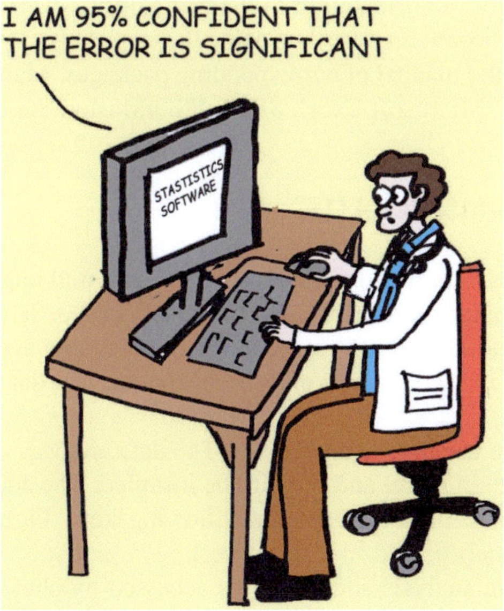

N. S. Nair (✉)
Professor and Head, Department of Biostatistics, Jawaharlal Institute of Postgraduate Medical Education and Research, Pondicherry, India

K. T. Harichandrakumar
Assistant Professor, Department of Biostatistics, Jawaharlal Institute of Postgraduate Medical Education and Research, Pondicherry, India

N. Ravishankar
Assistant Professor, Department of Statistics, Manipal University, Manipal, India

S. C. Parija, V. Kate (eds.), *Thesis Writing for Master's and Ph.D. Program*,
https://doi.org/10.1007/978-981-13-0890-1_26

Key Points

- This chapter provides a brief overview of the commonly used popular statistical packages for thesis or research project data analysis and report preparation.
- A comprehensive discussion on the strength, weakness and utility of packages namely Microsoft Excel, SPSS, PS, nMaster, Stata, Epi-info and EZR has been provided.
- The steps for installing data analysis add-in in MS Excel, using Master and gadgets of Epi-info have been described.

Background

This session deals with commonly available software packages for statistical analysis of health science research data. The main objective of this session is to sensitize the readers about various statistical packages which are regularly used for data analysis. This session introduces common packages, discuss various options available in each package and give an orientation to the difficulty level. However, this is not a manual to train you how to analyse data using these packages. For that purpose, you are advised to refer the manual of corresponding packages. Main packages included in the discussion are Microsoft Excel, SPSS, PS, nMaster, Stata, Epiinfo and EZR.

Microsoft Excel–MS-Excel [1]

MS Excel is the most common tool used for data entry and management. It is present in all the computers which possess Microsoft office. It features calculation, graphing tools, pivot tables, and a macro programming language called Visual Basic for Applications. It is used to store and retrieve numerical data in a grid format of columns and rows.

Excel can also be used for data analysis. The data analysis options are available as an add-in package in Excel and it has to be installed. The add-in package of data analysis in excel can be installed using the following steps. Figure 1 shows the steps for installing data analysis add-in in MS Excel.

The installed data analysis add-in can be accessed by clicking on '***Data***' in the toolbar.

The data analysis tools available in excel include descriptive statistics, t-test, Z-test ANOVA, Correlation, Regression, Covariance, moving average and random number generation. For a small set of data and simple analysis, this is a good package. However, the package does not have flexibility for more advanced options.

Excel is ideal to prepare different graphs and diagrams to summarize the data. It produces Line graph, Pie, Bar, Area, Scatter, Stack, Surface, Radar and Combo charts. The graphs and diagrams in excel are of high quality. Another advantage of the excel graph is that it can be edited as per the requirement. This is a good package for a beginner who does not have much knowledge about other statistical packages

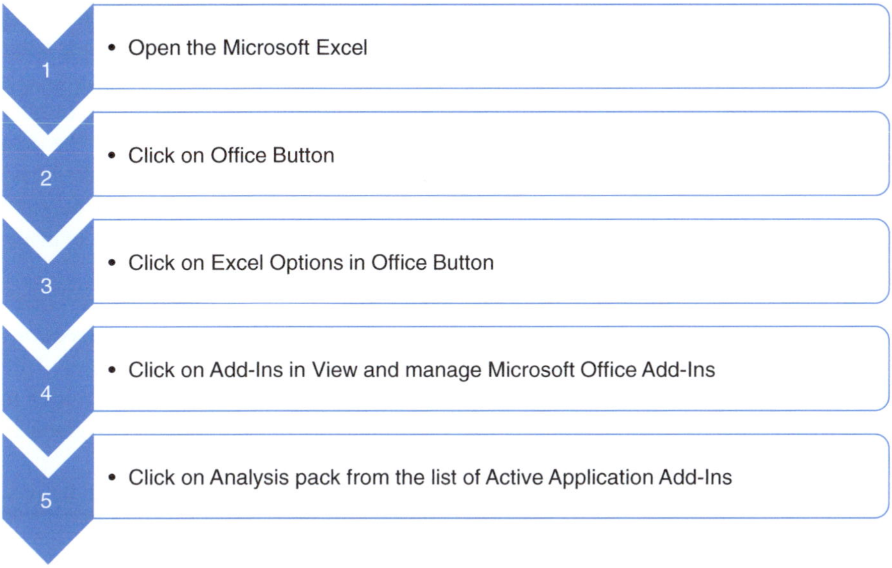

Fig. 1 Steps for installing data analysis add-in in MS excel

and required to do simple descriptive statistics, graphs and tests of significance. Data base prepared in Excel is compatible with many of the advanced statistical packages.

Statistical Packages for Social Sciences (SPSS) [2]

Statistical Packages for Social Sciences (SPSS) is one of the most commonly used statistical packages for data analysis by the health science researchers and Residents. The simple menu-driven characteristics, availability of most of the statistical methods and compatibility of the worksheet with other packages like excel make SPSS popular among medical researchers.

The SPSS basically consists of three windows namely Data editor/window, Output window and Syntax editor. The Data Editor is similar to Microsoft Excel and it consists of two sub-windows namely data view and variable view. Data view provides the complete view of the data set and variable view provides the characteristics of the variables. The variable characteristics such as type of variables, required width and decimal points, label of the variable name etc can be specified in the variable view. The coding for the categorical variables can also be defined through the values option in the variable view window. The characteristics of the variable should be clearly defined in variable view before entering the data. The Database for analysing the data in SPSS can be either created in SPSS or can be created in the worksheets of packages namely Excel, Systat, Stata, SAS etc. The database created in other formats can also be imported into SPSS for the analysis.

The spreadsheet in SPSS allows the user to split files, select cases based on specific characteristics of a particular variable, combine file, redefine variables, filter variables based on specific characteristic etc.

The different statistical analysis procedures available in SPSS are given under the drop-down menu '***Analysis***' in the data view. Descriptive Statistics for the data can be obtained through the drop-down '***Descriptive Statistics***' and '***Reports***' options respectively. The parametric tests such as one sample t-test, Independent Students t-test, Paired t-test and one-way Analysis of Variance (ANOVA) is available in '***Compare Means***' in the drop-down menu "*Analysis*".

Non-parametric tests are available under the menu '***Nonparametric Test***'. Correlation and regression analysis is given under '***Correlation***' and '***regression***' options respectively in '***Analysis***'. The analysis of time to even data such as Life Tables, Kaplan Meier estimates, Log Rank Test, Cox regression etc. are provided in '***Survival Analysis***'. The advanced statistical analysis is available and is given in respective options in the *Analysis* menu.

The output of the analysis is displayed in output window. The results will be produced in table format with extensive details. The SPSS output file will be saved in '***save***' format and it can be exported into other formats such as word document, excel etc. as per the requirement through '***Export***' option in '*File*' in the '*output*' window.

Overall SPSS is a user-friendly comprehensive programme used for statistical analysis. The resultant output requires editing and it requires a moderate level of statistical knowledge to choose items from the output.

Power and Sample Size Programme [3]

Power and Sample Size programme is abbreviated as PS, is an interactive program for performing power and sample size calculations. It is a free software and can be downloaded using the link (http://biostat.mc.vanderbilt.edu/wiki/Main/PowerSampleSize). PS software can be used for estimating the sample size and power for the studies with dichotomous, continuous, or survival response measures.

The PS software provides the sample size and power for the studies which involve independent and dependent groups with continuous outcome measure, for the studies related to survival times and hazard ratio, case-control and cohort studies, studies related to correlation and regression analysis and the studies involving independent and dependent groups with dichotomous outcomes. In PS, the explanation is provided for each of the items in the '***input***' menu.

Another merit of this package is that the output displays the sample size/power with a clear explanation of the calculation which will be helpful for users for writing the thesis or project report.

nMaster [4]

nMaster is another package which is exclusively meant for computation of sample size. This package is developed and marketed by Christian Medical College (CMC) Vellore, India. It provides a sample size for estimation and testing of hypothesis problems.

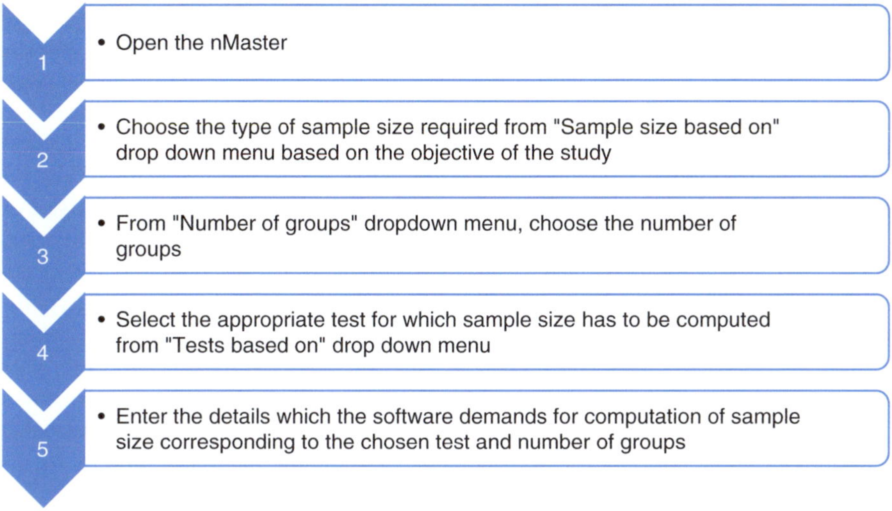

Fig. 2 Steps for using nMaster

Estimating and testing arithmetic means and Proportions. Further, sample size computations are available for Diagnostic test, Regression methods, Survival analysis, Cluster design, Clinical Trials, Epidemiologic Methods and Non-parametric methods.

Figure 2 provides the steps to compute sample size using nMaster.

In case of doubt, the users can click on the '***help***' button, which displays the assumptions of the concerned statistical test, the sample size formula along with an explanation for the terms in the formula and also an example.

Output from nMaster can be saved in different formats/printed.

STATA [5]

Stata is developed and marketed by "Stata Corp". It is the preferred statistical package for public health professionals and epidemiologists. Stata is a powerful statistical package with smart data-management facilities, a wide array of up-to-date statistical techniques and an excellent system for producing high-quality graphs. Stata is fast and easy to use package. It has both menu driven as well as command driven options.

The main window of stata consists of five sub-win dows. The "variables" menu displays the name and label of all the variables in the data-set. "Properties" displays the properties of variables as well as the dataset. Commands are typed in "Commands" window. The executed commands are displayed in "Review" window. Upon clicking a command in review window, it again appears in the command window, which can be re-executed by pressing the enter button to get the output.

Upon clicking the data editor in the main window (exactly below the "Statistics"), opens the data editor sheet, which provides access to the data.

Data can be imported into stata from different sources. The most unique feature of stata is that the value labels assigned to categorical variables can be saved as 'do files' and can be imported and used whenever required (Files ➔Do➔Save).

Stata performs a very wide range of statistical techniques (basic techniques to most advanced techniques like structural equation modelling, multi-level modelling, network meta-analysis etc.). Upon clicking the '***Statistics***' option on the main window, a drop-down of statistical techniques appears.

The options namely (Statistics ➔Summaries, tables and tests ➔ Other tables) compact table of summary statistics, flexible table of summary statistics, table of means, standard deviation and frequencies make stata an ideal choice for analysis of descriptive studies. Presence of calculators; CI calculator (Statistics ➔Summaries, tables and tests➔Summary and descriptive statistics), t-test calculator and effect size calculator (Statistics➔Summaries, tables and tests ➔Classical tests of hypotheses), odds ratio calculator, risk ratio calculator and matched case-control calculator (Statistics➔Epidemiology and related➔ Table for epidemiologists) are highlights of stata. Stata computes sample size for most of the statistical procedures (Statistics➔Power and sample size). It produces sophisticated graphs. Stata also provides example datasets for practice (File ➔ Example datasets), thereby facilitates self-learning of the users.

As stata is also command driven, it has the flexibility of providing customized outputs by executing appropriate commands. Results can be exported to word document/text document/excel.

Stata is a package with a lot of flexibility to customize the analysis based on individual requirement. However, it is not very user-friendly.

Epi Info [6]

Epi Info, as the name suggests it is meant for the analysis of data from epidemiological investigations. It is a freeware which works only in Windows and is developed by Center for Disease Control and Prevention (CDC), Atlanta. Epi Info is a user-friendly package that comes handy with key applications; (1) Creation of data entry forms (2) Data entry (3) Computation of sample size (4) Analysis and (5) Creation of maps. The most remarkable feature of Epi Info is that it is also available as a mobile application that works on smartphones and tablets, which makes it an ideal software for use during outbreak investigations and public health emergencies. The mobile application is endowed with "cloud services" which helps the investigators to collect the data from multiple sites and pool the collected data on a common platform for a combined analysis. An additional exiting feature of Epi Info is "Cloud Data Analytics" that facilitates handling and analysis of large-scale datasets.

Upon opening the Epi Info, it displays a set of six gadgets, which the users can choose based on their requirements. Figure 3 shows the gadgets of Epi Info.

Epi Info enables the creation of customized data entry forms (choose "Create forms"). It has provision for creating a facility for entering text, number, date and time, check-box, yes or no and choosing one among many options. Created data entry forms can be easily edited/modified. Data entry forms can be created only in Windows version. However, the created user forms can also be used in the mobile

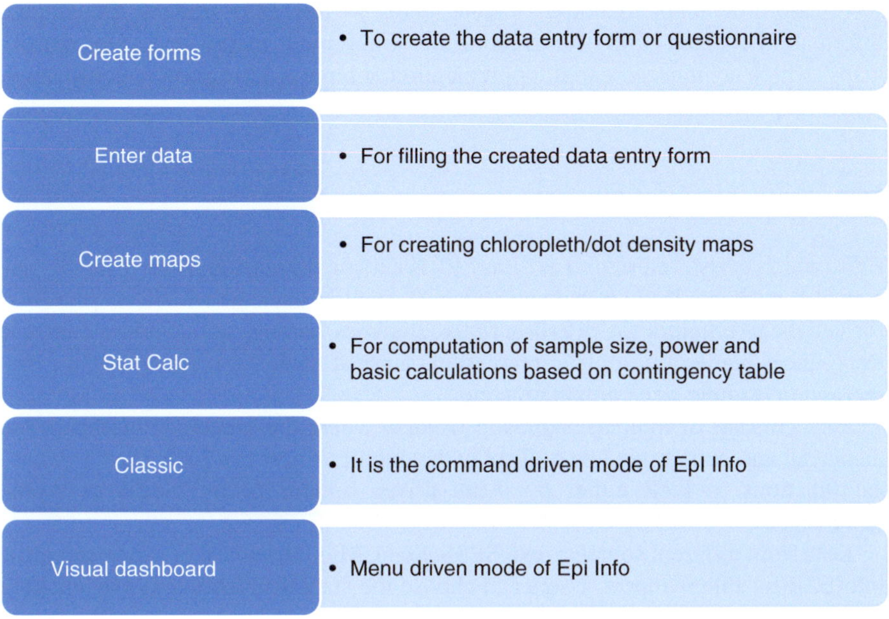

Fig. 3 Gadgets of Epi Info

version. Data can be entered either in Windows version or mobile version. The entered data gets saved in the database and can also be extracted in a Microsoft Excel data sheet.

Epi Info computes sample size for basic epidemiological study designs namely surveys, cross-sectional studies, cohort studies and unmatched case- control studies (choose "Stat Calc"). It is an easy procedure which requires entering the desired information in the checkboxes and in the fraction of a second, Epi Info displays sample sizes for different combinations of confidence levels/cluster sizes depending on the situations.

Epi info has the facility of calculators (choose "Stat Calc"). It has got a calculator for odds ratio, risk ratio, chi-square, Poisson probability, Binomial probability and matched case-control odds ratio.

Epi info has statistical methods that are sufficient for analysis of common epidemiological investigations (choose "Classic" or "Visual dashboard"). It includes descriptive statistics, linear regression, logistic regression and conditional logistic regression. Kaplan-Meier and Cox-proportional Hazards are available only in the classic (command-driven) version. Among graphical illustrations, Epi Info produces basic charts, aberration detection chart, Pareto chart and Epi curve. Additionally, Epi Info produces growth charts according to WHO and CDC standards for different anthropometric measurements. The Epi Info software permits importing of data from other databases; Microsoft access, excel, CSV files and My SQL. Output is displayed as ready to use tables. Outputs can be easily be exported to Microsoft word and excel.

Creation of maps (Choose "create maps")—Epi Info utilizes Geographic Information System (GIS) for creation of "Choropleth maps" and "Dot density maps" which are most essential for preparation of reports during outbreak investigations and public health emergencies

EZR [7]

EZR, which is also referred to as "Easy R" is a menu driven and a user-friendly version of R package. It is a free downloadable statistical package which has provision for statistical techniques such as descriptive statistics, parametric and non-parametric tests, linear regression, logistic regression, survival analysis, meta-analysis, meta-regression, sample size computation etc.

EZR consists of toolbar, command window where the executed commands are displayed and output window to display the output. A user can perform the statistical functions in EZR either by menu driven options or by means of typing commands.

Data from different sources; text, SPSS, Stata, Minitab and excel can be imported into EZR by File➔Import. Users can choose the statistical techniques by clicking on '***Statistical Analysis***'.

Output from EZR can be exported to text document by File➔Save output as.

Figure 4 shows the statistical packages and their utility.

Conclusion

Appropriate statistical analysis and interpretation is very crucial in any research. Numerous computer packages are available for statistical analysis of data. The choice of the statistical package for the preparation of data-base and data analysis depends on the ease, comfort, availability and flexibility. The knowledge in handling a particular package and the type of statistical analysis required also determine the selection. Many of the statistical packages require official licence to use. The researcher should have an idea about the computer packages going to be used for the preparation of data- base and data analysis and accordingly they can plan the format of the data- base.

Case Scenarios

1. You are a Resident in a Medical college and either you are in the stage of preparation of research proposal to be submitted to research monitoring committee in which sample size has to be computed or you have finished collecting the data and about to begin entry and analysis of the collected data.
   (a) Which will be your preferred statistical package for computing sample size?
   (b) Which package would you prefer for data entry?

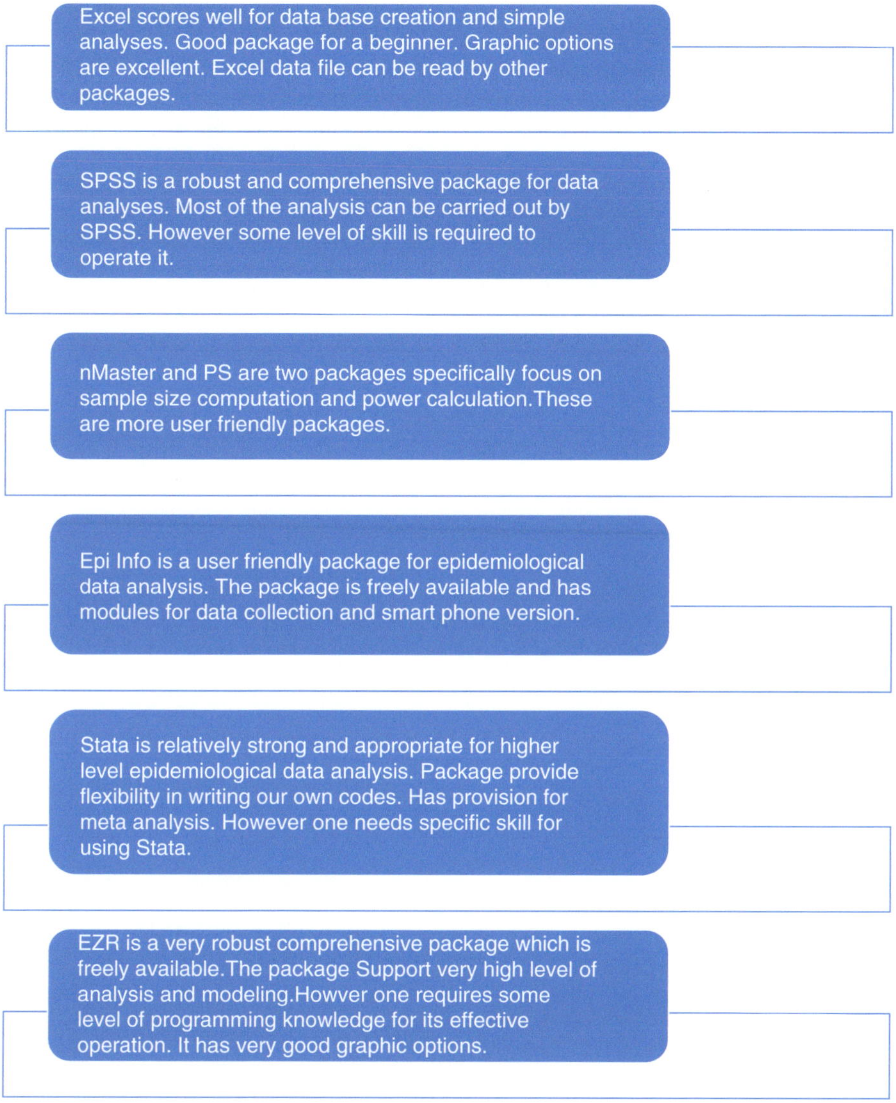

Fig. 4 Statistical packages and their utility

   (c) Which statistical package suits your data analysis requirement?
   (d) Which package would you use for producing graphs?
2. Your project is in evidence-based medicine and you have to finish meta-analysis as part of a systematic review.
   (a) Which are the statistical packages suits your meta-analysis requirement?
   (b) Which one you prefer among these and why?

References

1. About Microsoft Excel [Internet]. 2017 [cited 2017 Nov 12]. https://products.office.com/en-in/excel.
2. About SPSS [Internet]. 2017 [cited 2017 Nov 12]. https://www.ibm.com/analytics/us/en/technology/spss/.
3. About Power and Sample Size Programme [Internet]. 2017 [cited 2017 Nov 12]. http://biostat.mc.vanderbilt.edu/wiki/Main/PowerSampleSize.
4. About nMaster [Internet]. 2017 [cited 2017 Nov 12]. http://www.nmaster.cmc-biostatistics.ac.in/.
5. About Stata [Internet]. 2017 [cited 2017 Nov 12]. http://www.stata.com/.
6. About Epi Info [Internet]. 2016 [cited 2017 Nov 12]. https://www.cdc.gov/epiinfo/index.html.
7. About EZR [Internet]. 2017 [cited 2017 Nov 12]. https://www.r-project.org/about.html.

English Language and Other Software Used in Thesis

Ashutosh Mukherji

Don't use words too big for the subject. Don't say infinitely when you mean very, otherwise you LL have no word left when you want to talk about something really infinite.—CS Lewis

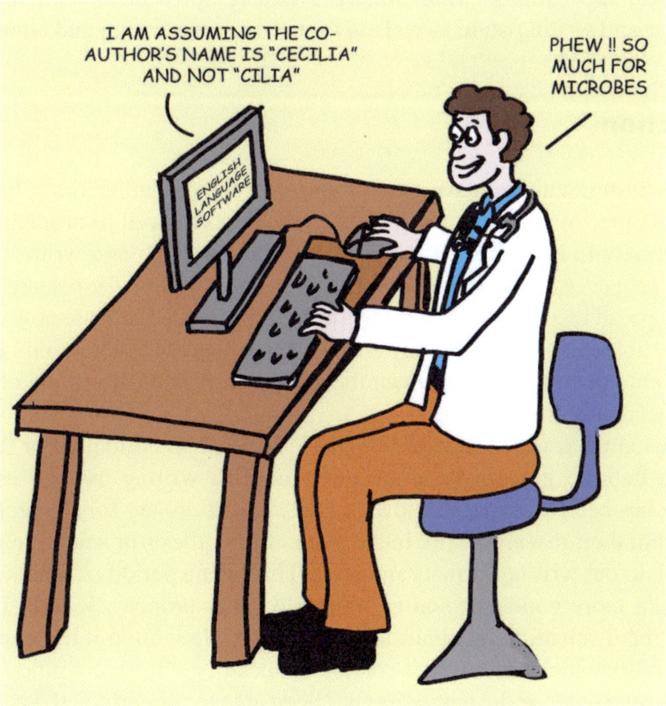

A. Mukherji
Additional Professor, Department of Radiation Oncology, Regional Cancer Centre, and Associate Dean Research, Jawaharlal Institute of Postgraduate Medical Education and Research, Pondicherry, India

S. C. Parija, V. Kate (eds.), *Thesis Writing for Master's and Ph.D. Program*,
https://doi.org/10.1007/978-981-13-0890-1_27

Key Points

- **Need for English language proficiency**: This chapter deals with the need for scientific writers to understand properly what they wish to convey, the necessity to be able to communicate with different researchers in a common language as well as the importance of proper presentation of their work.
- **Writing style**: Scientific writing differs from common writing and there are definite rules and language styles involved. It is important for an author to understand all this.
- **APA rules**: The sixth edition of the Publication Manual of the American Psychological Association has generally been considered the standard format for scientific writing style and structure. These rules govern writing styles, citations, references and help structure scientific writing.
- **Common mistakes in writing style people make in scientific writing**: This section deals with common mistakes non-native English speakers make while writing and suggests means to understand and avoid such mistakes.
- **Other language software used in thesis and scientific writing**: This section deals with the various commercially available software's, both for checking grammar and writing style as well as for correct referencing and citation.

Introduction

Scientific writing, with increasing focus on research and publications, has in recent decades become a necessary prerequisite for students as well as academicians. It is now a necessity to have a good knowledge of both spoken and written English as well as its proper usage in scientific writing. It is imperative for researchers if they want widespread recognition of their work. Modern researchers are now expected to not only be able to converse fluently and with confidence in "scientific" English but also to be able to correctly pen down their thoughts, conclusions and observations in proper academic English.

I have used the term "Academic English" rather than colloquial or the Queen's English as definite guidelines in scientific English writing as well as in verbal expression has been formulated and are in use. It is necessary for researchers to correctly present their research work in the form of their thesis or scientific publication following laid out writing formats and style. This over a period of time will not only make people more confident and comfortable using proper scientific English but also bring them scientific recognition and acclaim. How often it has happened that a research work which otherwise is sound but doesn't get the recognition it deserves because the presenter or the author has not been able to properly pen down his or her thoughts and findings. This chapter will deal with the use of correct scientific writing in English as well as use of necessary language software to help in language correction.

Writing Style

English has been the language of scientific expression in the modern age and this has posed problems for many non-native English users. Hence it is necessary for people not fluent in the language as well as for all general users to follow some common principles for scientific writing as well as maintain a common writing style. Insertion of references and citing sources in a paper or thesis should also follow well laid out rules. It is also important not to use phrases or colloquial slangs in writing as these may have different connotations in different cultures [1]. For example, "*Taking a call/asked to call*" in the US may mean making a telephone call to the required person. "*Taking a call*" may also mean taking a decision or making a choice. However, in countries such as in Ireland, these words may mean going to meet the required person. Thus the use of colloquial phrases may introduce an element of ambiguity in the sentence and may disturb the flow of the written matter [1].

A good scientific writing style should take into consideration the following points: linking words, use of apostrophes, use of linking sentences, use of pronouns and parallel structures, sentence lengths as well as the order of clauses [2]. Other points which are important include use of correct and if possible formal words; keywords have to be used repeatedly, using the precise word for the fact and proper use of voice and tense [2]. In the subsequent paragraphs, each of these aspects will be discussed in brief with examples.

Linking words are basically adverbs or adjectives which are used as a bridge or a link between two phrases or ideas. These words are used to connect ideas between various sections in a document or even different paragraphs or sentences. They can be used in different roles such as a summation, conclusion, negation, additive, correlation (whether temporal or spatial) or even illustrative. Examples of the use of such linking words include: *in conclusion to the above discussion; in a similar study; the results from the two previous studies; immediately preceding; adjacent to; study illustrates.*

Proper use of punctuation marks such as a comma or colon/semi-colon can add to or take away from the weight of the argument presented in a sentence. If a linking word or phrase is used before a clause, a comma should be present after the linking word. If this linking word is present in between a clause, then the comma should be present before and after the linking word. Use of a pronoun or an adjective can place an emphasis on the noun being described. Similarly, it may also be necessary to use parallel structures (sentences or words) in between phrases and sentences to show a linkage between different ideas [3]. Such as: *summer, winter and autumn in which the word "and" is linking word while the entire phrase can be used as a parallel structure. The linking word such as "and" in this case are usually called coordinating structures.* In the use of parallel structures, it is important not to unnecessarily add pronouns or adjectives inside the parallel structure; an example of the same case taken before: "*in summer, in winter and in autumn*" in which the various "*in's*" are not required.

An important aspect of writing style is the flow achieved during reading the manuscript. This can be achieved by ensuring proper use of language, varying the length of sentences, using proper tense and person. Sentence lengths are an important determinant of the ease of readability of a manuscript. It is necessary not to create sentences which are too long as this will disrupt the thought flow and increase the chances of error. It is also necessary not to have very short sentences line after line as then the manuscript will resemble a collection of bullet points and read like a collection of telegrams. Variation in the length of sentences in a paragraph will keep the reader interested and involved.

In addition to variations in sentence length; variations can also be inserted in the clauses used which would make a paragraph interesting to read; again rather than as a collection of bullet points from a presentation. What is important is the need to ensure that there is some sort of connection between the various ideas put forth in a paragraph. Example: a simple paragraph with similar clauses will read as "*Volcanic soil is found in the Deccan Plateau. This is located in central India. This soil is made of magma seeping up through cracks in the crust. This magma then dries and undergoes degradation to form soil.*" This could be re-written as "*Volcanic soil is commonly seen in the Deccan Plateau area of central India. This soil is produced by the drying magma which has exited the crust and degrades later*".

As mentioned in the previous sections also, scientific writing is not an exercise in showing off the author's command over language or literary creativity. The manuscript language should be clear, focused, precise and easy to comprehend. It is necessary to repeat the key words through the text to drive home the importance of these words. It is important to use the exact keywords throughout the text and to avoid the use of synonyms or similar sounding phrases. Use of synonyms will confuse the reader to the intent or the importance of the keywords. Also it is important to use a single tense throughout the manuscript and changes in the tense if they are required should match the language. For example; it is the convention to use *past tense* to describe the hypothesis, methodology, results and observations as these constitute work already completed. Discussion and conclusion can be written in the *present perfect tense*. This signifies work already done in the past and which is relevant in the present time and may continue into the future. The review of literature can also be written in the present perfect tense [3].

Another important component of the language of the written draft is the voice. People frequently switch over from an active to passive voice and vice versa within the same paragraph. This has an adverse effect on the flow of ideas and reading ease and may even result in rejection of such manuscripts by good publishers. In general, it is better to write in short sentences in an active voice in a formal language than to introduce twists and turns in the language through the use of a passive voice. Passive voice generally reflects "*what has been done*" and hence may be more objective. But it results in winding sentences, increasing the risk of grammatical errors and plagiarism and is boring to read. On the other hand, the active voice is now preferred by most scientific publishers and represents "*what is being actively performed by the researcher*". It is also more clear and unambiguous [3]. Readers for further reading can refer to the websites such as http://www.americanscientist.org/issues/pub/the-science-of-scientific-writing/99999 or http://www.nature.com/scitable/ebooks/english-communication-for-scientists-4053993/contents.

Use of the American Psychologist Association Guidelines for Writing Style [4]

The sixth edition of the Publication Manual of the American Psychological Association has generally been considered the standard format for scientific writing style and structure [4]. This guideline includes formats for citations, references, page structuring, and thesis structuring as well as writing style. This chapter however, will concentrate only on the English writing style and structure according to this guideline. According to this guideline (Table 1) [4], the page is formatted as follows: Language format in Times New Roman, font size 12 with double spacing between the lines; page margins all around are set at 1″ while the top margin is set at 0.5″; the text is aligned left for all headings and paragraphs except for major section headings which are centered; the first line of each paragraph is indented half an inch to the right from the left margin.

Also according to these guidelines, the draft should be written in the manner as prescribed: full sentences should be used with complete independent clauses; use of

Table 1 APA checklist for correction of writing style [4]

Check list	
Feature	Recommendation
Font size	Times New Roman 12 size
Line spacing	Double spacing
Spacing after punctuation	Two spaces after punctuation at the end of a sentence; else use one space after punctuation
Alignment	The text is aligned left for all headings and paragraphs except for major section headings which are centered;
Margin	Page margins all around are set at 1″ while the top margin is set at 0.5″;
First line of paragraph	The first line of each paragraph is indented half inch to the right from the left margin
Sentences	Full sentences should be used with complete independent clauses
Punctuation—commas	After each item when more than three items in a sentence; as a coordinating conjunction before independent clause
Punctuation—colons	Separate a grammatically complete clause from an extension
Punctuation—semi-colons	Connect two independent clauses not connected with a conjunction
Voice	Active voice preferred
Tense	Past tense for methodology, results and discussion; present perfect tense for introduction, review of literature and conclusions
Pronouns, linking words, parallel structures	Prefer to use
Sentence subject and verb	Both should match each other
Contractions	Are not recommended
Words	Use precise, formal and scientific words; gender—neutral pronouns preferred; male and female used as adjectives.

parallel structures is encouraged as it is expected to improve the clarity of the sentence (**example**: consider this sentence—"*the people at the cricket match were cheering, playing music and thus had engagements around the field*" which could be shortened and clarified further with parallel structures, "*the people at the cricket match cheered, sang, played music and enjoyed*"); check for conformity of the sentence subject with the verb used as well as the noun with pronoun; proper use of apostrophes and synonyms; use of active voice; correct use of punctuations such as commas, colons and semi-colons; proper use of abbreviations. Commas are used in sentences before a coordinating conjunction connecting two independent clauses (***Example:*** *He wanted badly to win the game, and played his heart out*) [4] or before the main independent clause or in a series of three or more items after each item. They should not be used to divide a sentence or affect a pause. A semi-colon is used to connect two independent clauses not connected with a conjunction (***Example:*** *Many people come to the city; some come for work; others come for leisure*); while a colon is used to separate a grammatically complete clause from an extension (***Example:*** *The study involved three groups: the young, the middle aged and the old*). These rules also recommend using the minimal possible words to convey the message; recommend use of standard abbreviations where required and do not encourage the use of word contractions (use complete words such as "do not" instead of "don't").

Common Mistakes in Scientific Writing Style

"*Much of the common mistakes many non-native English speakers make during scientific writing happen because of their trying to introduce unwanted complexities in their writing styles in an effort to show off their writing skills and language proficiency*". This sentence itself denotes what we usually don't want our writers to do. A lot of mistakes happen when we try to make sentences complex and sound scientific. Some common do's and don'ts have been enumerated in Table 2. It is better to make shorter and to the point statements rather long rambling arguments. Shorter statements also help putting across the message more clearly and keep the reader interested. A book or thesis with long winding statements usually written in the third person is often the first reason for readers losing interest. Another common mistake many non-native English speakers make is in the use of the words "the"; "while" and "since". Many authors use "the" as a form of expression of the importance of the word; but this usually ends up looking as broken sentence hastily put together. Therefore use of this "the" results in the word appearing singular and usually out of context. People also use the words "since" and "while" as a form of reasoning or comparison. However, according to the APA rules these words are to be used only to refer to events occurring in relation to time. (***Example***: "*Since my friend did not pick me up I could not perform*", is wrong usage and here "since" should be replaced with "because"; the correct usage of "since" would be, "*They have been sitting together since the show started*"). Similarly, other common mistakes people make while drafting a document is mixing up the active and passive voices; the recommendation is to write as far as possible in the active voice only. To minimize errors it is better to create algorithms (Fig. 1) and Checklists (Tables 1 and 2) during writing a manuscript.

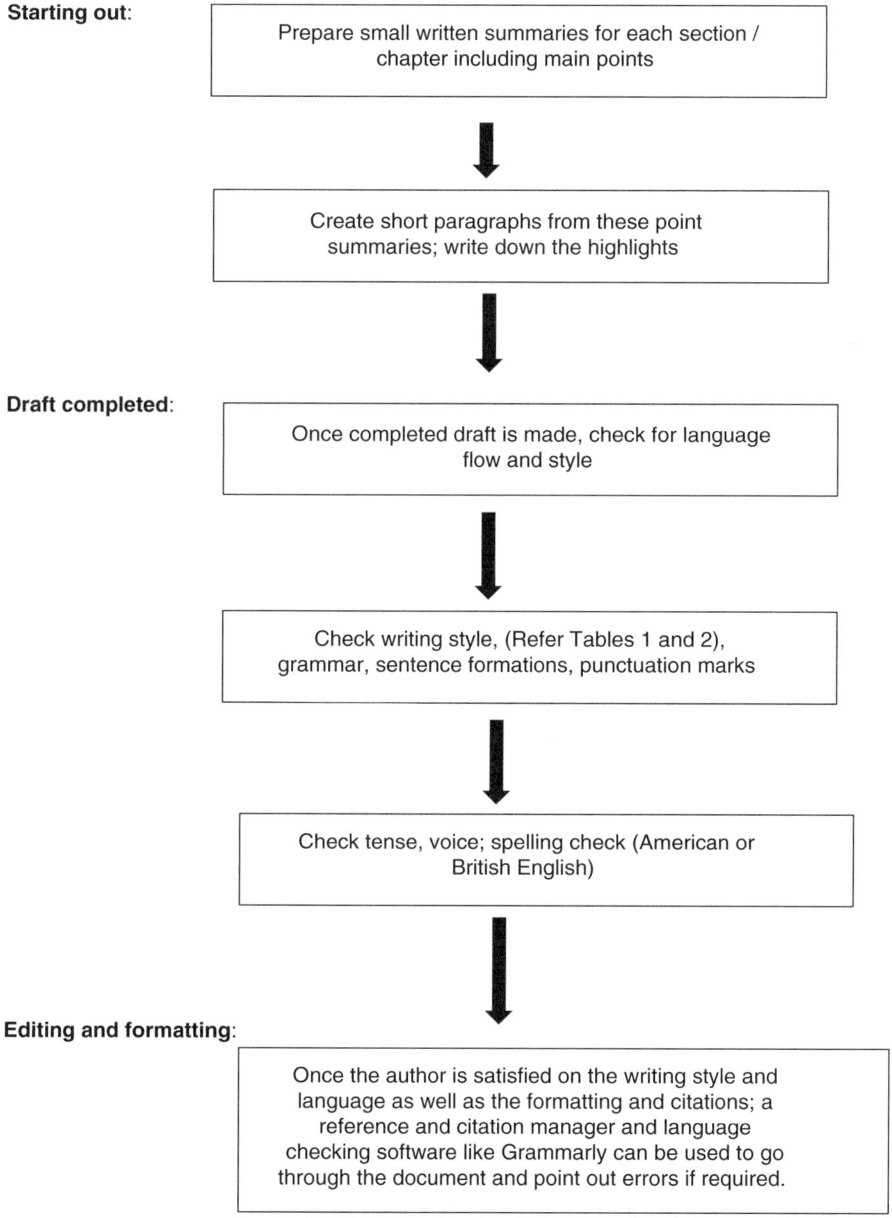

Fig. 1 Algorithm for language and literature review of the scientific manuscript

Table 2 Writing style for scientific writing; do's and don'ts

Do's	Don'ts
Short sentences	Long rambling arguments
Use active verbs	Using indirect passive verbs and phrases
Use first person	Using third person
Each paragraph should communicate 1–2 ideas	Multiple points elicited in each paragraph
Short paragraphs	Long paragraphs
Use formal words	Use of informal words
Proper use of linking words and sentences	Unnecessary use of parentheses and apostrophes
Using similar tense throughout the document	Change in tense and person in different portions of the document
	Unnecessary use of words such as "the" to place emphasis where not required
Use complete words	Do not use non-standard contractions or abbreviations
Use proper scientific and precise descriptions	Avoid clichés and subjective words
Use single type of spelling (British or American English)	Do not use slang
Past tense used for methodology, results and observations and related discussion	
Present perfect tense used for introduction, review of literature and conclusions	

Other Language Software Used in Thesis and Scientific Writing

Commonly used language software include Microsoft Word, LaTex, LyX and Scrivener. MS word is one of the most simple and easy to use templates for writing scientific documents. However, when the job requires more complex tasks or there is requirement for insertion of graphics or multi-media, MS word is frequently difficult to handle. Editing for completed drafts can also be easily done in this template using the track changes mode. LaTeX [5] is an open-source document preparation system which was specifically designed for scientific writing and can easily handle large and complex documents; its benefit being that it is able to separate content and document design. This system also has BibTex which is an online reference manager and provides good support. This system needs however practice and there is a learning curve. This system is freely available online. LyX [6] uses the LaTex system for page setting and formatting in the background but uses a user interface similar to MS word. It has the computing abilities of LaTex and is integrated with BibTex. It is also freely available online. Scrivener [7] acts well as a reference manager and a citation manager but does not have the type-setting and document formatting abilities of MS word or LaTex.

Other useful software available includes Grammarly and Reference Manager. Grammarly helps go through the MS word or Mac/Linux document and points out the various types of typographical as well as grammatical errors in each sentence of the draft and suggests changes as well. It is customer friendly and the learning curve is not steep. Similarly, Reference Manager helps identify the various citations used in a draft and cross-checks these from the various citation indices present and provides the correct citation. It also helps by highlighting each of the selected citations in the body of the text helping considerably the author in numbering the citations.

Case Scenarios

Consider the following paragraphs and identify the errors in language, style or grammar

1. Consider the following paragraph and identify the errors in language, style or grammar: "*This study has been performed in an attempt to correlate the levels of exercise with that of blood cholesterol sampled in the studied individuals. The authors note that there is an increase of 10%–20% in blood cholesterol levels for every 2 h of less exercise done on an average. Also, the cholesterol tends to increase with the decrease in the grade of exercise done and the total duration of the exercise done; and it was found that our results were consistent with standard clinical data available worldwide. This study also illustrates the relationship between the type of exercise done and the level of cholesterol in the blood and thus by detecting this important correlation, we, the authors, would like to contribute to the importance of maintaining a healthy life style.*"
2. "*We the authors did this study to categorise, functionally and biochemically the active elements of the drug being studied. We found that in the 55 gents and 83 ladies we examined; there was significant discrepancy of results in 35% of the subjects. We determined what was the cause of this discrepancy and it was seen to be a minor calibration error in the newer batch of reagent used.*"

References

1. Martin C. 5 Ways to improve scientific writing for non-native speakers. http://www.nextscientist.com/scientific-writing-non-native-english-speakers/.
2. Hopkins WG. Guidelines on style for scientific writing. Sportscience. 1999;3(1). sportsci.org/jour/9901/wghstyle.html, (http://www.sportsci.org/jour/9901/wghstyle.html).
3. van der Perk M. A guide for scientific writing. Guide Manual, Utrecht University, April 2015.
4. Publication Manual of the American Psychological Association (6th ed.). Washington: American Psychological Association; 2010. Copyright (c) 2010 by the American Psychological Association.
5. http://www.latex-project.org/.
6. http://www.lyx.org/.
7. http://www.literatureandlatte.com/scrivener.php.

Plagiarism Software

C. Adithan and A. Surendiran

Originality is undetected plagiarism.—William Ralph Inge

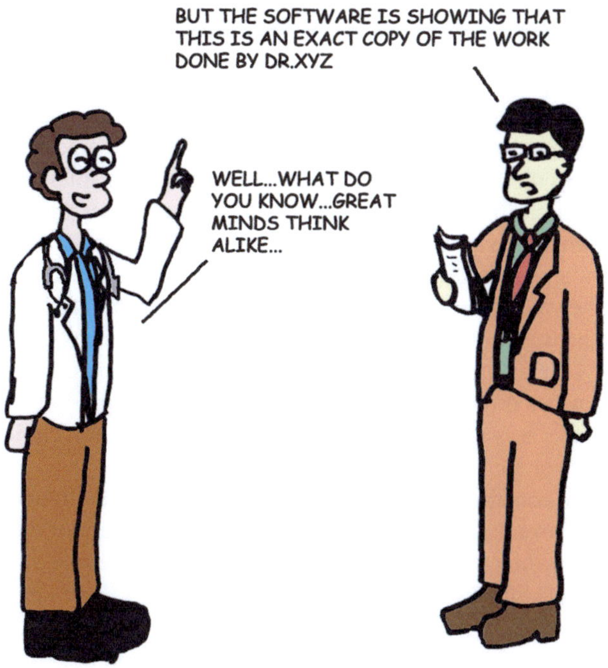

C. Adithan (✉)
Dean (Research), Sri Balaji Vidyapeeth, Pillaiyarkuppam, Pondicherry, India

A. Surendiran
Associate Professor, Department of Pharmacology,
Jawaharlal Institute of Postgraduate Medical Education and Research, Pondicherry, India

S. C. Parija, V. Kate (eds.), *Thesis Writing for Master's and Ph.D. Program*,
https://doi.org/10.1007/978-981-13-0890-1_28

Key Points

- Plagiarism checking software identify similarities in manuscript with existing literature by comparison of texts. The working algorithms in each software vary in effectiveness, thus producing differences in similarity reports. All similarities are not plagiarism.
- Plagiarism software reports require manual scrutiny to assess potential plagiarism and its nature of seriousness.
- Free and paid software are available for checking plagiarism. However, reliability is poor in most free software. The nature of the plagiarised content is as important as the quantity plagiarised. In certain instances, a single plagiarised phrase can be a more serious offence than a plagiarised paragraph.
- Software service packages can be chosen based on the nature of requirement—student, instructor or institutional activity.
- Plagiarism checking softwares cannot check images and their copyright violations.

Introduction

Plagiarism refers to the act of taking credit for ideas or content that were originally created by another individual [1]. Plagiarism has been found to occur in various fields in addition to science. Even famous people such as the Nobel Prize winner and civil rights activist Dr. Martin Luther King Jr. has been accused of plagiarism [2]. Historically, as far as the times of the Roman poet Marcus Valerius Martialis who lived between 38–40 AD to 102–104 AD plagiarism had been a common practice where he was the victim of plagiarism and other poets copied his work [3]. With the advent of the internet, plagiarism can occur with ease. In the past, detecting plagiarism was a difficult task. Although, it is easier at present to detect plagiarism using software, it is still a challenging task due to several techniques used to mask plagiarism from the software.

Plagiarism constitutes an academic fraud that can occur intentionally or unintentionally. To prevent plagiarism, researchers must be aware of the concept and have clear idea regarding the guidelines that govern this concept. However, unintentional plagiarism can still be found to have crept into the literature. Lack of understanding of the concept of plagiarism is not an acceptable excuse for an instance of plagiarism. This makes it imperative for every student to be able to understand and avoid plagiarism. Merely placing citations does not always necessarily mean that plagiarism has been avoided.

Several software can check a manuscript for plagiarism. Software that check for plagiarisms are merely similarity detecting tools, which uses a vast database of scientific journals, magazines, books, and other e-resources including database of webpages, against which the manuscript is compared to look for similarities. The detected similarities in the choice of words or sentence frames are described in the form of numerical percentage or highlighted in the report. The algorithms used in different software vary along with their database resources. Thus, there can be differences in the results of various plagiarism checking software [4]. A knowledge of efficiency of commonly used software and their costs would help researchers and institutions to choose the most appropriate software for their need. In this chapter, we shall discuss some of the commonly used paid and free software that can be used to check for plagiarism (Table 1).

Paid Software

Turnitin

Turnitin Revision Assistant and Turnitin Feedback Studio are products for the purpose of use by the instructor. They can serve several purposes such as writing assistance, feedback, and checking of plagiarism. The software uses a vast collection of resources in its database which includes 62 billion indexed webpages, 734 million student papers, and 160 million scholarly journals and articles [5]. Manuscripts submitted in Turnitin will be stored in the student database. This is to identify plagiarism of one student by another. Turnitin matches similarities with its database and produces a similarity report. This report displays the sources from which similarities have been identified. The subscription price of Turnitin is not available for public in its website and can be obtained only by request for quotation. The database of Turnitin are also used by two other products of the same company namely, WriteCheck and iThenticate.

WriteCheck

WriteCheck is a product of Turnitin that is designed for the purpose of use by the student to self-check manuscripts for plagiarism and grammar correctness. WriteCheck is not intended for evaluation purpose. WriteCheck cannot be used for commercial purpose by the subscriber. This software helps the student to predict the outcome of a plagiarism check by Turnitin when it is evaluated by the instructor. WriteCheck does not store the scanned manuscripts in its database, due to which, resubmissions of a corrected manuscript do not get flagged by the similarities from the earlier submission. If a student scans the manuscript with Turnitin first, followed by WriteCheck, then WriteCheck will identify similarities with the same manuscript scanned earlier with Turnitin, since the manuscript has been saved in student database of Turnitin. Hence the student must not scan his manuscript in Turnitin before checking with WriteCheck or before submission to the instructor [6].

Although, it may be helpful if used with the right intention, this may also become a setback if the intention of checking for plagiarism is not to screen for unintentional plagiarism, but rather to ensure evasion of detection of intentional plagiarism. In this tool, the software shows the detected similarities in the submitted manuscript, but

Table 1 Comparison of features between plagiarism checking software

Feature	WriteCheck	Turnitin & iThenticate	Check for Plagiarism. net	Grammarly	Plagramme	Viper	Plagtracker	Dustball	Duplichecker	Paper rater
Free/paid	Paid	Paid	Paid	Paid	Free & Paid	Free & Paid	Free & Paid	Free & Paid	Free	Free & Paid
Database used	Journals, Books, Magazines, Abstracts, Webpages	Journals, Books, Magazines, Abstracts, Webpages	Journals, Books, Magazines, Abstracts, Webpages	Webpages	Journals, Books, Magazines, Abstracts, Webpages	Journals, Books, Webpages	Webpages, University databases	Webpages	Webpages	Webpages
Report nature	Similarity only	Similarity and sources	Similarity and sources	Similarity and sources	Similarity and sources	Similarity and sources	Similarity and sources	Similarity only	Similarity and sources	Similarity and sources
Offline report	No	Yes	Yes	No	Yes	Yes	No	Yes	No	No
Storing/ reuse of file	No	Stored. Not reused	No	No	Stored. Not reused	No	No	No	No	No
Languages supported	English	English	Multiple	English	Multiple	English	Multiple	English	English	English
Input method	Upload file Copy paste	Upload file	Upload file	Upload file Copy paste	Upload file	Upload file	Copy paste (free) Upload (paid)	Upload file Copy paste	Upload file Copy paste	Copy paste (free) Upload (paid)
Format supported	doc, docx	txt, doc, docx, rtf, pdf, html	txt, doc, docx, rtf, pdf, html	txt, doc, docx, rtf	doc, docx	doc, docx	doc, txt	doc, docx	doc, txt	doc, docx, txt, rtf
Grammar check	Yes	No	Yes	Yes	No	No	No	No	Yes	Yes

does not provide the source of matched similarity. WriteCheck partners with ETS® to provide e-rater grammar checking service. This is a comprehensive tool which is linked to the Writers Handbook, which tutors the students to understand their grammatical errors and improve their writing skills. In addition, WriteCheck also includes Professional Tutoring service by Pearson Tutor Service (PTS), which can be used by students to submit their manuscripts to get critique and constructive feedback from PTS tutors [7].

WriteCheck subscription prices are available as single paper plan at 7.95 USD for a single document, semester plan at 19.55 USD for three documents and graduate plan at 29.95 USD for five documents [8]. A word count of 5000 is taken as one document. WriteCheck does not offer institutional subscription packages.

iThenticate

Turnitin provides iThenticate as a tool to evaluate manuscripts for plagiarism by means of identifying similarities and calculation of similarity index. Contrary to WriteCheck, iThenticate is intended to be used for evaluation purpose by the instructor. iThenticate uses a vast collection of resources in its database namely, Crossref Similarity Check, against which the submitted manuscript gets screened for potential similarities in text. It includes enrolment of 1300 publishers, including the top 15 influential publishers with 182 million articles including conferences proceedings from 226 thousand scientific journals, periodicals, magazines, encyclopedias, and abstracts and 60 billion webpages [9]. In addition to the difference in purpose, iThenticate offers certain additional features as compared to WriteCheck. When a manuscript is evaluated with iThenticate, it shows the matched similarities and can take the instructor to the sources of detected similarities. This function is not present in WriteCheck. However, iThenticate does not evaluate grammar of manuscripts, which is done by WriteCheck and it does not provide writing support and feedback as given by Turnitin. The evaluated reports are stored in a secure database for retrieval when required. The scanned manuscripts can be accessed only by the user. In iThenticate, the scanned manuscripts are not used for other purposes. iThenticate allows the admin to create multiple user accounts within a single subscription. Further, there are options to upload documents in the form of MS Word file or PDF file. Multiple files can also be compressed in zip format for upload.

iThenticate offers flexibility in choosing the subscription plan. For instance, to check a single document for plagiarism with iThenticate, one credit point is required which costs 100 USD. One document in this case refers to a document with less than 25,000 words. If a larger document with less than 75,000 words or three single documents needs to be checked, then the subscription cost of three credit points would be 300 USD [10]. Institutional subscription is possible with iThenticate and the cost varies upon the requirement. With a larger institutional subscription, the cost for one document will be calculated at a much lower rate.

Check for Plagiarism.Net

The online tool CheckForPlagiarism.net is a paid software that uses 'sentence structure assessment and synonym identification technology', a patented approach, to check manuscripts for plagiarism. It scans the manuscript across its database which contains billions of academic journals, magazines, and books. Further, its database also includes a vast number of webpages in internet. Further, it supports multiple languages (more than 100), and supports documents in multiple language scripts. This software claims to detect even subtle plagiarism and offers a money back guarantee with terms and conditions. It also enables comparison of two documents for similarities. In addition, it also has features of correcting grammatical errors [11]. The submitted manuscripts will not be stored in any database of the software and will not be available for any third party. In addition, plagiarism correction service and proofreading service is available underpayment, where the manuscript is submitted to the company, where it is processed by experts and delivered back to the account holder with corrections for plagiarism and proofreading [12].

This software offers three types of subscription plans namely, account for students and researchers, academic accounts and professional accounts. Under account for students and researchers two offers are available. The basic plan costs 20 USD which provides five submission slots (25,000 words per slot). This is suitable for high school students to check assignments. The advanced plan costing 39.95 USD provides 15 submission slots (30,000 words per slot) and is more suitable for college or university students, and the database used for checking is larger than basic plan. Under academic accounts, two offers are available. The academic plan for 99 USD per month is billed annually, and supports unlimited document submission with applicable fair usage policies. This is suitable for institutional setup, where free accounts can be given to faculty and students. The second plan is for individual teachers who screen limited number of documents. This plan is available at a cost of 350 USD valid for 1 year which can be used for screening 400 documents with 25,000 words constituting one document. The professional account can be for monthly use costing 95 USD or for annual use which costs 850 USD. The monthly plan offers screening of 20 documents per 24 h with a 30-day validity. The annual plan offers screening of 50 documents per 24 h with a validity of 1 year and a higher word count of 50,000 constituting per document [13].

Grammarly

This software which can be used online encompasses the features of checking a manuscript for grammar mistakes as well as for potential plagiarism. Grammarly can be used free of charge for the purpose of checking grammar in a manuscript. This software can also be added to Microsoft Word as an add-on and can be used in real time to check the manuscripts for grammar. However, the feature of plagiarism checker can be activated only by means of subscription. Grammarly claims use eight billion webpages to scan for potential plagiarism [14]. It must be remembered that the primary purpose of Grammarly is to check for grammatical errors. Grammarly cannot be used for evaluation of plagiarism by an instructor in an institutional setting, since there is no function of storing of generated reports. Subscription to Grammarly is available as monthly, quarterly and annual plans, at the rates of 29.95 USD per month, 19.98 USD per month, and 11.66 USD per month, respectively [15].

Free Software with Paid Features

Plagiarism checking tools are available free of cost as online webpage and as software that can be downloaded to a computer for installation. The manuscript can be uploaded or copy pasted in the webpage, which will then be screened for plagiarism. Many of the free online software may perform the function of scanning the manuscripts only against a limited database of webpages. The homepage of the plagiarism checking software usually provide information on the databases against which the software will evaluate the manuscript. Many competing plagiarism checking webpages may provide a faulty report incomplete report, resulting in issues of plagiarism at the time of submission to a journal or instructor.

Plagramme

Plagramme plagiarism checker claims to check plagiarism in documents by matching with texts over 640 repositories and 14 trillion webpages, articles, books and periodicals [16]. The software runs online without a need for installation in the computer. The basic function of scanning a manuscript and producing a preliminary report of similarity score, paraphrase score, improper citation and plagiarism risk is free. However, to see details of the report, payment is needed in the form of credit points. Credit points may be purchased with payment. It costs around 2.4 USD to view the report of a single document. Paraphrasing score refers to the extent of paraphrasing in the entire manuscript. Risk of plagiarism indicates the probability that the detected similarities could amount to potential plagiarism. This software supports multiple languages for checking plagiarism [17].

Viper

Viper is a free online software which can be used for scanning manuscripts for plagiarism. It claims to be easy, fast and it uses around ten billion resources to scan a manuscript for plagiarism. The software generates a report after scanning the manuscript which can be downloaded. This software in its free version stores the manuscript after scan in its student database and 3 months later, uses it as a resource for subsequent scanning of other manuscripts. This stored file can be deleted from their database upon individual request. The scanned document may be subsequently published in their study sites (UKEssays.com, LawTeacher.net and Uniassignment.com) as a model for other students which can be deleted upon request. There is a limit of scanning to only two new documents in a 24 h period [18]. Currently Viper is not available for users in India. However, Viper Premium for international students, has been announced to be available soon, with additional features. In the premium version, there will be no limit in the number of new documents scanned per day and the documents will not be stored in any databases. The price of subscription for premium version is not available as of date.

Plagtracker

Plagtracker is an online plagiarism checking tool that scans the manuscript with more than 14 billion webpages and four million academic papers. It supports six languages namely, English, French, German, Spanish, Romanian and Italian. Though, in the free version, the word limit in a document is restricted to 5000, word count will be unlimited in the paid premium version. Similarly, additional features such as uploading a document in a word file, saving the report as PDF file, grammar checking, exclusion of references and scanning multiple documents will be available only in the premium version. This software does not save a copy of the scanned document. The premium version is available at a price of 7.49 USD for the first month followed by a rate of 14.99 USD per month [19].

Dustball

Dustball is an online based plagiarism checking tool that scans the document with internet webpages. Based on the similarities detected, it creates a similarity report. The current version of dustball provides a downloadable similarity report with the similarity percentage. The software is also available in a paid version which claims to be three times as accurate as the free version. The document to be checked for plagiarism can be copy pasted online in the free version or uploaded in the webpage in MS Word format in the paid version. The free version is limited to checking only 1000 documents per day worldwide, which can be overcome by payment. Further, the paid version has the function of ignoring texts which are given in quotes which is absent in the free version. The premium version costs at the rate of 8 USD per month for 50 uses. Each additional uses costs 25 cents [20].

Duplichecker

This tool is another online plagiarism checking software that requires that the users register to create a free account. Registered users can check up to 50 documents per day, where as guest users can check only one document per day. This software also scans a manuscript against billions of internet webpages and identifies similarities in the manuscript. It can also be used to screen a webpage in internet for plagiarised content. It provides the options of copy pasting a document content in which case it has a word limit of 1000 words, or a MS Word document can be uploaded in the webpage [21].

Paper Rater

Manuscripts can be checked for plagiarism with this online software free of cost. This software has functions of checking for grammatical mistakes and proofreading. The system for plagiarism detection splits the manuscript into smaller parts which is then matched against more than 20 billion webpages in books and journals, indexed by search engines such as Google, Yahoo and Bing [22]. The report is shown in the form of originality percentage in contrast to other software which produce report in the form of similarity percentage. However, in the free version, no matching report is generated. This means that the student will not be able to know which sentences were flagged for plagiarism. This feature is available in the paid version. Further, there is a limit of five pages per submission in the free version which gets expanded to 20 pages per submission. This software considers 300 words as one page. Therefore, the total words that can be screened per submission is only 6000 words in the paid version. However, there is no limit on the number of submissions. The premium version costs 14.95 USD per month or 95.40 USD per year [23].

The free software discussed above are a few of the many software available in internet. They have mostly similar features of checking plagiarism by means of matching against webpages. Free plagiarism checking software may be useful for students who wants to check small manuscripts or essays on general topics. However, for specialised contents such as medicine, the database and methods used by free software may not be adequate. It must be understood that, plagiarism of even a single phrase can sometimes be a serious issue, depending upon the significance of the phrase and the context in which it has been used. Paid versions are expensive but they are exhaustive in their matching database. Publication agencies and universities/institutions mostly use paid software to screen manuscripts for plagiarism owning to the seriousness of the issue of plagiarism.

Similarity Index and Interpretation of Similarity Report

It must be remembered that a software can detect only similarities in text, ranging from phrases to paragraphs. Plagiarism checking tools such as iThenticate provide a score of similarity called as similarity index. Similarity index is proportion of number of word in a given manuscript that is found to be occur similar to other published content. There are instances where similarity index can be high, yet the manuscript may not have been plagiarised. For example, when a medical student mentions a criteria used for classification of a disease in the study, the wordings in the criteria will be identified by the software similar to the other publications of the criteria. In a small scale study manuscript, the criteria may constitute a significant share of the word count. This results in a high similarity index. Yet, standard criteria used for classification of diseases cannot be changed in the medicine.

This shows the need to carefully scrutinise each similarity report. The identified similarities can provide an idea regarding the extent of plagiarism that we can expect. If a scientific manuscript on screening has a large similarity index, there is a higher probability that there would be one or more instances of plagiarism in the large document. Thus, similarity report can be a screening tool which alerts the instructor to scrutinise manuscripts that have a higher probability of potential plagiarism. The similarity report must be manually evaluated by the instructor in order to rule out 'acceptable similarities' from plagiarised content [24].

Exceptions to be Considered in a Similarity Report

All plagiarisms will be similarities, however, all similarities are not plagiarism. For instance, definitions are not to be changed from their original source. Similarly, diagnostic criteria, classification of diseases or drugs, and in some instances, guidelines of disease management may be required to be reproduced verbatim. Though it may be indicated as a similarity in the software, it may not be considered as a plagiarism, as long as the authors have cited the original source with reference. Verbatim copy of lines, phrases or a paragraph may require to be given within quotes to indicate that they are reproduced from a different source. In iThenticate, it is possible to change the settings so as to instruct the software to ignore contents given within quotes, to ignore contents that appear below the word 'references' and to exclude certain customised phrases from the similarity report.

The subscription cost for plagiarism checking software varies with the available functional features and the nature of subscription such as single document, individual account, or institutional subscription. Process of evaluating a manuscript with plagiarism checking software is given in Fig. 1.

Limitations of Plagiarism Checking Software

- Copyright violation is another major concern that very often accompanies instances of plagiarism. When an author publishes a manuscript, very often, the copyright for the entire content is given to the publisher. Hence, when plagiarism occurs, it may also violate the law of copyrights to a variable degree. Young researchers and students, unaware of this fact, tend to copy paste images in their manuscript, which are also often copyright protected. The plagiarism checking software will not be able to screen images in a manuscript which are in violation of copyrights.

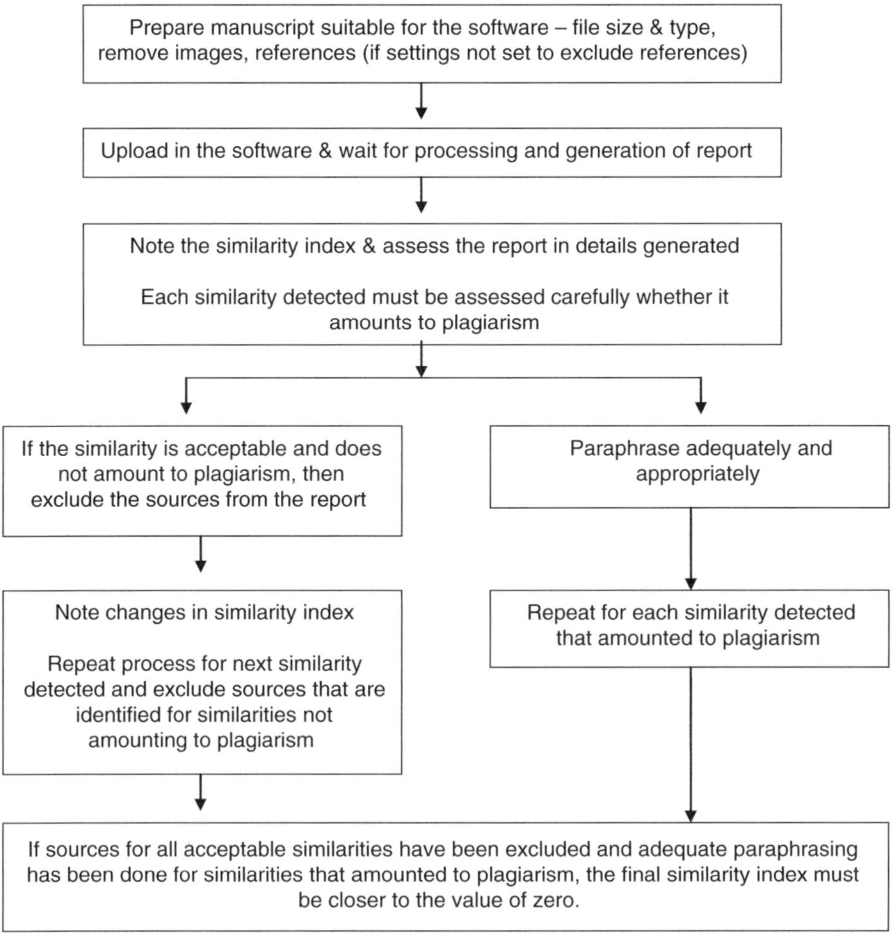

Fig. 1 Process of evaluating a manuscript with plagiarism checking software (e.g., iThenticate)

- Unpublished data will not be available in the databases of plagiarism checking software and hence will not be included in the screening of manuscripts for plagiarism. These include unpublished content delivered in a lecture, unpublished PhD thesis documents, research protocols, etc. Similarly, plagiarism of ideas or style may also go undetected.
- The paid software such as WriteCheck and iThenticate are very efficient but expensive which makes it unusable by many on an individual subscription basis. However, with institutional support they may be affordable.
- Plagiarism checking softwares are helpful if used with the right intentions. However, they are not fool proof and several cheats are available to overcome the similarity detection by the software.
- The process of scrutinising a large number of manuscripts for potential plagiarism as in an institutional setup would be cumbersome and time-consuming since every report must be carefully evaluated to rule out acceptable or ignorable similarities.

Summary and Conclusion

Plagiarism checking software help in maintaining ethical standards of academics, research and publications. Utility of the software require investment of funds which is required for all educational institutions, research centres and publishers. Although the cost of paid software high, it is valuable due to the vast database used by them in evaluating a manuscript. This results in a trustworthy report that can be used for correction. All students and young researchers should be encouraged to learn scientific writing and principles of ethics in academia and research. Yet, it is imperative to self-check one selves to avoid unintentional lapses in ethical conduct in the form of plagiarism or copyright violation.

Case Scenarios

1. You are authoring a chapter for a textbook to be published by a renowned publisher. Your manuscript contains references to several studies and you have provided citation for all of them. Do you still need to check your manuscript for plagiarism with a software?
2. You are an editor for a newly launched journal. You started receiving manuscripts for publication. Which software would you use to screen the manuscripts for potential plagiarism?

References

1. Gasparyan AY, Nurmashev B, Seksenbayev B, Trukhachev VI, Kostyukova EI, Kitas GD. Plagiarism in the context of education and evolving detection strategies. J Korean Med Sci. 2017;32:1220–7.
2. Boston U. Panel finds plagiarism by Dr. King. The New York Times [Internet]. 1991 [cited 2017 Aug 25]. http://www.nytimes.com/1991/10/11/us/boston-u-panel-finds-plagiarism-by-dr-king.html.
3. The Pragmatics of Quoting Now and Then [Internet]. 2015 [cited 2017 Aug 25]. https://www.degruyter.com/view/product/457182.
4. Živković D. Anti-plagiarism software: usage, effectiveness and issues. Synth 2015—Int Sci Conf IT Bus-Relat Res. 2015;119–22.
5. Turnitin—Home [Internet]. Turnitin. 2017 [cited 2017 Aug 25]. http://turnitin.com/en_us/.
6. WriteCheck. Frequently Asked Questions [Internet]. Plagiarism Checker | WriteCheck by Turnitin. 2017 [cited 2017 Aug 25]. http://en.writecheck.com/faq/.
7. WriteCheck. Features [Internet]. Plagiarism Checker | WriteCheck by Turnitin. 2017 [cited 2017 Aug 25]. http://en.writecheck.com/features/overview/.
8. WriteCheck—Home [Internet]. Plagiarism Checker | WriteCheck by Turnitin. 2017 [cited 2017 Aug 25]. http://en.writecheck.com/.
9. Crossref Similarity Check [Internet]. iThenticate. 1998 [cited 2017 Aug 25]. http://www.ithenticate.com/products/crossref-similarity-check.
10. Packages [Internet]. iThenticate. 1998 [cited 2017 Aug 25]. https://app.ithenticate.com/en_us/signup/individual.
11. Unique Service Features [Internet]. Checkforplagiarism.net. 2004 [cited 2017 Aug 25]. https://www.checkforplagiarism.net/service-features.

12. Professional Proofreading Service [Internet]. Checkforplagiarism.net. 2004 [cited 2017 Aug 25]. http://www.checkforplagiarism.net/proofreading.php.
13. Plagiarism Checking, Document Correction and Comparison Services [Internet]. CheckForPlagiarism.net. 2004 [cited 2017 Aug 25]. https://www.checkforplagiarism.net/services.
14. Grammarly—Home [Internet]. Grammarly. 2017 [cited 2017 Aug 25]. https://www.grammarly.com/.
15. Grammarly Premium [Internet]. Grammarly. 2017 [cited 2017 Aug 25]. https://www.grammarly.com/premium.
16. General questions on our plagiarism tool [Internet]. Plagramme. 2011 [cited 2017 Aug 25]. https://www.plagramme.com/plagiarism-tool-faq.
17. Multilingual Plagiarism Checker [Internet]. Plagramme. 2011 [cited 2017 Aug 25]. https://www.plagramme.com/.
18. Viper Plagiarism Checker [Internet]. Viper. 2017 [cited 2017 Aug 25]. https://www.scanmyessay.com/.
19. PlagTracker—Home [Internet]. PlagTracker.com. [cited 2017 Aug 25]. http://www.plagtracker.com/.
20. Plagiarism Checker [Internet]. Dustball. 2002 [cited 2017 Aug 25]. http://www.dustball.com/cs/plagiarism.checker/.
21. Dupli Checker [Internet]. Duplichecker. 2017 [cited 2017 Aug 25]. https://www.duplichecker.com/.
22. PaperRater—Home [Internet]. PaperRater. 2017 [cited 2017 Aug 25]. https://www.paperrater.com/page/plagiarism-detection.
23. PaperRater—Pricing [Internet]. PaperRater. 2017 [cited 2017 Aug 25]. https://www.paperrater.com/pricing.
24. The Similarity Report [Internet]. Turnitin. 2017 [cited 2017 Aug 25]. https://guides.turnitin.com/01_Manuals_and_Guides/Student_Guides/Turnitin_Classic_(Deprecated)/17_The_Similarity_Report.

MIX
Papier aus verantwortungsvollen Quellen
Paper from responsible sources
FSC® C105338

If you have any concerns about our products,
you can contact us on
ProductSafety@springernature.com

In case Publisher is established outside the EU,
the EU authorized representative is:
Springer Nature Customer Service Center GmbH
Europaplatz 3, 69115 Heidelberg, Germany

Printed by Libri Plureos GmbH
in Hamburg, Germany